ADOLESCENT PSYCHIATRY

DEVELOPMENTAL AND CLINICAL STUDIES

VOLUME 13

Annals of the American Society for Adolescent Psychiatry

ADOLESCENT PSYCHIATRY

DEVELOPMENTAL AND CLINICAL STUDIES

VOLUME 13

Edited by
SHERMAN C. FEINSTEIN
Coordinating Editor

Senior Editors
AARON H. ESMAN
JOHN G. LOONEY
ALLAN Z. SCHWARTZBERG
ARTHUR D. SOROSKY
MAX SUGAR

The University of Chicago Press
Chicago and London

The University of Chicago Press, Chicago 60637
The University of Chicago Press, Ltd., London

International Standard Book Number: 0-226-24059-2
Library of Congress Catalog Card Number: 70-147017

CONTENTS

PART II. PSYCHOTHERAPEUTIC ISSUES IN ADOLESCENT PSYCHIATRY

PART III. AN OVERVIEW OF EATING DISORDERS
ARTHUR D. SOROSKY, Special Editor

PART IV. TODAY'S ADOLESCENT PSYCHIATRY: WHICH ADOLESCENTS TO TREAT AND HOW?
FRANÇOIS LADAME AND PHILIPPE JEAMMET, Special Editors

IN MEMORIAM

Dedication to Hilde Bruch (1904–1984)

This volume is dedicated to the memory of Hilde Bruch, who was a contributor to this series; a friend of the American Society for Adolescent Psychiatry; the William A. Schonfeld Award honoree in 1978, when she addressed us on "Island in the River: The Anorexic Adolescent in Treatment"; and a world figure in the field of the study and treatment of eating disorders.

Dr. Bruch was born in Germany on March 11, 1904. She earned her medical degree at the University of Freiburg in 1928 and trained in physiologic research and pediatrics. She left Germany in 1933, spending a year in London at the East End Child Guidance Clinic. She was then invited to join the staff at Babies Hospital in New York, where she developed a pediatric endocrine clinic and focused her attention on childhood obesity.

Theodore Lidz has described how Dr. Bruch first gained prominence in 1939 by eliminating a famous syndrome, named after Froehlich, said to consist of excessive obesity, small genitalia, and sluggish behavior in young boys and thought to be due to an unknown disturbance in pituitary activity. She demonstrated that the boys were fat from overeating and underactivity and that the genitals were of normal size but appeared tiny owing to pads of fat.

After recognizing the importance of emotional and familial influences in eating disorders, Dr. Bruch began psychiatric training at The Johns Hopkins Hospital and simultaneously undertook psychoanalytic training at the Washington-Baltimore Institute of Psychoanalysis with Frieda Fromm-Reichmann as her analyst.

In 1943 she started her practice in New York City, taught at Columbia University's College of Physicians and Surgeons, and served as the director of the children's service at New York State Psychiatric Institute from 1954 to 1956. Dr. Lidz states that "her work, particularly her studies with Stanley Polumbo, led to recognition of how parental misconceptions of the child's needs could lead to misinterpretations and confusions of bodily sensations and physiologic messages in schizophrenic, obese, and anorexic patients."

In 1964 Dr. Bruch accepted an appointment as professor of psychiatry at Baylor University in Houston, where her talents as teacher, therapist, and researcher were enthusiastically recognized.

In addition to many papers, Dr. Bruch published six books; her last, *Conversations with Anorexics*, is in press. Other titles include *Don't Be Afraid of Your Child: A Guide for Perplexed Parents; The Importance of Over-Weight; Eating Disorders: Obesity, Anorexia Nervosa and the Person Within; The Golden Cage: The Enigma of Anorexia Nervosa*; and *Learning Psychotherapy*.

Dr. Bruch raised a nephew whose parents had perished in the Holocaust. She was a keen listener, a great teacher, a superb therapist, and a devoted searcher after truth, with a tremendous zest for life. After developing severe Parkinsonism, Dr. Bruch died in Houston on December 15, 1984.

BERTRAM SLAFF

PREFACE

This thirteenth volume of the *Annals of the American Society for Adolescent Psychiatry* celebrates a rite de passage, the psychological entry into adolescence of this series of clinical and developmental studies of adolescence. As with any celebration, there are many who helped and supported this effort, and it is to our devoted contributors, audience, and publisher that the editors of these volumes are most appreciative.

During the early years of the development of the American Society for Adolescent Psychiatry, Daniel Offer had the foresight to have a sociologist, Paul Dommermuth, study the organizational efforts of a group of young, devoted psychiatrists with a growing interest in adolescence. Dommermuth observed that segmenting and branching in a valid profession is continuous and involves redefining the divisions of labor and developing new missions. This would attract new members and result in new groupings.

This volume of *Adolescent Psychiatry* reflects the fulfillment of the prediction that new subgroups or segments within the Society would emerge, emphasizing a wider range of clinical and research issues. The arrival at psychological manhood, after thirteen years of presenting an overview of the best clinical and research studies on adolescence, reflects the segmenting and branching foreseen. The volume represents a panoramic display of the many vicissitudes of adolescent development: normative and pathological; family reactions and supports; cultural aspects; creativity; regression; contributions and hindrances to diagnosis; and treatment whether inpatient or outpatient.

During the United Nations Year of Youth 1985, the International Society for Adolescent Psychiatry was organized to carry forward throughout the world the segmenting and branching earlier performed by the American Society for Adolescent Psychiatry and its predecessors. The American Society for Adolescent Psychiatry itself is undergoing important internal changes as a task force studies and redefines the Society's function.

So growth and development proceed, the new a reflection of the old but always, if true to itself, experimenting, segmenting, and branching, resulting in new challenges.

SHERMAN C. FEINSTEIN

PART I

ADOLESCENCE: GENERAL CONSIDERATIONS

EDITORS' INTRODUCTION

The chapters in this section document the wide range of issues germane to the practice of adolescent psychiatry in the 1980s. It is clear that the development of adolescents, both normal and exceptional, is shaped not only by internal forces but by a vast array of sociocultural influences. A historical perspective is a valuable adjunct to the usual clinical and sociological frames of reference for an adequate understanding of the role of these multiple factors, and these chapters consider adolescent issues from the Golden Age of Greece to the "culture of narcissism" of the present.

Donald B. Rinsley presents a psychosocial commentary on influences on personality formation in the past decades. He reiterates that the family remains the nuclear socializing factor for the oncoming generation and recommends a number of qualities: biparenthood, full-time mothering, differential parent roles, proper discipline, articulation with the wider extrafamilial culture, and adequate achievement of developmental tasks. Lamenting the presence of a rather narcissistic culture, Rinsley examines a number of social phenomena that he believes have influenced its emergence: the Vietnam conflict, demystification of social archetypes, demystification of sexuality, environmentalism, feminism, rock music and drugs, the civil rights movement, leveling, and the demise of quality. The author concludes that parents and society must permit the full growth and development of psychic structures and sees hope for the future.

Jerry M. Lewis reports his study of the impact of adolescent children on family systems. He describes the varieties of family structures from the perspective of a continuum of family competence as an important determinant of the family's response to the adolescence of their children. He describes family interactional processes in highly competent, competent but pained, dysfunctional (dominant-submissive and chronically conflicted), and severely dysfunctional families. Lewis concludes that parents with effective relationships can have difficult problems with their adolescent children, but parents who have resolved the relationship issues of closeness, intimacy, and power minimize that risk.

Herman Sinaiko discusses courage, expertise, psychotherapy, and adolescence from a Socratic viewpoint, as recorded in Plato's *Laches*, from the *Dialogues*. Socrates first establishes that knowledge, not majority rule, should dominate decisions and that teaching should be carried out by a doctor of the soul, not an expert in technique. After an exploration of virtue, human excellence, courage, and wisdom, Socrates applies these values to parenting techniques and attitudes and concludes that "care of the soul" is of great importance. Professor Sinaiko believes that this is the first mention of psychotherapy in the literature and traces the value of courage in achieving action (creativity) rather than predictable behavior.

Aaron H. Esman explores the literature on gifted and creative children. He reviews the development of intelligence testing and attempts to measure creativity; psychoanalytic perspectives, including constitutional, developmental, and parenting influences; and the studies of lives of creative geniuses. Esman cites some specific case examples—Mozart, Schubert, Mendelssohn, Raffaelo, Bernini, Picasso, and Chatterton. From these examples he concludes that the early flowering of creative genius in adolescence is favored by an intense supportive relationship and identification with the father figure. Practical suggestions for psychiatric help with the gifted and creative are discussed.

Richard L. Munich argues that the self-consciousness of adolescents and young adults, while a painful consequence of normal development, illustrates many elements of pathological narcissism. The author examines consolidation of the self-concept and identity formation and demonstrates through clinical material the development of a grandiose self and other forms of pathological narcissism. Munich discusses various treatment approaches and emphasizes the importance of the therapeutic alliance and its management.

Elisa G. Sanchez, in her research award–winning paper, examines the factors complicating the psychiatric diagnosis of adolescents. Viewing adolescence as a stage of life that implies growth, change, and intricate

4

adaptive processes, the author believes that there is a lack of conceptual consistency in the field. Sanchez discusses characteristics of adolescence (developmental tasks, clinical manifestations), the therapist's conceptual framework (psychoanalytical or empirical), the personality of the therapist (countertransference reactions to adolescent behavior and values), sociocultural factors (the struggle for identity), and familial factors (the adolescent as delegate) and concludes that it is necessary to evaluate the adolescent as a whole, in context.

1   THE ADOLESCENT, THE FAMILY,
AND THE CULTURE OF NARCISSISM:
A PSYCHOSOCIAL COMMENTARY

DONALD B. RINSLEY

What follows is a distillate of inferences and conclusions drawn from intensive psychotherapeutic work with children, adolescents, and their families during the 1960s and 1970s. More generally, it is derived from merely having lived during those years in the United States in a society that to many of us seemed for all the world to have been descending into decadence and anomie. It will please some, and it will offend others. However that may be, the topic itself constitutes a challenge to anyone who thinks that he knows something about personality development and who has not been oblivious to what has happened in this country during the past quarter-century.[1]

What I shall present now is leavened by my belief that man is by nature greedy, egocentric, and territorially aggressive and expansive and that the virtues of altruistic love and empathy emerge only after many years of disciplined training within the optimal context of the healthy biparental family. It is fair to say that adolescence comprises a period and an experience integral to a further narcissistic muting that accompanies a reworking of the separation-individuation process (Blos 1962, 1967, 1979; Mahler, Pine, and Bergman 1975). Should society as a whole lack coherence and stability, however, these will essentially fail to occur.

Finally, I make no excuse for not being expert in sociology. By the same token, I report here no large-scale statistical studies or other quantitative data that convey domestic behavioral science's preoccupa-

7

tion with the numerology of the *Naturwissenschaftlich* rather than the essentiality of the *Geisteswissenschaftlich*. I am convinced that value judgments must be made in respect to the matters I shall be taking up, that there is no such thing as treatment devoid of values, and that in the end one's values are shaped by those articulated by and within one's wider sociocultural context.

The Wider Sociocultural Context

In the musical *Fiddler on the Roof*, the Russian Jewish peasant, Tevye, sings of the importance of tradition. He discovers that his beloved daughter desires to marry a *goy*, and in great anguish, in accordance with orthodox Jewish law, he must disown her even to the point of considering that she has perished. For Tevye, individual and communal life could be understood only within the context of religious law and tradition. For him and for those akin to him, it was impossible to live apart from that body of Jewish life and the basis for the survival of the Jewish people in a world that had long been hostile to them and to their beliefs.

I select this example from the Judaic-Hebraic tradition to highlight not religious narrow-mindedness but rather the ages-long and ineluctable conflict that arises between the wants and needs of the individual and those of the group or collective. For it has long seemed to me that the Ashkenazic Jews serve as quintessential examples of intelligence, tough-mindedness, creativity, and survival both before and after the biblical exodus precisely because of their immensely coherent and consistent religiocultural traditionalism, centering on a cohesive family life that maintains intergenerational continuity and thereby amply provides for the progressive socialization of the young. Much the same could indeed be said in the case of other family-oriented and family-centered ethnoreligious groups. My point is simply and basically to reiterate here the truism that the family remains the nuclear socializing factor for the oncoming generation. In order to fulfill this fundamental function, the family must possess certain characteristics to catalyze the passage of its young through the successive stages of separation-individuation so that they will ultimately assume the responsibilities that mature adulthood requires.

Growing children require the presence of both a father and a mother for optimal development. By the same token, the uniparental family will raise and produce a significantly greater number of mentally disturbed and socially deviant youth—a specter that haunts the future of this country as well as much of Western culture. Thus, barring the exigencies of accident or illness, the family should, indeed must, be biparental.

The average-developing child achieves object constancy (Fraiberg 1969; Mahler et al. 1975; Rinsley 1982) and the beginning of a coherent sense of self and separateness only by three years of age. It is evident, therefore, that the mother should be freely and continuously available to the young child throughout this critical period and, hence, should not be employed outside the home on anything approaching a full-time basis.

Despite the sometimes strident protests of assorted self-styled androgynists and unisexists, respective paternal and maternal roles within the nuclear family, although reasonably flexible, are not interchangeable. Especially during the preschool years, the paternal role is basically executive and administrative, while the maternal role is basically alimentary and nurturant. Traditionally and appropriately, therefore, the mother serves to maintain the nest while the father serves to support and protect it. In fact, in the healthy functioning family a sensitive awareness and acceptance of these differential roles precludes their becoming rigid to the point of stifling communication and growth.

Of course, related directly to the healthy operation of these differential parental roles is the matter of sexual or gender identity. The nuclear family serves as growth promoter for parents and children alike. In the case of the parents, the experience of family life generates the basis for the achievement of genuine intimacy. Within the conjugal bond, the husband achieves increasing comfort with his need to nurture within the context of his masculine identity, while the wife progressively and healthily integrates her aggressiveness within the context of her feminine, maternal identity.

The healthy family sympathetically but firmly imposes due and proper discipline in accordance with the child's needs for equitable guidance and limit setting. In curbing the youngster's natural egocentrism and grandiosity, the parents properly divert raw instinctual needs and demands into progressively effective sublimatory channels, thereby providing the child with expanding opportunities for emotional growth and cognitive and social learning. So-called laissez-faire approaches to child rearing, allowing the immature child to control and even dominate the parents and the overall family structure, produce ill-socialized and learning-deficient adolescents and adults, just as such approaches in the school produce "graduates" who are notably deficient in literate cognitive skills.

Especially important are the family's extrafamilial relationships and

9

commerce, particularly during the child's latency or primary school years. As the child's intellectual horizons progressively expand throughout this period, the family's ties to outside individuals, families, and agencies afford him multiple opportunities to compare and contrast the specifics of his family's modus vivendi with that of others, to diffuse and displace the infantile grandiosity he or she has projected onto his or her parents, and to demystify them. This fundamental step toward eventual adulthood is optimally taken only if the nuclear family is meaningfully articulated with the wider extrafamilial culture. At the same time, it is inhibited or even precluded if the wider culture is in a state of disarray.

Paraphrasing Erikson (1963), we may say that the three major "tasks" of the preschool years are: the establishment of the foundations of self-identity ("I am, I exist"); the mastery of self and of the environment ("I can, I am able, I have impact"); and the beginning consolidation of gender identity ("I am boy, I am girl"). Their achievement in turn testifies to the attainment of a degree of separation-individuation that is appropriate for this time of life. It includes the consolidation of the sense of ownership or property, the control of one's eliminative sphincters, the beginning of early peer-group identifications, and the development of evocative memory that signifies the inception of preoperational cognition (Piaget 1937). These and numerous other related developmental attainments attest to the preschooler's preparation for definitive entrance into what has been termed the child's "occupation," namely, the experience of attending school, which for the next twelve-odd years will occupy between one-fourth and one-third of the child's time. By the time the child begins school, the nuclear family must have brought him to a degree of socialization that will permit and stimulate his efficient and expanding use of the range of cognitive and psychosocial experiences that constitute his education toward the goal of healthy, literate adulthood.

Few students of the domestic cultural scene would dispute that these and numerous related traditional values and mores had come into serious question during the 1960s and well into the 1970s—if, indeed, they had not been scrapped altogether. In the United States, a complex of social dynamisms and their visible public effects portrayed a society profoundly at odds with itself, driven by internecine conflicts, and increasingly characterized by situational ethics that amply justified the application of Christopher Lasch's (1978) label, "the culture of narcissism." Although the history of this benighted period remains to be written, and our temporal proximity to it is ever conducive to inferential distortion, I shall

DONALD B. RINSLEY

nonetheless have the temerity to list and briefly discuss a number of social phenomena I believe to be related to, if not etiologic for, this trend.

1. THE VIETNAM CONFLICT

No other single factor than this country's bellicose involvement in Southeast Asia seemed more to divide the American people throughout the 1960s and even beyond its ignominious end in 1975. Of the many social divisions it spawned, none seemed more significant than the split between youth and adults, epitomized by the tragedy at Kent State University. During this time the phrase "generation gap" came into popular use, and the exhortation, "Don't trust anybody over thirty!" became the chief platitude of the disaffected young. The conflict itself served as arena for every conceivable error in the use and deployment of men and material; a grand exercise in self-defeat. Its veterans returned, not as heroes, but as pariahs whose high frequency of posttraumatic psychopathology will haunt society for decades to come.

2. DEMYSTIFICATION

As I am using it here, the term "demystification" is roughly equivalent to demythologization, encompassing several social trends with considerable national impact. One of these involved a falling away from traditional religion, including what is often termed the Protestant work ethic. The avant garde demythologizers proclaimed that "God is dead" or else that he was living in Argentina. A new realism pervaded the populace, including elementary and secondary school textbooks, in effect debunking our traditional heroes as flawed, inept, or misguided personalities. The inspirational clichés long employed to provide the basis for juvenile identifications, hence for later identity consolidation, were characterized as empty phrases or even as hoaxes. Who could then believe, much less behave, in accordance with such platitudes as "honesty is the best policy" and "a penny saved is a penny earned"?

Along with the demystification of traditional religious and cultural values and figures proceeded a similar demystification of parental surrogates. The confused, dysfunctional family portrayed in the 1950s movie *Rebel without a Cause* seemed increasingly to characterize middle-income and affluent America. Schism and skew (Lidz, Fleck, and Cornelison 1965, 1968) and the "rubber fence" (Wynne 1961) appeared more

11

and more to typify families whose parents (if, indeed, there were two of them) suffered from parental perplexity (Goldfarb 1961)—they seemed not to know what to do with or how to raise their offspring. The latter floundered in a domestic atmosphere replete with parental ambivalence and inconsistency articulated by an attitude of laissez-faire.

3. DEMYSTIFICATION OF SEXUALITY

During the 1960s the demystification process progressively included the sexual relationship, encompassing the sexual aspect of parental bonding. Sex emerged "from the closet" and "went public." The so-called sexual revolution had arrived, its hedonistic ethic expressed in what came popularly to be known as the Playboy Philosophy that, in its most elemental form, held that "If it feels good, do it!" In accordance with this point of view, only the most egregiously bizarre or revolting forms of human sexual behavior could be considered abnormal, perverse, sick, or unhealthy. And since sexual interaction was considered to be little more than another of various forms of human communication, then the sexual relationship could indeed bear no fundamental relationship to marriage, child rearing, or family building. I shall illustrate this sexual state of affairs by briefly comparing the respective features of the traditional and the so-called evolving contemporary pattern of parental sexual relations (Rinsley 1980):

Traditional Pattern	*Evolving Contemporary Pattern*
a) Sexual intercourse is legitimized only within the marital relationship and is accepted, if not as an inevitable relationship, to the birth and rearing of children.	*a*) Because sexual intercourse or, for that matter, any form of sexual behavior is merely another variety of human communication, and since almost all forms of sexual behavior are completely private and equally normal or healthy, sexual activity bears no ultimate relationship to child rearing or family building.
b) The family's task is the intergenerational transmission of	*b*) The family cannot serve as transmitter of wider sociocultural

traditional, wider, sociocultural values and norms, thereby providing for the socialization of the next generation's members.

c) Children are not merely little adults. Their progressive and effectual socialization require careful, nurturant parental attention to their age-graded developmental needs and capabilities throughout childhood and adolescence. Such nurturant attention is predominantly supplied by the mother.

d) The basic task of childhood is separation-individuation from the infant's early symbiotic tie to the mother, the significant implementation of which is performed by the father, whose basic familial role is that of nest protector, breadwinner, administrator, and planner.

e) The basic parent-child relationship, later expressed in the teacher-student relationship, is therefore asymmetric. In decreasing degree as the child matures and progressively socializes, he submits to the parents' benevolent but firm authority and support and "rewards" the parents by identification with and acceptance of their standards of conduct and belief and by successful performance of the child's "occupation," namely, successful use of the school. The parents' responsibilities to the child include successful promotion

norms and values since these are subjective and situational.

c) Because children cannot be expected to conform their thought and behavior to such norms and values, the basic parent-child relationship is essentially symmetric; as a corollary, children will enjoy the same constitutional and civil rights as adults.

d) The nurturing of children may be equally shared or delegated between the father and the mother and parental roles are largely if not fully interchangeable.

e) The parents' laissez-faire attitude toward their children, reflected in the symmetric parent-child relationship, seeks no "rewards" in terms of the child's ultimate separation-individuation and eventual emancipation, in turn expressed in marriage and child rearing. The parents' grandparental role vis-à-vis their children's children no longer legitimizes the parents' parenthood. How the child eventuates is his own affair and no business of the parents.

of the latter's emancipation and assumption of independence, the last in turn expressed through the child's own marriage and family building. The parents' grand-parenting of their children's children serves as metaphor for the ultimate success of their own child-rearing efforts.

Little needs to be added concerning that particular component of sexual demystification known as gay or homosexual rights. Publicly touted as a major aspect of a purported advanced wave of sexual libera-tion, the homosexual movement witnessed assemblages of torch-bearing and placard-wielding male and female homosexuals vociferously pro-claiming their health and demanding the enactment of ordinances and statutes recognizing them as a valid "minority" and guaranteeing protec-tion against all forms of discrimination.

4. DEMYSTIFICATION OF THE SCHOOL

Nor was the school exempt from the demystification process. Growing numbers of alienated, disaffected, drug-suffused students turned to teachers and professors for the emotional sustenance their parents had proved incapable of providing, only to be frustrated again. For indeed, the schools had since evolved into glorified baby-sitting agencies inca-pable of imparting literate cognitive skills, beset with violence, and producing graduates unable to read, write, or reckon. Johnny couldn't perform because he had been exposed to a congeries of pseudoeduca-tional folderol typified by the "open" classroom, the ungraded curricu-lum, and the infamous social promotion administered by cadres of teachers graduated from college-level educational programs that had taught them little or nothing.

5. ENVIRONMENTALISM

Taking their departure from Rachel Carson's (1962) book, *Silent Spring*, vocal environmentalists and self-styled consumer advocates trumpeted throughout the land that Americans were poisoning them-selves with a variety of toxic wastes, smokestack and automobile exhaust

14

fumes, detergents, and other morbid effluents, effluvia, and miasmas. Although by no means without a basis in fact, these accusations led to a rash of legislation and judicial pronouncements that further added to an already bloated, wasteful governmental bureaucracy, fueling inflation and compounding the view that the United States had developed into a grand pestilential sinkhole. The psychoanalyst would be tempted to consider these phenomena as symbolic of a progressive accumulation of bad internal objects with the results expressed in accumulated rage, depression, and alienation. And what should otherwise have served as a ready outlet for the aggression associated with these objects, namely, a winnable shooting war with a despised "bad external object"—our traditional "solution" for accumulated excremental representations—turned out to be the self-defeating, no-win debacle of Vietnam.

6. FEMINISM

Related to the so-called sexual revolution of the 1960s and 1970s was the emergence of what came to be known as the feminist or women's movement with its roots in women's suffrage during the early years of this century. Terms and phrases such as "androgyny," "sexism," "unisex," and "sex role stereotype" were pressed into service in connection with demands for "equal rights" for women but often going well beyond that in asserting that "women can do anything men can do" and even advancing the claim that the numerous assumed and evident differences between the genders were the products of social learning and had nothing to do with biology. Operating with this point of view and beginning in many cases as early as in the nursery school, so-called unisex teachers attempted to jettison the traditional gender-related approach to boys and girls in order to preclude the young students' acquisition of what the teachers regarded as sexist attitudes and to minimize gender-related differences. This approach generally took the form of pushing girls into "male" attitudes and activities while often not unsubtly denigrating the latter in an attempt to effeminize boys. The more strident feminists viewed women as "nigger," exploited and enslaved by unscrupulous, exploitive, strutting, and prancing "macho" men beset with "womb envy," the presumed male counterpart of the hated "penis envy," a concept derived from the "sexist" Viennese, Sigmund Freud.

The feminist movement received increasing impetus from the economic inflation that extended throughout this period and witnessed in-

15

creasing numbers of single and married women entering the full-time work force, competing with men as breadwinners, and serving as heads of fatherless households. At the same time, these women consigned their preschool children and, in increasing numbers, their infants to assorted baby-sitters and group care facilities, the dire effects of which are only now becoming evident. Male-female role reversal likewise witnessed the emergence of what came to be known as the "househusband." Again, as one female author put it, "We don't need men—we can have better orgasms by masturbating, we can get pregnant through artificial insemination, and the State will protect our nests!"

7. ROCK MUSIC AND DRUGS

Of widespread appeal to the adolescent and young adult population during the 1960s and 1970s was that particular variety of strident, often cacophonous, and rhythmically stereotyped aural phenomenon known as rock music. Rock music had its inception in a late 1950s precursor termed "rock-and-roll," epitomized in the work of its acknowledged master, the late Elvis Presley, a talented and musically versatile artist whose successful career peaked and rapidly receded during and after the last few years of the 1950s and the first few years of the 1960s. Presley's replacement, the Beatles, whose often nonmelodic style and offbeat life-styles established a trend that continues to the present, came to be slavishly mimicked by a seemingly endless array of bizarrely named and often outlandish appearing and acting rock groups. Rock lyrics often typically consisted of nonrhyming expostulations of misery and alienation coupled with occasionally precocious insights into mankind's meaninglessness and depravity, and they often touted the use of illicit drugs. Many of rock music's practitioners were themselves drug addicts, and some of them eventually drugged themselves to death. From this ilk emerged the youth idols of the last score of years, the symbols of the alienated young who tastelessly adored them, culminating in the latter-day so-called punk rockers whose entertainment consisted of scatology and obscenity.

The burgeoning social disaster that was the 1960s, with racial riots and cities afire, also witnessed the emergence of what came to be known as the "drug culture." Timothy Leary exhorted youth to "tune in, turn on, and drop out"; others such as Richard Alpert, who gratuitously renamed himself Baba Ram Dass, embraced various forms of culture-alien guruism, immersing themselves in the purportedly superior wisdom and

16

higher consciousness of Eastern mysticism that had been wrenched from its context. Communes, sometimes called ashrams, burgeoned while some of the period's aberrant pseudoreligions reacted to the period's sexual and pharmacological disasters by extolling abstinence and celibacy.

8. THE CIVIL RIGHTS MOVEMENT

Receiving powerful early impetus from the 1954 Supreme Court decision in *Brown* v. *Board of Education*, the expanding civil rights movement of the 1960s served as a powerful attraction, a cause célèbre, to which alienated youth and adults could attach themselves idealistically to terminate all "discrimination," eliminate all "inequalities," and provide "equal opportunity" for all. Much of the movement's dynamic witnessed concerted and not rarely violent efforts by young people to disempower the "privileged" and to redistribute their holdings or vitiate their effect among the poor and the downtrodden. Easily discerned in many of their responses within this movement are the dynamics of the egocentric, megalomanic child who would greedily appropriate the strength, possessions, and privileges of the parent. Thus did teachers, policemen and fire fighters, politicians, administrators, health-care professionals, corporate executives, and others of influence and achievement acquire the collective title "establishment." They came to be viewed as representatives and entrepreneurs of a supposedly inequitable, decadent system symbolic of the home and the parents. The resurgent egalitarianism and antielitism inherent in this movement spawned a situational and hierarchy-free ethics devoid of rules, legitimate distinctions and differences, academic tests, course grades, and other supposed indicators of privilege and uniqueness.

9. LEVELING

As employed here, the term "leveling" has to do with the process of effacement of distinctions and differences, the unstated objective of which is to banish or eliminate individuality, uniqueness, and excellence through a reduction to a minimal if acceptable degree ("level") of mediocrity of whomever or whatever is subjected to it. In contemporary America, leveling came to be reflected in a pervasive sense of entitlement, ranging from the guaranteed annual income to the guaranteed high school diploma and, in some settings, the guaranteed—hence meaning-less—college degree. The demystification of parents, of teachers, of national leaders, and of authorities of all sorts reflected that literal misinterpretation of the Declaration of Independence to the effect that everybody was "equal to" everybody else. Thus, we were told that there were really no differences between male and female, between parent and child, between teacher and student, between manager and worker. And as if that were not all, we were told that there was really no difference between the mentally healthy and the mentally ill; we were informed that psychotic thinking and behavior could indeed represent a higher form of conscious awareness; that the civil commitment of the severely mentally ill was nothing more than imprisonment without due process of law; that such persons were a minority of people whom other people could not bear to have around. We were advised that mental health professionals should disband, join the ranks of social activists, shut down the mental hospitals, and proceed to correct social injustices, including the stifling partriarchism, from which that variety of human unhappiness and oppression mislabeled mental illness purportedly arises (Brown 1959; Laing 1967; Marcuse 1955; Szasz 1965, 1974).

10. THE DEMISE OF QUALITY

Related to the shibboleths of the civil rights movement and its associ-ated processes of leveling was the general demise of quality. Along with the steady decline of quality public education went a concomitant decline in the quality of domestic manufactured products, most evident but by no means limited to electrical appliances and the once-vaunted American automobile. Indeed, so sleazy were our manufactured products consid-ered to be in the world marketplace that the Japanese, once viewed as makers of the cheap and the shoddy, turned up their noses at anything marked "Made in the U.S.A." while their automotive vehicles estab-lished high marks for quality and reliability. Throughout the 1960s and 1970s American consumers became inured to, if not satisfied with, that state of affairs, while the measurable productivity of the American worker proceeded inexorably to fall. And, indeed, Mr. Average Amer-ican became increasingly aware of an adversarial economic system ener-vated by repetitive conflicts between labor and management, between workers and owners, between employees and employers. It seemed as if in their headlong rush to generate a society that guaranteed womb-to-

tomb security, the work force had lost sight of the quality of the goods and services it was supposed to provide; "What's in it for me?" became the worker's catch phrase, while his employer, the corporate executive, likewise proceeded to sabotage quality in a singleminded pursuit of short-term profit.

Of course, quality is strongly related to frustration tolerance, the capacity to postpone gratification in favor of longer-term goals. And frustration tolerance disappears amidst a national atmosphere that lionizes the immediate, the here-and-now, the ruthlessly individualistic, and the hedonistic. It comes as no surprise that in such an atmosphere there came to the fore a host of individuals, groups, and publications devoted to "self-realization" and "self-actualization," to strategies for "how to win," "how to gain the upper hand," "how to be creatively aggressive" and "self-assertive," and how to "do your own thing." It is as if these proffered pathways to influence and affluence were indeed defenses against deeply felt ineffectuality, emotional poverty, and alienation (Vitz 1977).

A Comment on Social Pathogenesis

Having in mind the pitfalls of analogical reasoning, I shall nonetheless put forward the inference that the leveling to which I have made reference reflects the wider sociocultural expression of the sort of dynamics and structure that typifies dysfunctional families. Numerous studies, beginning with that of Healy and Bronner (1936) and extending to the contributions of Bateson and his colleagues (Bateson 1972; Bateson, Jackson, Haley, and Weakland 1968; Lidz, Fleck, and Cornelison 1968; Wynne 1961), have demonstrated the baleful effects on growing children's identities of the sort of familial aimlessness, pseudomutuality, narcissistic self-absorption, and inconsistent or absent self-discipline that seemed to characterize significant segments of our society during the period under discussion (Lasch 1977, 1978). As I noted elsewhere (Rinsley 1978), even the healthy family would experience significant difficulty in raising its offspring while attempting to articulate itself with a wider sociocultural nexus characterized by anomie, drugs, and violence. Thus, with what coherent, meaningful, and predictable extrafamilial educational and wider cultural standards would the latency-age child be expected to compare those of his nuclear family in such an atmosphere? To what extent could such a wider culture be expected to further the child's need to broaden his self-concept and successfully traverse the stages of preoperational thought toward fully developed abstract-categorical cognition? Within such a context, how could the early and middle adolescent be expected to defer heterosexual intercourse, for which he or she is unprepared, in the interest of ongoing age-appropriate emotional and intellectual development? And what of the child "raised" in a uniparental, female-dominated household, early given over to the care of assorted baby-sitters, devoid of the intimate, growth-promoting maternal bond that is essential for healthy separation-individuation?

I have no doubt that three significant phenomena characteristic of the period of the last quarter-century are intimately related to the sort of individual and wider sociocultural leveling I am discussing, namely, the documented increases in juvenile delinquency, the rate of crime, and the rate of divorce. It can be argued that a society characterized by a widespread public feeling of entitlement, of earning without producing, of academic advancement without study, of sex without responsibility sets the stage for the increasing emergence of those who would take without earning, who would rob and assault without concern for their victims, and who would regard the marital contract as a readily terminable cohabitation akin to a contract to purchase and exchange commercial merchandise. Their deficient socialization reflects an infancy and childhood deficient in healthy parenting, and their narcissism drives them in repetitive and futile attempts to fill in the gaps in their identity (Balint 1968), to make good the losses they have never worked through with little or no regard for the consequences. Those who become criminals from a sense of guilt, as Freud (1916) so cogently put it, unconsciously seek in the experience of apprehension, trial, and imprisonment to reembrace and recapitulate the symbiotic mother-infant tie from which they never extricated themselves, to recapture at last the longed-for state of primitive fusion through incarceration behind concrete walls and iron bars.

Effects on Adolescent Identity

As is well known, the consolidation of one's identity as a mature, socialized, stable, and productive individual represents a coalescence of self and object representations that begins with what Winnicott (1950–1955) aptly termed "good enough mothering" and continues throughout life (Erikson 1963). Good enough mothering represents the precursor of *good enough parenting* in accordance with the optimally flexible functional differences between the roles of mother and father; it likewise defines the goodness of fit, as it were, between the evolving needs of the growing child and the communicatively matched needs and responses of the parents.

By the time the child reaches and enters adolescence, this goodness of fit should have provided him with the perceptual, cognitive, affective, and interactional foundations of separation-individuation—of the three basic tasks of the preschool child to which I have already made reference. Where these tasks have effectively been accomplished, the child's transit of the adolescent period and experience is largely devoid of the so-called storm and stress that psychoanalytic writers were earlier wont to associate with that period (Rinsley 1980).

However much the regressive-recapitulative aspects of adolescence were overemphasized by devotees of the so-called turmoil view of the adolescent experience, they nonetheless exert a not inconsiderable effect on the adolescent's search for identity; in them we note an amended recapitulation of the three basic tasks to which I have referred. The earlier "I am" becomes for the adolescent "Who am I?" and "What am I to become?" The earlier "I can," "I am able," and "I have impact" become for the adolescent the important matter of occupational choice, of commitment to work and to produce. The earlier "I am boy" or "I am girl" becomes for the adolescent the salient matter of consolidation of polymorphous-perverse pregenital aims within an emerging genitality conveyed in respective manhood and womenhood. Another feature of adolescence, the consolidation of abstract-categorical, hypothetico-deductive, or circular operational thinking gives expression to the end point of the ever-widening intellectual scope that typified the adolescent's preadolescent years. The adolescent, as it were, falls in love with this powerful cognitive tool and, yet retaining much of the narcissism of his prior childhood years, concludes that others, most notably his parents, should think and act as does he: as he often oppositionally embraces unpopular causes, seeks and finds myriad "injustices," and waves assorted flags and banners, in many cases well into young adulthood.

Case Example

Debra, a bright thirteen-year-old borderline adolescent who was drawing close to a successful termination of a three-and-one-half-year full-time, residential treatment program, said to me in the 325th hour of her individual psychotherapy:

Well . . . I know I've been sick and now I'm almost well—but the world is a mess . . . people killing each other, countries at war, crooked politicians, crazy families like mine was . . . wow! . . . how do you make it out there? . . . if that's all crazy then why get well, why not just stay sick . . . ?

Debra's anxiety over her future, over her as yet untested ability to cope extramurally, was, of course, evident in her cogent statement and question. As well, her question concerned my own integrity and believability as well as those of the intensive therapeutic program in which she had for so long been involved; and, of course, the projective implications, inherent in her question in terms of viewing "out there" as a macrocosm of what was once her own pathology, were also evident. In response, I reminded Debra of one of our previous discussions regarding "options," a term and concept that had served her well during the course of her treatment. She replied, "Oh, I remember . . . you told me that the sicker you are the fewer your options . . . like when you're in the hospital with a broken leg, you can't even get up to go to the bathroom and you have to have a nurse bring you a bedpan . . . like when you're well you're free to choose. . . ." In affirming her statement, I added, "Right, there's a lot of craziness out there but there's a lot of the opposite too . . . we've got to see both and be free enough to make the right decisions for ourselves and those we love . . . options again!" Debra replied, "Well, I've got some more of those now than I had when I first came in here. . . ." We could agree!

Quite apart from the evidently defensive aspect of her view of the world as a "mess" was a deeper awareness of the degree of dysfunctionality, of stress and strain, as it were, that had typified the intrafamilial and extended social milieu within which her illness had been spawned. She could not have known that sociocultural disintegration constituted the key variable of the Stirling County Study (Leighton, Harding, Macklin, MacMillan, and Leighton 1963) and degree of "stress and strain," a key variable in the Midtown Manhattan Study (Srole, Langner, Opler, and Rennie 1962; Langner and Michael 1963). Both studies pointed up the relationship of prevalence of mental disorder and socioeconomic determinants deleterious to human development. One implication of these studies, consonant with the earlier findings of Faris and Dunham (1939) in the Chicago area, was to the effect that delapidated, disintegrated social milieus are conducive to a higher rate of psychopathology. Such milieus constitute environments that are less than "average expectable," hence are pervasively unsupportive for healthy human development and adaptive capacity. At the same time, they serve as attractants for numbers of distracted and disorganized individuals essentially devoid of meaningful human relationships ("downward drift"). We thus come full circle in realizing that these milieus are deficient in tradition. Those very characteristics of what Winnicott called the facilitating environment characterize the microcosm of the healthy family that functions in accordance with rules and principles on which its members may confidently depend and from which the next generation's mature adults may be expected to emerge.

A major issue for everyone, which the adolescent experiences with particular poignancy, has to do with the relationship and necessary balance between authority and responsibility, between the exercise of one's effect on and control of others in relation to the mature awareness and sensitivity that must temper them. In his effort to define himself, the adolescent is wont to attempt to exert the former with a deficient awareness of the latter. And whether he is well or ill, he readily finds reinforcement for his often thoughtless exercise of authority, for his narcissistic expectation that others will think and act as he does, within a wider narcissistic culture that mirrors, hence that justifies, his egocentrism. For of what value and significance is the rule of law in a society where people are endlessly exhorted to "do their own thing," where, in the time-honored prisoner's cliché, "Nobody is a crook until he is stupid enough to get caught"?

A Comment on Borderline Disorder

It comes as no surprise that the concept and the clinical syndrome labeled borderline should have come into prominence during the past quarter-century and particularly in this country. I relate its emergence to the dethronement of the male. Its origin is to be found in the era of the Great Depression that extended throughout the 1930s when up to 20 percent of male workers, the families' father figures, were unemployed. Its emergence was facilitated by World War II, during which the nation's viable men were off to war, leaving behind them female-dominated, uniparental families into which their children were born, later to become the adolescents and young adults of the disastrous 1960s and 1970s. From that war, numerous combatant men returned with various degrees of what we now term posttraumatic stress disorder to resume their places in society and among their welcoming families—bearing the psychological scars from which many would never adequately recover. During that war, women assumed the roles of both parents, for the first time donning jeans and trousers, entering the factories and armed forces in support of the war effort, and experiencing a new if ambivalent "liberation" from domesticity.

I relate the social upheavals of the 1960s in substantial measure to the attainment of adolescence and young adulthood of the damaged offspring of wartime families, antecedent to which had been the more extended erosion of strong masculine authority and leadership during the Depression years. The various rights "movements" of the last quarter-century symbolized challenges to the attenuated authority of the white male, the symbolic plantation owner, by assorted minority subgroups who perceived opportunities to get for themselves what they believed the symbolic Simon Legrees had long denied them. The associated vacuum of national leadership found graphic expression in this nation's post–World War II military operations: the ill-starred, politicized "police action" in Korea, the failed action at the Cuban Bay of Pigs, and, last and most horrendous, the debacle of Vietnam—from which those who managed to survive returned, not as welcomed gladiators, but as scapegoated pariahs.

As Masterson and I have attempted to show, the pathogenesis of the borderline personality and its close relative, the narcissistic personality, is to be found in failure of separation-individuation with persistent, unresolved symbiotic needs (Masterson 1981; Masterson and Rinsley 1975; Rinsley 1982). The recognized effects of this persistent, infantile "tie that binds" include symptoms that result from failure to negotiate the infantile depressive position (Klein 1935, 1940): persistent depression and underlying or overt rage; persistent infantile megalomania admixed with feelings of emptiness, helplessness, and worthlessness; inability to work through (mourn) separations and losses; persistence of part and transitional object relations; persistence of the splitting defense and failure adequately to replace it with normal repression. As the father serves as the major factor in assisting the mother and the child to desymbiotize (Abelin 1971), the absence of the father or the presence of a weak, ineffectual, or otherwise immature and inadequate father deters the process of separation-individuation. It may be concluded that a major determinant of the upsurge of personality or characterologic disorders and of the borderline concept during the past twenty-five years has been the relative dearth of male functional leadership, both in the home and on the national scene.

Conclusions

Four centuries before Christ, the pre-Socratic, hylozoist philosopher Anaximenes wrote that the world consists of an ongoing series of rarefactions and condensations, analogous to the endless cycle of the vaporization and precipitation of water. Twenty-five hundred years later, Melanie Klein taught us that, in effect, life is a series of affiliations and separations of comings and goings and that much of what we call psychological health is based on coping with them and, in particular, with separations. Throughout mankind's countless generations there has occurred the similarly endless cycle of birth, death, and rebirth, of one generation's preparation of its children to take their place in the next, to guarantee a vital sequence symbolic of the continuity that represents immortality. To do this successfully, each of us must have acquired that degree of selfhood that permits us healthily to mourn—hence, however reluctantly at times, to separate. This is the quintessential legacy that parents must leave to their children and that a sane society must assist its many families to carry out. For to bid goodbye to our loved ones, not to mention our enemies, is the hallmark of mental health, and those who are unable to accomplish this are forever doomed to live their lives in the past from which they will, paradoxically, learn little or nothing.

The sociocultural phenomena to which I have made reference here have, in my view, essentially precluded this important working through for many people. By so doing, they have precluded the relinquishment of infantile grandiosity that characterizes the healthy transformations of puberty. The reaction to them, however, has now set in; a widespread revolt against the excesses and aberrations of the 1960s and 1970s is evident. More and more people are demanding a return to traditional, basic values, to a reestablishment of meaningful norms, to a rediscovery of faith. The national cry is for the public schools to teach rather than to baby-sit; the so-called Playboy Philosophy no longer serves as leitmotiv for the alienated; and there is mounting evidence of the disaffection of youth with the self-serving bizarreness of these decades.

I shall close this discussion with a fond return to Tevye the Jew, whose traditionalism is expressed in the wise words of Sir Francis Bacon, who

25

said: "Nature is often hidden:/Sometimes overcome:/Seldom extinguished."

NOTE

1. Revised from an address originally delivered at the Central States Conference of the American Society for Adolescent Psychiatry, Galveston, Texas, September, 1980.

REFERENCES

Abelin, E. L. 1971. The role of the father in the separation-individuation process. In J. McDevitt and C. F. Settlage, eds. *Separation-Individuation: Essays in Honor of Margaret S. Mahler.* New York: International Universities Press.

Balint, M. 1968. *The Basic Fault: Therapeutic Aspects of Regression.* London: Tavistock.

Bateson, G. 1972. *Steps to an Ecology of Mind.* New York: Ballantine.

Bateson, G.; Jackson, D. D.; Haley, J.; and Weakland, J. H. 1968. Toward a theory of schizophrenia. In D. D. Jackson, ed. *Communication, Family and Marriage.* Human Communication, Vol. 1. Palo Alto, Calif.: Science and Behavior Books.

Blos, P. 1962. *On Adolescence.* New York: Free Press.

Blos, P. 1967. The second individuation process of adolescence. *Psychoanalytic Study of the Child* 22:162–186.

Blos, P. 1979. *The Adolescent Passage.* New York: International Universities Press.

Brown, N. O. 1959. *Life against Death.* Middletown, Conn.: Wesleyan University Press.

Carson, R. 1962. *Silent Spring.* Boston: Houghton Mifflin.

Erikson, E. H. 1963. *Childhood and Society.* Rev. ed. New York: Norton.

Faris, R. E. L., and Dunham, W. H. 1939. *Mental Disorders in Urban Areas.* Chicago: University of Chicago Press.

Fraiberg, S. 1969. Libidinal object constancy and mental representation. *Psychoanalytic Study of the Child* 24:9–47.

Freud, S. 1916. Some character types met with in psychoanalytic work. *Standard Edition* 14:311–333. London: Hogarth, 1957.

Goldfarb, W. 1961. *Childhood Schizophrenia.* Cambridge, Mass.: Harvard University Press.

Healy, W., and Bronner, A. F. 1936. *New Light on Delinquency and Its Treatment*. New Haven, Conn.: Yale University Press.

Klein, M. 1935. A contribution to the psychogenesis of manic-depressive states. In *Melanie Klein: Love, Guilt and Reparation and Other Works, 1921–1945*. New York: Delacorte/Seymour Lawrence, 1975.

Klein, M. 1940. Mourning and its relations to manic-depressive states. In *Melanie Klein: Love, Guilt and Reparation and Other Works, 1921–1945*. New York: Delacorte/Seymour Lawrence, 1975.

Laing, R. D. 1967. *The Politics of Experience*. New York: Pantheon.

Langner, T. S., and Michael, S. T. 1963. *Life Stress and Mental Health: Volume 2 of the Midtown Manhattan Study, T.A.C. Rennie Series in Social Psychiatry*. New York: Free Press.

Lasch, C. 1977. *Haven in a Heartless World: The Family Besieged*. New York: Basic.

Lasch, C. 1978. *The Culture of Narcissism: American Life in an Age of Diminishing Expectations*. New York: Norton.

Leighton, D. C.; Harding, U. S.; Macklin, D. B.; MacMillan, A. M.; and Leighton, A. H. 1963. *The Character of Danger*. New York: Basic.

Lidz, T.; Fleck, S.; and Cornelison, A. R. 1965. *Schizophrenia and the Family*. New York: International Universities Press.

Lidz, T.; Fleck, S.; and Cornelison, A. R. 1968. Schism and skew in the families of schizophrenics. In N. W. Bell and E. F. Vogel, eds. *A Modern Introduction to the Family*. Rev. ed. New York: Free Press.

Mahler, M. S.; Pine, F.; and Bergman, A. 1975. *The Psychological Birth of the Human Infant: Symbiosis and Individuation*. New York: Basic.

Marcuse, H. 1955. *Eros and Civilization*. Boston: Beacon, 1965.

Masterson, J. F. 1981. *The Narcissistic and Borderline Disorders: An Integrated Developmental Approach*. New York: Brunner/Mazel.

Masterson, J. F., and Rinsley, D. B. 1975. The borderline syndrome: the role of the mother in the genesis and psychic structure of the borderline personality. *International Journal of Psycho-Analysis* 56:163–177.

Piaget, J. 1937. *The Construction of Reality in the Child*. New York: Basic, 1954.

Rinsley, D. B. 1978. Juvenile delinquency: a review of the past and a look at the future. *Bulletin of the Menninger Clinic* 42:252–260.

Rinsley, D. B. 1980. *Treatment of the Severely Disturbed Adolescent*. New York: Jason Aronson.

Rinsley, D. B. 1982. *Borderline and Other Self Disorders: A Developmental and Object-Relations Perspective*. New York: Jason Aronson.

Srole, L.; Langner, T. S.; Opler, M. K.; and Rennie, T. A. C. 1962. *Mental Health in the Metropolis: The Midtown Manhattan Study.* Vol. 1. New York: McGraw-Hill.

Szasz, T. S. 1965. *Psychiatric Justice.* New York: Macmillan.

Szasz, T. S. 1974. *The Myth of Mental Illness.* Rev. ed. New York: Harper & Row.

Vitz, P. C. 1977. *Psychology as Religion: The Cult of Self-Worship.* Grand Rapids, Mich.: Eerdmans.

Winnicott, D. W. 1950–1955. Aggression in relation to emotional development. In *Collected Papers: Through Paediatrics to Psycho-Analysis.* London: Tavistock, 1958.

Wynne, L. C. 1961. The study of intrafamilial alignments and splits in exploratory family therapy. In N. W. Ackerman, ed. *Exploring the Base for Family Therapy.* New York: Family Service Association of America.

2 THE IMPACT OF ADOLESCENT CHILDREN ON FAMILY SYSTEMS

JERRY M. LEWIS

While emptying the pockets before washing a sixteen-year-old son's jeans, Mother discovered a condom. "You've got to talk with him," Mother said to Father. "What do you think I should say?" was the response.

Awakening in the middle of the night parents heard footsteps and whispers in the hall. A daughter's boyfriend is an overnight guest. "We need to do something," the father said to the mother. "I agree," she replied. "What did you have in mind?"

A sixteen-year-old daughter received two speeding tickets in the same week. "She needs to be grounded," Father said. "I'm not sure," Mother responded. "How will she get to school and her after-school job?"

"They are B's not D's," Mother said. "He's an A student, and we need to do something," was Father's quick response.

These brief parental exchanges are commonplace (at least in middle-class families) and reflect the uncertainties and difficulties involved in having adolescent children. Each of the vignettes poses a challenge to the parental relationship. Do the parents agree on what their response should be? If they differ, how do they characteristically resolve such disagreements? Will these brief (and obviously not golden) moments in their parenting experience serve as a launching pad for yet another escalating conflict?

I wish to explore the impact of family structure and, in particular, the parents' marital relationship on the family's experience of its children's adolescent years and the reciprocal influence of the children's adolescence on the family structure.

Olson, McCubbin, and Associates (1983) report that parents report greater stress when their offspring are adolescents than at other times in the family life cycle and that adolescents themselves may be the least satisfied of all family members with their family situations. Careful studies are rare, however, and little is known about the factors that influence the way normal families react to the adolescence of their children. A large number of variables are almost certainly involved. Some relate to the adolescents, and some of these are biologic in nature (for example, gender and the role of physical maturation). More recently, the almost exclusive emphasis on male development has been corrected, and we are beginning to understand crucial differences involved in female adolescent development. Although such differences may reflect primarily the operation of cultural values regarding gender roles, the parental anxieties and stress are different for boys and for girls. Another issue is that of the adolescent's physical development. Parents may be concerned about the eleven-year-old daughter whose breasts are well developed and whose menstruation has started, but parents can also be concerned about a sixteen-year-old daughter whose development does not include breast development and the menarche. There are comparable concerns about developmental extremes in boys.

Another group of critical variables involves the nature of the child's experience of adolescence. Because they were drawn from clinical samples, early models presented normal adolescence as tumultuous, but research has established that there is considerable variation in how youngsters experience their adolescent years (Offer 1965). For some it is a relatively quiet and smooth process, and anxiety and other affects are dealt with, for the most part, internally. For others, however, there is more intense affective expression and greater lability. For some families the nature of their adolescent's experience is critical. The relationship between the adolescent's experience and family variables is, however, complex. Family variables can influence, often decisively, the nature of the child's experience of adolescence.

Peer group norms and the degree to which a particular adolescent is a part of such groups can influence the family's experience of its child's adolescence. Socioeconomic and cultural variables can also influence the adolescent's experience and its impact on the family decisively. Growing up poor or being a member of an ethnic minority can distort the adolescent developmental process beyond belief, and in combination their effects can be devastating.

Some family variables, in conjunction with adolescent variables, play a crucial role in determining the impact of adolescence on the family. Whether a family is biologically intact, single-parent, or recombined, the family's economic circumstances, religious orientation, and ethnic membership mold the family's hopes and expectations and contribute decisively to its experience. The amount, duration, and severity of stress attributable to other issues that the family faces may overburden the family's coping capacity.

The family as an entity passes through a sequence of developmental stages, and the impact of adolescent children may be very different for a couple in their late fifties than it is for thirty-five-year-old parents. Although various adolescent and family variables interact in ways that give form and substance to the family's experience, I wish to focus this presentation on the ways in which a family's basic organizational structure influences its children's experience of adolescence and on the impact of that adolescent's experience on the family, considering in particular the often critical role of the parental alliance in determining the quality of the reciprocal relationship between adolescent experience and the family.

In describing the parental relationship as a central family variable, my focus is transactional and macroscopic. At a more microscopic level and from a self-psychology perspective, Weissman and Cohen (1985) have provided a description of the parenting alliance as a component of the marital relationship, an adult life-course process that both amplifies and is amplified by the self-psychology concept of self-selfobject relationships orginally developed by Kohut (1971, 1977). What seems needed to bridge the levels between their work and my own is the systematic study of parenting alliances with the different characteristic marital relationship structures that occur across the continuum of family competence.

The Braxtons appeared to be a well-functioning family who were middle-class, churchgoing, and had three active little boys, a brick home, and a carefully tended lawn. When their eldest son, Bobby, reached age fourteen, however, the family seemed to change. Bobby began to fail courses in school, smoke marijuana, associate with a tough group of boys, and was arrested for breaking and entering.

The parents began to disagree openly—often violently—about how to manage Bobby. Father favored a stern, discipline-oriented approach, and Mother pleaded the need for greater understanding and counseling; their disagreements and conflicts grew in frequency and intensity. The two younger sons began to distance themselves from the family and spend more time with peers. Bobby's antisocial behavior became more pronounced, and ultimately a sentencing judge gave the parents the option of either admitting Bobby to a treatment program or remanding the boy to the state juvenile justice system. The Braxtons chose treatment, and the family was evaluated, as one facet of the son's assessment.

The data that emerged broaden our understanding of the many interacting factors that played crucial roles in Bobby's and the family's behavior. I wish to focus particularly on a more private view of the Braxton family and to introduce the concept that the organizational structure of the family is an important determinant of the family's response to the adolescence of its children. By organizational structure I refer to those more or less enduring patterns of interaction among family members and between the family and the outside world that are so much a part of life within the family that they are unnoticed by family members.

Behind a facade of conventionality, the Braxtons were a clearly dysfunctional family, and the assessment data suggest that the family's dysfunction existed long before Bobby entered adolescence. Bobby's struggle with adolescent developmental challenges, however, had altered the expression and the pattern of the family's dysfunction. Life in the Braxton family strongly reflected the quality of the parents' relationship, which involved a controlling and domineering role for Mr. Braxton and a more passive and subservient—but clearly resentful—role for Mrs. Braxton. This unequal distribution of power began early in the parents' relationship and echoed the family organizational structure of both of their families of origin. Mrs. Braxton's resentment was clear to the observer, but it was not expressed directly; it erupted in a variety of forgetful, omitting, and other passive-aggressive mechanisms. Mrs. Braxton, whatever her contribution to her dominant-submissive marriage, was chronically lonely, and it was easy for her to enter into a very special relationship with her firstborn son. The relationship seemed innocent enough when Bobby was younger, but it became destructive as Bobby entered adolescence. Bobby's antisocial behavior reflected Mrs. Braxton's anger at her husband. She subtly encouraged her son's behavior and enjoyed a vicarious satisfaction when her husband, not being able to control him, suffered much anguish.

Three observations of the Braxton family's organizational structure are important: (1) the family structure had been dominated by the father prior to Bobby's adolescence, (2) a long-smoldering conflict between the parents had intensified and become overt as the cadence of Bobby's symptoms increased, and (3) Mrs. Braxton and Bobby had an important alliance that came to be oppositional to Mr. Braxton's attempts to dominate and control the family. What is the meaning of these three observations? To what body of data and theory of family functioning do they relate most clearly? What relevance do they have for the clinician as he or she constructs a treatment plan? In order to approach these issues I wish to outline briefly certain of our research findings as they relate to the issues of family organizational structure and family competence.

Our research demonstrates that families with different organizational structures can be located at different points on a continuum of family competence. Family competence is measured by the extent to which a family both facilitates the developing autonomy in children and provides a psychosocial medium in which parental personalities can grow. These two cardinal tasks of the family are themselves value judgments regarding that which families "ought" to do, and they are influenced by sociocultural variables. Our data suggest, however, that families from two different socioeconomic and ethnic samples demonstrate striking similarities at different points on the continuum of family competence (Lewis, Beavers, Gossett, and Phillips 1977; Lewis and Looney 1983). Families that accomplish the two cardinal tasks well are termed highly competent, optimal, or healthy. Such families demonstrate a parental coalition characterized by flexibility, shared power, and considerable psychological intimacy. Together the parents provide strong, effective leadership of the family, but they are not authoritarian; rather, they listen to their adolescent children's ideas and feelings and seek solutions through negotiation. Communication in healthy families is clear and spontaneous. Family members are responsive to each other and take responsibility for individual opinions and actions. (Our research suggests that psychological intimacy is more prevalent in middle- and upper-middle-class than in lower-income, working-class families.) All kinds of feelings are clearly expressed, and empathy is commonplace. Roles are flexible, and differences acceptable. Such families use a wide range of processes to deal with novelty, change, and stress.

Competent but pained families are seen as being between healthy and dysfunctional families on the continuum of competence. Although as many of the adolescent children in these families are as psychologically healthy as is the case in optimal families, the parental coalition is not as strong—more specifically, the parents are anxious and fearful of closeness in their relationship. On the surface it is usually the wives who are dissatisfied and blame their husbands' remoteness for their own affective starvation. The husbands, in turn, blame their wives' unhappiness for the lack of closeness, and each participant fails to see his or her role in the shared dilemma. Because of their underlying anxiety about intimacy, the marital partners focus their relationship on the children and the children's activities. Such families lack the spontaneity, warmth, and affective openness of optimally healthy families. It is important to recognize, however, that the parental differences are reasonably contained in the parental relationship—they do not draw the children into their conflict.

Dysfunctional families are of two basic types: the dominant-submissive and the chronically conflicted. Dominant-submissive families are characterized by a skewed balance of power in the parental relationship. One parent controls the family in a strongly authoritarian way. He or she is in charge of all family decisions, and frequently the family has an oppressive tone. A discriminating variable is the degree to which the submissive spouse accepts his or her lack of power. If powerlessness and lack of responsibility are acceptable, the relationship is complementary, and there is little, if any, conflict. If the submissive spouse resents his or her position, however, one or more of the children may be drawn into the parental conflict. The child can be drawn into a coalition with the submissive spouse in opposition to the powerful parent, and the submissive spouse may subtly encourage rebellious behavior of the child whom the dominant spouse is unable to control and who brings the latter considerable grief (as with the Braxtons).

A different pattern, scapegoating, may be seen, in which both parents rivet their attention on the disturbing behavior of a child in order to deflect their focus from their marital conflict. Regardless, however, of whether the dominant-submissive marital relationship is complementary or conflicted, the family's characteristics are decisively influenced by the controlling of the dominant parent. Such families are rigid; they are not affectively open, and often there is underlying fear or resentment. Children have a difficult time moving toward autonomy because their own decision making is not encouraged, and the late-adolescent developmental challenges of increased separation from the family system are associated with an increased potential for regression.

Chronically conflicted families are characterized by the parents' battle for power as each tries unsuccessfully to dominate the marital relationship. In many chronically conflicted families the conflict serves the purpose of helping the parents avoid closeness that is desired but feared. The endless rounds of conflict create a disagreeable emotional climate in the family. Manipulative power plays are common; other persons are used for one's own gain. The children are often used as pawns, first by one parent, then the other. Children often leave such families prematurely and have difficulty establishing enduring relationships.

Severely dysfunctional families appear disorganized and chaotic. Family members cling together without clear personal identities. Projective maneuvers, primitive object relationships, and symbiotic processes are common. Exchanges with the surrounding world are reduced, and, with the exception of the parents' families of origin, there is little openness to others or tolerance for differences. Communication in such families may reflect such a high level of disorganization that the clinician has difficulty understanding the family themes. Many children in chaotic families cannot develop a cohesive sense of self, and they retreat from challenges that demand that they be autonomous. They often receive projections of fragmented self- and object representations from the parents and often are bound by parents' defensive economy.

These brief descriptions illustrate how the organizational structures of families from the most competent to the severely dysfunctional ends of the continuum of family competence differ from flexible to rigid to chaotic. These structures can also change in response to severe family stress (Lewis 1984). The work of Anthony (1970) and Reiss (1981) and our own clinical observations suggest that under circumstances of severe stress many flexible families undergo a change in structure, becoming more rigid. Most often one parent plays an increasingly dominant role in the family. Unless the stress abates or is contained by this structural alteration, the dominant-submissive structure can become increasingly conflicted, and this change may progress to disorganization and, ultimately, disintegration of the family. At any phase of this disintegration process, however, the family may reintegrate—and, in some instances, at a higher level of competence than that at which it was functioning prior to the stress. I wish to emphasize, however, that the changes in the structure of a family under severe stress can be understood as being parallel to the basic organizational structures of families across the continuum of family competence. It is helpful for the clinician to keep in mind the impact that severe stress may have on family organizational structure because some families respond to particular aspects of their children's adolescent experiences as stressful and undergo an alteration in basic family organizational structure. Indeed, the Braxtons' previously stable dominant-submissive family structure became increasingly conflicted as Bobby entered adolescence and became symptomatic. In planning treatment it is important for the clinician to be aware both of the family's basic organizational structure and of its recent changes.

To ask the question, What is the impact of adolescence on family systems? is to make the level of specificity too general. A more useful question might be, What is the impact of adolescence on families with a particular organizational structure?—and its corollary, What is the impact of a particular family organizational structure on a child's experience of adolescence? Because our definition of family competence includes the family's capacity to facilitate the autonomy of children and because autonomy is such an important dimension of psychological health in this culture, it is no surprise that healthy families produce more psychologically healthy adolescents than do families at the more dysfunctional end of the continuum of family competence. However, let us examine more closely some of the family interactional processes that appear to be involved across the continuum.

Healthy families facilitate the development of children who have both the capacity for independent, autonomous functioning and the capacity for close connectedness with other persons. Autonomous functioning is facilitated by a number of family characteristics. It is clear that the parents' relationship presents the children with a model of both autonomy and connectedness. From a different perspective the parents' capacities to encourage the development of the children's individual interests and their tolerance of (or pleasure in) differences also aid the development of autonomy. To experiment with autonomy is simply easier if there are few (if any) parental prescriptions about how one must be. Certain of the healthy family's communication characteristics also facilitate autonomous development. Encouraging clarity in the expression of thoughts and feelings can augment autonomy because it is through clear communication that individuals define themselves and learn how they differ from others. In a comparable way, attention to messages from others is a characteristic of healthy families and contributes to the growing capacity for self-other distinctions that are the anlage of autonomy. Healthy families accept mistakes as part of being human, and there is relatively little blaming. Children find it easier in such a family system to "own" their own behavior than to deny and project, responses that are so commonplace in some dysfunctional families.

Other family characteristics play a central role in facilitating the capacity for connectedness as well. Obviously, the parents' ability to share feelings openly and to express affection to each other is a powerful message to the children that closeness and psychological intimacy are desirable and not to be feared. The healthy family's openness with affect and capacity for empathy are other processes that facilitate closeness, for it is most often through shared affective experiences that closeness and intimacy develop.

I believe that it is through these and other characteristics that well-functioning families produce a very high percentage of healthy children who are capable of making age-appropriate steps toward increasing autonomy. Such families seem well designed for the task of facilitating adolescent development. Indeed, our research suggests that, even in adverse socioeconomic circumstances, such family characteristics are associated with the high probability of psychological health in adolescent children (Lewis and Looney 1983; Looney and Lewis 1983).

What happens to healthy families, however, if they are presented with the stress of an adolescent child in a tumultuous adolescence or with a clear-cut psychiatric syndrome or a severe and chronic physical illness or disability? There is much to suggest that healthy families utilize a variety of coping mechanisms while maintaining their basic organizational structure. These coping mechanisms range from active information gathering to the appropriate use of friends, relatives, and experts. The family's capacity for sharing thoughts and feelings—and, hence, for involving all family members in the exploration and possible redefinition of a problem—is an asset. Despite its assets, however, the coping capacity of a healthy family can be exceeded, and a structural realignment of the family begins. Most commonly these flexible systems move toward rigidity or that which Reiss (1981) describes as the loss of the implicit level of function and the appearance of explicit rules. This alteration may then evolve as a rigidly tyrannical structure, then become increasingly conflicted, then chaotic, and then the family may even disintegrate. Most healthy families, however, are able to contain stress without disintegrating, but when stress begins to alter a basically open and egalitarian parental coalition and a family moves toward a dominant-submissive structure, conflict, chaos, and disintegration can ensue. For this reason, the parental coalition is the family subsystem with the greatest relevance for maintaining the family's basic organizational structure. Elder's (1974) report of the impact of the Great Depression on families underscores this point. He demonstrates that when the father's unemployment resulted in a breakdown in the parental relationship and the mother assumed an increasingly powerful role, very young male children (not older males or any of the female children) were more likely subsequently to develop adolescent identity conflicts. However, if the father's unemployment did not result in a structural change in the parents' relationship (a relationship evaluated previously as being an effective and committed coalition), the young sons did not develop the adolescent identity problems. Elder supports the centrality of the parents' relationship in determining the nature of the children's adolescent experience, at least for boys.

Competent but pained families illustrate a related point. In these families the parents' dissatisfaction is contained within their relationship. The children are not brought into the conflict, as so frequently occurs in more dysfunctional families. A number of experts emphasize the importance of containment of conflict. Engel's (1979) biopsychosocial model of illness posits that the spread of problems from one level of the system hierarchy to other levels is paradigmatic of illness. In this instance, the involvement of the children in the parental conflict represents an expansion from the marital pair to the family. Bowen's (1982) theory postulates that the spread of marital conflict to the children plays a destructive role in their development. In these competent but pained families, clinical evidence supports these premises, for the adolescents from such families show high levels of psychological health in prevalences equal to those of healthy families. It seems clear that during both childhood and adolescence children have a high likelihood of psychological health if the family context, however flawed, provides them with affection, support, and the encouragement of individual identity. It is when children are caught up in parental conflicts that developmental risks are increased.

Competent but pained families have fewer resources with which to handle stress—including the stress arising from a difficult, disturbed, or disabled adolescent child—than do healthy families. When the parental coalition is already strained by an unresolved conflict regarding regulation of the distance between them, these families are vulnerable to the development of patterns of clear dominance, overt and intense conflict, chaos, and disintegration.

Although psychologically healthy and autonomous children can develop in dominant-submissive dysfunctional families, there are fewer such children than there are in either healthy or competent but pained families. The family interactional characteristics make autonomy more difficult to achieve and augment the development of both excessive dependency and adolescent rebelliousness that so often appear to evolve from conflicts about dependency. Growing up in a family dominated by a powerful parent—even if this domination is acceptable to the submissive parent—often means learning indirection, obliqueness, and secrecy in order to hide thoughts and feelings that may lead to the dominant parent's disapproval.

Children of such families may be comfortable only to the extent that they avoid direct encounter. Their inhibited expression may be seen as shyness; their passivity may be interpreted as reticence. At the same time, intrusion of the dominant parent into inappropriate areas of the adolescent's decision making hampers the adolescent's confidence in his or her capacity for autonomous functioning. After years of this type of parent-child interaction, the adolescent may come to be excessively dependent on the dominant parent and, consequently, vulnerable to anxiety when the dominant parent is unavailable. These dynamic factors are intensified and complicated in the presence of underlying resentment and conflict between the parents, and in one common pattern the adolescent "learns" that his or her behavior, although distressing to both parents, diverts the parents from their conflict.

An alliance may develop between one or more of the children and the submissive parent, or, as with Mrs. Braxton and Bobby, an alliance from early childhood may be intensified and have a tone that is distinctly oppositional to the dominant parent. The child may be used by the submissive parent as a confidant, often with vastly inappropriate sharing of intimate marital details and dissatisfactions. If, within the context of this alliance, the submissive parent subtly encourages the adolescent to behaviors that the dominant parent cannot control, patterns of rebellious "acting out" may be learned and become ingrained.

There are, then, multiple ways in which the dominant-submissive family structure may impair the development of both the adolescent's confidence and sense of autonomy and also his or her ability to relate to others without excessive dependency, passivity, or rebelliousness.

The rigidity of the dominant-submissive family structure does not tolerate a disturbed or disturbing adolescent very long without the appearance of parental conflict. The submissive spouse may become increasingly direct—first imploring and then demanding that his or her dominant spouse ease up on their adolescent child. Arguments may evolve, and the previously submissive spouse may find greater courage in fighting for the adolescent child than he or she had in establishing respect for himself or herself. The dominant-submissive family structure may erode slowly or break quickly, and the ensuing conflict may lead to increasing family disorganization and, ultimately, to disintegration of the family. Better outcomes are possible, however, and the parental conflict may lead to a redefinition of the parental relationship and a move toward a less skewed marital system. But the more dysfunctional the basic organizational structure of the family, the greater the likelihood of further regressive structural change in the family in response to the presence of a symptomatic adolescent.

Chronically conflicted families can produce psychologically healthy children, but it is not usual and often occurs only when other adults have played prominent parenting roles. Children from chronically conflicted families are apt to develop severe relationship difficulties. They are frequently narcissistically exploitative and manipulative. They avoid closeness at all cost because of the attendant vulnerability. The mood of these families is angry, and there is a tendency for some of the children to leave prematurely via teenage marriages.

These families have very few resources with which to handle additional stress. Usually stress leads to more conflict, disorganization, and chaos; but occasionally a difficult, disturbing, or disturbed adolescent may serve as a distance regulator in the parental relationship, and the parental conflict may diminish.

In either the dominant-submissive or the chronically conflicted family a difficult or symptomatic adolescent may diffuse or divert parental conflict. It is, therefore, no surprise that clinicians working successfully with adolescents (separate from their families) note that improvement in the adolescent may be followed by disintegration of the parent's relationship and then by divorce.

40

Growing up in a severely dysfunctional, chaotic family seriously impedes the development of a clear sense of self, sharply defined ego boundaries, and knowledge of sharp differences from others—all of which are necessary precursors of autonomy. There is such blurring of personal boundaries, so much invasiveness, such elaborate projective systems that children have greatly reduced opportunities for the development of autonomy. That a small percentage of children raised in chaotic families turn out to be clearly defined, autonomous, and often unusually creative (the so-called invulnerables) begs clarification for better understanding of human development.

If one lives in a human system that has difficulty maintaining a focus of attention, views all change as precarious, assumes that outsiders are dangerous, and does not encourage clear expression, one may cling to one's family, without motivation to move out into a more independent life.

Chaotic families are apt to deal with a disturbed adolescent by relying on primitive denial mechanisms, saying, for example, that a psychotic, delusional, and hallucinating adolescent is "nervous because of vitamin deficiency." Refusal to acknowledge the reality of a child's distress is commonplace in such families. Indeed, early family theorists speculated that one function of adolescent psychosis was an attempt to separate from a severely dysfunctional, enmeshed family—a hypothesis which, if valid, explains the family's denial. A child cannot be trying to separate (albeit through psychosis) if nothing is "wrong" with him or her.

At the core of chaotic families is an enmeshed and frequently symbiotic parental relationship. If a child is incorporated, a classic severely dysfunctional family is apt to evolve, and the child is at risk for severe disability in his or her sense of self. This disability may be one pathway to late-adolescent vulnerability to schizophrenic regression. Or, as Gunderson (personal communication, 1981) has suggested, children excluded from the parental symbiosis may develop borderline personality disorders.

Conclusions

These observations about family organizational structure and the impact of adolescent children on the family constitute but one piece of a complex puzzle consisting of many variables. There are, for example, families who respond specifically to one or another aspect of their child's adolescence, as, for example, the child's emerging sexuality. There are adolescents whose rebellious behaviors are not internalized pathology but can be most parsimoniously understood as behavioral messages informing parents of the need to clarify and strengthen family rules regarding certain issues.

Even parents with very effective relationships can have difficult problems with their adolescent children, but parents who have resolved between themselves the relationship issues of closeness, intimacy, and power minimize that risk. If, in addition, they are highly committed to the marital relationship as the central axis of the family structure, if they genuinely care for each other, and if they understand how confusing and difficult adolescence may be for their children, they lay the bedrock for their own continuing development and present a model for their children's futures.

REFERENCES

Anthony, E. J. 1970. The impact of mental and physical illness on family life. *American Journal of Psychiatry* 127:138–146.

Bowen, M. 1982. *Family Therapy in Clinical Practice.* New York: Jason Aronson.

Elder, G. H. 1974. *Children of the Great Depression.* Chicago: University of Chicago Press.

Engel, G. L. 1979. The biopsychosocial model: resolving the conflict between medicine and psychiatry. *Resident and Staff Physician* 25(7):72.

Kohut, H. 1971. *The Analysis of the Self.* New York: International Universities Press.

Kohut, H. 1977. *The Restoration of the Self.* New York: International Universities Press.

Lewis, J. M. 1984. Family structure and stress. Paper presented at the meeting of the Marriage Council of Philadelphia, Inc., Division of Family Study, Department of Psychiatry, The University of Pennsylvania School of Medicine, November 3.

Lewis, J. M.; Beavers, W. R.; Gossett, J. T.; and Phillips, V. A. 1977. *No Single Thread: Psychological Health in Family Systems.* New York: Brunner/Mazel.

Lewis, J. M., and Looney, J. G. 1983. *The Long Struggle: Well-functioning Working-Class Black Families.* New York: Brunner/Mazel.

Looney, J. G., and Lewis, J. M. 1983. Competent adolescents from different socioeconomic and ethnic contexts. *Adolescent Psychiatry* 11:64–74.

Offer, D.; Sabshin, M.; and Marcus, D. 1965. Clinical evaluation of normal adolescents. *American Journal of Psychiatry* 121(9):864–872.

Olson, D. H.; McCubbin, H. I.; and Associates. 1983. *Families: What Makes Them Work*. Beverly Hills, Calif.: Sage.

Reiss, D. 1981. *The Family's Construction of Reality*. Cambridge, Mass.: Harvard University Press.

Weissman, S., and Cohen, R. S. 1985. The parenting alliance and adolescence. *Adolescent Psychiatry* 12:24–45.

3   PLATO'S *LACHES:* COURAGE, EXPERTISE, PSYCHOTHERAPY, AND ADOLESCENCE

HERMAN SINAIKO

The *Dialogues*, written by Plato in the fourth century B.C., are for the most part narrative or dramatic accounts of conversations of Socrates, an older contemporary of Plato who was executed for impiety and corrupting the young by the city of Athens when he was seventy and Plato was about twenty-seven. During his life, Socrates apparently wrote nothing and founded no schools. There is considerable debate among ancient scholars as well as modern ones about whether he developed or espoused any particular philosophical doctrines. He seems to have spent most of his time talking to people in the streets and markets of Athens, delighting the young and frequently infuriating their elders. Yet he also seems to have revolutionized Greek thought, and, even in antiquity, Greek philosophy was divided into pre-Socratic and post-Socratic periods. After his death it became quite the fashion for philosophers to write Socratic dialogues. This seems quite natural, since most of the ancient schools of philosophy claimed to be intellectual descendants of Socrates. Almost all of these so-called Socratic writings have been lost through the centuries; only the dialogues of Plato and his contemporary Xenophon have survived intact. Much of what we know about the intellectual life of Athens at the time we know only from these dialogues of Plato.

It seems clear that Socrates was a seminal thinker of enormous importance for the whole history of Western thought, though we really know very little about him apart from Plato's writings. Plato's *Dialogues* have been recognized from antiquity as philosophical and literary masterpieces of the highest order. The *Dialogues* are rooted in the history of a particular time and place, the city of Athens in the last quarter of the fifth century B.C. With perhaps one exception, every character in the *Dialogues* seems to have been a real historical figure, and some of the occasions of the dialogues were also real. But we have absolutely no evidence as to whether any of the dialogues actually occurred or whether Plato's literary account is historically accurate.

My own private judgment is that none of the dialogues, as we have them, could be fully accurate renderings of historical events. My reason for believing this is quite simple: the dialogues are too perfect as literary works to be historically accurate. No events in the real world are as perfectly formed, as coherent, as devoid of irrelevancy and accident as Plato's *Dialogues*. It must be said here, however, that Plato's artistic powers are so great, his control of this material so complete, that his works frequently appear to the unwary as artless, even clumsy. Shakespeare's plays are similar in this respect: to unsophisticated audiences or critics they often seem shapeless, full of digressions, and sprinkled with unnecessary detail. It takes a good deal of experience even to begin to see how perfectly crafted the plays are. The same is true of Plato's *Dialogues*, and the *Laches* is a perfect example of this effect.

In many respects the *Laches* is a typical Platonic dialogue: it is short, it seems to be an attempt to define a virtue (in this case, courage), it fails in that attempt, and thus ends inconclusively. I would like to start with the notion, however, that if the *Laches* is inconclusive, that is because Plato wanted it that way—that is, we are intended to be genuinely puzzled by the dialogue.

Let me summarize in some detail the action of the dialogue to remind you of what happens and in what order. The dialogue opens with Lysimachus explaining to Nicias and Laches why he and Melesias have invited them to watch an exhibition by a reputed expert on fighting in armor. Lysimaches and Melesias each have an adolescent son who has reached the age at which he needs formal training to equip him for adult life and an active career. Lysimachus explains that he and Melesias need help in deciding what training to give to their boys, because they feel inadequate to the task. These two rather elderly fathers are the sons of two of the most eminent figures of the previous generation, the generation that fought and defeated the Persians in defense of Greek freedom and then went on to found the Athenian empire and initiate the golden age of Greece. Lysimachus explains that the two statesmen/fathers were so busy founding an empire that they had no time for their own sons, and consequently he and Melesias have had unusually mediocre and undistinguished careers. Now, they feel, their sons (who are named after their grandfathers, as was the tradition) should have careers like their grandfathers and not like their fathers. They have asked Nicias and Laches, two eminent generals-statesmen, for their advice. Nicias agrees to help, and so does Laches, with the added remark that they should invite Socrates, who is also present at the exhibition, to join the consultation. Lysimachus, who knew Socrates' father, invites him to join the conversation, mentioning that the two boys have recently been talking about their conversations with someone named Socrates. He asks them if this is the same Socrates. In the only remark they make in the entire dialogue, the boys say that it is. And so Socrates joins the group, as Laches adds a compliment about his sterling performance as a soldier during the Athenian defeat in the battle of Delium.

Socrates begins by deferring to the views of the older, more knowledgeable Laches and Nicias. Nicias presents a careful, ordered argument that learning to fight in armor is the first step toward mastering the art of the general and will also make the boys braver and give them a fine martial appearance. Laches then argues, in sharp contrast, that the Spartans, the acknowledged masters of the art of war, have nothing to do with this sort of newfangled skill. He asserts that this man, Stesilaus, made a laughingstock of himself in battle with some absurd new weapon he invented and that the so-called art he now teaches will merely make cowards more rash and brave men more cautious.

With the two experts in open and flagrant disagreement, Lysimachus turns to Socrates to cast the deciding vote. Socrates, surprised, asks whether Lysimachus intends to go with the majority. Lysimachus asks what the alternative is. Socrates then turns to Melesias, and in the only part of the dialogue where Melesias joins in, Socrates leads Melesias through an argument that is almost a commonplace of Socratic conversation. If the question is whether Melesias's son should practice a particular kind of exercise, asks Socrates, should Melesias follow the advice of the greater number of those who happen to be on hand or the advice of one who has been educated under a good trainer? Melesias agrees that it should be the latter. Thus, says Socrates, it is by knowledge that one ought to make such decisions and not by majority rule. Melesias agrees. Having established the supremacy of the knowledgeable expert over the ignorant majority, Socrates then points out that what they are talking about is not some small thing but perhaps the greatest of all their possessions—their sons. The question is whether their sons will turn out to be worthwhile persons or the opposite, and on that outcome the whole of the fathers' reputations and estates are staked. And so the question becomes, Who is the expert? Who is the man who has studied and practiced the art?

But first Socrates raises the question of what exactly is the art that they are looking for someone to teach. Now Nicias joins the conversation and asks, Aren't they discussing the art of fighting in armor and deciding whether young men ought to learn that? Using the example of medicine, Socrates asks whether, if the eyes are diseased and one takes counsel, one should take counsel about the medicine or about the eyes? Nicias agrees—one should take counsel about the eyes. Therefore, says Socrates, in the case that they are discussing, the question is not about fighting in armor but about that for which one might learn to fight in armor. What they are looking for is not an expert skilled in the art of fighting in armor but an expert skilled in the care of the souls of young men. What they need is a doctor of the soul, not a doctor of the body.

Now that the general subject matter of the dialogue—the care of the soul—has been defined, the question becomes one of methodology: how to investigate it; that is to say, how to find the expert who understands the art and who can instruct them. And to mark this shift, Laches now replaces Nicias as Socrates' interlocutor. The mark of the good craftsman, says Socrates, is not the touting of his own skills but the well-executed product of his art. What Laches and Nicias and he should do for Lysimachus and Melesias is to point out those good teachers who have tended the souls of the young and have taught them well. If one of the three of them claims to have the skill without having had a good teacher, says Socrates, let him show which Athenian or which foreigner, which freeman or which slave, is recognized to have become good through his influence. In this context Socrates notes that he himself has had no teacher, because he has had no money to pay for one (though he has wished that he had had one). On the other hand, Nicias and Laches, who are wealthy men, have had plenty of opportunities to get educated. So, says Socrates, Lysimachus and Melesias should not let Laches and Nicias go until they reveal who is cleverest at educating young men and from whom they learned the art, unless they taught themselves. In that way, if Nicias and Laches are too busy, the two fathers can go to the teachers of Nicias and Laches and get advice.

The question of who is the expert in the art of improving the young has turned into a process of investigating Nicias's and Laches' strong but conflicting claims to be experts in this art. Lysimachus picks up on Socrates' suggestion and now requests that Laches and Nicias jointly answer Socrates' questions. This matter, he points out, is important not only to Melesias and himself but to Nicias and Laches also, because they too have sons who are nearly of an age to be educated.

And so Socrates has subtly managed to transform the conversation from one in which two humble laymen request advice from experts to one in which he, Socrates, as the agent of the humble laymen, will examine the supposed experts on an issue in which they themselves have a direct stake. Nicias now explains to the two old men that they are obviously unacquainted with Socrates except as the child of his father—as an adult, Socrates conducts conversations in an unusual way. In the first place, says Nicias, when one converses with Socrates one is led by his arguments to answer questions about oneself until one's whole life is subject to investigation, and Socrates does not let a person go until he has been tested in every detail. Nicias professes to know Socrates well: he says he has been put through this treatment before, and he knows to what he is about to submit. He says that he likes Socrates and that he does not run away from such things because he values learning, as Solon once said, as long as he lives. But he cautions the old men that, in an examination by Socrates, the conversation will not be about the boys but about themselves. Nicias is obviously sophisticated and well aware of the effect of Socrates on a conversation.

Not to be outdone, Laches now chimes in with his views about discussions. He has two opinions; in some respects he loves discussions, and in others he hates them. The difference, he says, depends on the character of the man with whom he is talking. If he is talking with a man about virtue and such matters, says Laches, and there is a harmony between the speaker and his words, then he is a lover of discourse and delights in the conversation. But, he says, if he is talking with someone for whom there is a deep disjunction between words and deeds, then he becomes a hater of discussion. Laches is not, he says, familiar with the words of Socrates; all that he has experienced hitherto is Socrates' deeds, and these have been such as to ensure the nobility of his words. Laches claims that he, too, like Solon, wishes to grow old learning many things—but only, he adds, from good men. The fact that Socrates is younger than he makes no difference to Laches. Because of his respect for Socrates' valor, he says, he is prepared to allow Socrates to cross-examine him.

On account of what he says is his failing memory, Lysimachus now turns the entire conversation over to Socrates. From here on the dialogue is basically a three-part conversation among Socrates, Nicias, and Laches. And—characteristically—Socrates begins by redefining the question once more. Instead of asking about teachers, Socrates pushes back still another step to a more fundamental issue, returning to his medical metaphor. If we did not know, he says, that sight added to the eyes improves the eyes, we would hardly be good doctors or worthy counselors about the health of the eyes. We not only have to know that it is sight that improves the eyes—we also have to know what sight is. Analogously, he says, is it not virtue or human excellence that we wish to add to the souls of the young? Do we not, he asks, therefore have to know what virtue is? Laches quails at this task, so Socrates narrows it somewhat. Perhaps we do not have to explore the whole of virtue—that would be too great—but perhaps we can get sufficient knowledge of a part. Laches eagerly agrees, and Socrates asks which of the parts of virtue they should choose. Is it not obvious, he remarks, that the one that seems to be involved in fighting in armor is the virtue of courage? So, says Socrates, let us undertake first of all to state what courage is.

With this remark—halfway through the dialogue—Socrates has finally got around to defining the subject of the investigation. The rest of the dialogue consists mostly of alternating arguments between Socrates and first Laches, then Nicias, and then Laches again. Each general tries his hand at defining courage but finds himself unable to withstand the rigors of Socrates' cross-examination. Nevertheless, it may be instructive to look at their attempts to define courage—even if they fail, we may learn something from those failures.

Laches starts by defining courage in an extremely simple, straightforward way—a courageous man is a man who remains at his post to defend himself against the enemy without running away. Socrates attacks this view by citing a certain sort of tactical situation. For example, he notes that in their battles against the Persians, the Scythians, instead of remaining at their posts, feigned retreat in order to draw the Persians after them; then, when the enemy was disarrayed in pursuit, the Scythians turned, attacked, and defeated them, thereby gaining great reputation for valor. Even Laches' beloved Spartan hoplites, Socrates points out, behaved in a similar manner at the battle of Plataea. In sum, says Socrates, we are not trying to discover what constitutes the courage of a hoplite or a horseman only but what also constitutes the courage of other sorts of warriors and of people who are not warriors: those who are in danger at sea; those who show courage in illness, poverty, affairs of state, and in the face of pain or fear; and those who fight desire and pleasure—in all these aspects of life, says Socrates, we want to find out what it is that makes some brave and others not.

With some help, Laches gets the point and now redefines courage in a fully generalized way: courage is not standing one's post in the physical sense but is an endurance of the soul. Socrates next goes after the notion of endurance. Is it any and every kind of endurance, he asks, or only some instances of endurance that are courageous? Is it not always endurance accompanied by wisdom that is the virtue, the human excellence, that they are looking for? So not endurance but "wise endurance" becomes the definition of courage. And so Socrates explores this new definition. What about the man in battle who wisely calculates that his position is stronger than the position of his enemy, that he outnumbers the enemy, that he is better armed and better trained? Would the endurance of this man, based on this wisdom, be courage? Or, says Socrates, is it the man in the other camp, the man who is willing to hold out against great odds, who is the brave one? Laches, predictably, prefers the man in the opposite camp. Thus, not "wise endurance" but "foolish endurance" becomes the measure of courage. At this point Laches, understandably, gets confused. Socrates points out that their deeds are not in harmony with their words. Laches seems discouraged by this turn of the argument, but Socrates exhorts him by urging that they endure in the investigation— that they should not become ridiculous in the face of courage itself by being cowardly in their search for it. Laches responds with great enthusiasm and expresses a powerful desire to pursue the conversation. He insists that he knows what courage is but cannot understand how it has escaped him; he can not quite pin it down in words. The disjunction in Laches, according to himself, is not between words and deeds but between understanding and words.

At this point Socrates turns to Nicias and asks if he can help out. Nicias starts by saying that he thinks that their whole approach has been wrong. He uses an observation that he has heard from Socrates on previous occasions: every one of us is good in respect to the things in which he is wise and bad in respect to those in which he is ignorant. This means, says Nicias, that if a man is really courageous it is clear that he is wise, and so courage is not endurance but some kind of wisdom. What kind of wisdom? asks Socrates. Nicias replies that it is knowledge of the fearful and hopeful in war and in every other situation.

Laches breaks back in with the observation that Nicias is talking nonsense, because wisdom is quite a different thing from courage. Nicias retorts that Laches wishes to accuse him of talking nonsense merely because Laches has been shown to be doing that sort of thing himself. Laches now briefly takes on the role of Socrates and attempts to demonstrate to Nicias the absurdity of his definition. He points out that farmers know what is to be feared in farming, and every craftsman knows what is to be feared in his craft; but these people are in no way courageous for all of that. Nicias responds that doctors know what can make a person sick or healthy but that they cannot tell when it might be better for a person to be sick than to be healthy. Laches is confused by this answer and accuses Nicias of twisting about in trying to avoid contradicting himself. And so, with Laches' approval, Socrates takes over the questioning again to see if they can find out what Nicias is really saying.

According to Nicias, says Socrates, courage is knowledge of the grounds of fear and hope; Nicias agrees. Socrates observes that this knowledge can be possessed by very few and that Nicias must necessarily deny courage to any wild beast or else admit that these beasts have a kind of knowledge that can be attained by very few men. Laches joins in, delighted by what he sees as Nicias's difficulty, saying that all these wild beasts—the lion, the wild boar, the leopard—that we all agree are courageous, would also have to be described as wise, which would be absurd. Again, Nicias, in his sophisticated way, avoids the trap. They are not courageous, he says, because they lack understanding; they are merely rash or mad. Children, he says, who fear nothing because they have no sense, can hardly be called courageous. Laches objects and accuses Nicias of logic chopping.

Again Socrates takes up the argument, first getting Nicias to agree that courage is only one part of virtue, the other parts being such things as justice and moderation. He then explores further the definition of courage as the grounds of hope and fear. Fearful things are things that produce fear; hopeful things are those that do not produce fear. And fear, says Socrates, comes not from evils that have happened or are happening; it comes from evils that are anticipated, because fear is the expectation of evil; and knowledge of these things is what is called courage. Socrates then argues that there is not one kind of knowledge about the past, another about the present, and a third about the future. The knowledge of what is fearful and what is hopeful—whether it has already happened, is happening, or will happen— is the same in each

51

case. In the case of health, he says, there are not separate arts related to the present, past, and future. Medicine is a single art of what was, what is, and what is likely to be. But if the fearful and hopeful things are future goods and evils, then knowledge of these things must also be knowledge of present and past goods and evils. To define courage as wisdom or knowledge about the grounds of fear and hope, about future goods and evils, says Socrates, is thus to define only a part of courage, since the whole of courage, according to Nicias, is knowledge of practically all goods and evils—past, present, and future. Socrates goes on to say that the man with this kind of knowledge would seem to have virtue. And so Nicias's definition also fails to convince; they still have not discovered what courage is.

Again Laches cannot restrain himself from taking a dig at Nicias, and Nicias reciprocates. Both men agree, however, that Lysimachus and Melesias would do well to retain the services of Socrates rather than the services of either of them; Nicias further says that he would be delighted to entrust his own son to the care of Socrates, if Socrates did not seem to be unwilling and did not always recommend someone else for the job. Lysimachus now returns to the discussion and joins in a general appeal that Socrates help them make the young men good. Socrates agrees that it would be a terrible thing to be unwilling to assist such an undertaking. The trouble is, he says, that he is no better than Nicias and Laches—he too is essentially ignorant of what they are searching for. What he suggests instead is that they all search for the best possible teacher for themselves—because they really need one—and then for a teacher for the young men. Even if they should become ridiculous in the eyes of others— searching for such a thing at their age—they should do so anyway. Lysimachus then ends the dialogue by inviting Socrates to come to his house on the following day in order to plan this search. Socrates accepts, and the dialogue ends.

I have summarized this dialogue at such length not only to remind you of the mass of detail and the complexity of the arguments that are packed into a relatively short space but also to bring home to you as vividly as I can the fact that the *Laches* is, like all of Plato's works, a genuine dramatic dialogue and not merely a disguised treatise. Let me point out that the dialogue is half over before Socrates even gets to focus on the question of the nature of courage. The inconclusive arguments about courage, then, occur in a larger context—that of the conversation between Socrates and the two fathers. Let us begin by looking a little more closely at these two gentlemen and their situation.

Discussion

There is a peculiar poignancy and irony in the way the two fathers define their own condition. Lysimachus is the son of Aristides, nicknamed "The Just," who was a peer of Miltiades, the hero of Marathon, and of Themistocles, the hero of Salamis. Melesias is the son of Thucydides the admiral (not related to Thucydides the historian), who was among the leading figures who, following the Persian wars, converted the league of Greek cities into the Athenian empire, which dominated the whole of the eastern Mediterranean during most of the fifth century B.C. What are we to make of the attitudes of Lysimachus and Melesias toward *their* fathers? On the one hand, it is clear that they deeply resent their fathers, who were so busy doing great deeds that they had not time to give their own boys the kind of attention that they needed in order to have glorious careers of their own. The resentment and anger that Lysimachus and Melesias feel are still palpable. At the same time, of course, like hurt little boys they want nothing more than that their own sons—namesakes of their famous grandfathers—should grow up to have careers like their grandfathers. And I suppose that we have a right to ask, If the two boys were to grow up like their grandfathers, would they in turn neglect *their* sons? By seeking to give their children careers like those of their illustrious grandfathers are Lysimachus and Melesias merely perpetuating the pain and resentment that has marred their own lives? By their own admission, Lysimachus and Melesias are mediocre men who have led lives that are largely wasted. And yet, why should we accept their judgment of themselves? In the brief passage in which Socrates talks to Melesias, Socrates gets the reticent fathers to agree that their sons are the greatest of all their possessions and that the father's estate—what he bequeaths to posterity—will be managed well or poorly depending on how his sons turn out. By that standard, Aristides the Just and Thucydides the admiral, fathers of Lysimachus and Melesias, were failures because they did not do well by their sons. Lysimachus and Melesias, despite their mediocrity by conventional standards, at least are devoting their lives to the care of their children. By Socrates' standards they may be better than they think—a good deal better, in fact, than their illustrious fathers.

All of the ambivalence and irony reflected in Lysimachus's and Melesias's relationships to their fathers and their sons are mirrored in the next generation by the attitudes of Laches and Nicias. Laches and Nicias are, as it were, the Aristides and Thucydides of the present generation. They are, at the moment, the experts in valor, the winners of battles, the builders of the empire. They are also so concerned with public affairs that they seem at the present to be neglecting their own children; they seem prepared simply to turn them over to teachers, without further thought.

And yet, for all the ironies implicit in the situation, the generations do not merely repeat the patterns of the past. The actual situation is far more complicated than that. Plato was born and grew up in the last quarter of the fifth century B.C., but he lived the bulk of his adult life and wrote during the first half of the fourth century B.C. The immediate audience for whom the *Laches* was written, therefore, would have been about as distant from and as familiar with the events to which the *Laches* refers, as we are distant from and familiar with the sequence of events from the First World War through the Second World War into the postwar period up to the debacle of Vietnam.

Much of the irony that informs the *Laches* should now be apparent. Both Laches and Nicias—as portrayed in the dialogue, two eminent, confident, and successful generals— were known to the original readers of the dialogue as generals who presided over two of the most costly defeats ever suffered by the city of Athens. Laches, the uncritical admirer of Spartan valor, came to know the full value of that valor. Nicias, the man who defines courage as a kind of wisdom, died at Syracuse because he observed the superstitious custom of not moving an army following an eclipse. And yet, perhaps we should not judge these men so harshly. After all, if Lysimachus and Melesias can be wrong in their evaluations of themselves, who is to say that because Laches and Nicias died in defeat they were not courageous? There may be courage in defeat as well as in victory. But before we tackle the question of courage, let me point out that the consequence of the defeats of Nicias and Laches was, ultimately, the destruction of the Athenian empire. When the two young sons of Lysimachus and Melesias reached manhood, there simply was not an empire left for them to maintain with glorious deeds. And so to the original audience of the *Laches*, all of the ironies and ambiguities attendant on the rise and fall of the Athenian empire in the fifth century B.C. are encapsulated in this charming little inconclusive conversation about courage. The mythical glories of the founding generation, the mediocre nonentities of the succeeding generation, the pompous certainty of the third generation that will lead the city to defeat, and the sad realization that all the anticipation of the coming generation will come to nought— all this is built into the very structure of the *Laches*.

You will note that almost everyone we have been discussing occurs in the *Laches* as a member of a pair—the two founding fathers, the two mediocre elderly men, the two young sons, and the two eminent generals. Each pair represents a different polarity. Of the founding fathers, Aristides was a land general, Thucydides an admiral. Of the two mediocre men, Lysimachus talks at great length, Melesias hardly at all. As I noted, there is only one passage in which Melesias talks, and then only because Socrates addresses him directly. And yet that is the passage in which the central subject of the dialogue is first articulated. One wishes that Lysimachus had talked less and Melesias more. The two generals, of course, stand in the sharpest possible contrast to each other—in character, in what they say, in their relation to Socrates, and in their understanding of courage. Laches believes in deeds more than in words; Nicias has a love of argument. Laches believes in old-fashioned virtues of obedience and endurance; Nicias is a follower of the newfangled rational study of strategy and of modern weapon development. Laches admires the Spartans; Nicias, the Athenian style of warfare. Laches is quick to anger; Nicias is calm and sophisticated. Laches knows the deeds of Socrates the warrior; Nicias knows the words of Socrates the supersophist. Whereas Laches identifies courage with endurance—a stolid, even foolish or mindless holding on—and is prepared to claim that wild beasts may be courageous, Nicias identifies courage with a special kind of arcane knowledge, available only to the elite few who can grasp its rational principles.

We will return to the contrast between Laches and Nicias shortly, but for the moment let us turn to two other figures in the dialogue who do not occur as a pair but seem to stand out as singular, even unique. I refer, of course, to Stesilaus, the man who gave the exhibition of fighting in armor, and to Socrates. Stesilaus is unique in that he seems to be something of an inventive genius: he invents new weapons and techniques of fighting. Unfortunately, the weapons do not work very well, and it is uncertain whether the method of fighting in armor has anything to recommend it either. Socrates too is something of an innovator—not in the martial arena but in ways of arguing and procedures for investigating the truth. The original occasion for the dialogue is Stesilaus's exhibition of martial skill, a kind of skill that the two fathers think may help their sons to become brave. The dialogue itself consists of an exhibition by Socrates of the unprecedented art of investigation through argument—an art that, ironically, the two boys have already discovered for themselves because they have known Socrates for some time. We go to watch Stesilaus, but we stay to listen to Socrates. What we hear from him is that we do not understand courage.

There remains, I think, one other rather extraordinary fact about the dialogue. Socrates says, "Then the question whether any one of us is expert in the care of the soul and is capable of caring for it well and has had good teachers, is the one we ought to investigate." That sentence, as I have suggested, is the moment at which Socrates defines once and for all the fundamental issue of the dialogue. I wish to point out that the phrase in Greek that is translated by the English "expert in the care of the soul" is τεκγικος περιψυχης θηραπιογ, "skilled in the treatment of the soul." The phrase "treatment of the soul" is ψυχης θηραπιογ, "psychotherapy." To my knowledge this is the oldest and perhaps the first use of the term "psychotherapy" in Western literature. So, if any of you has been wondering what a lecture on the *Laches* has to do with psychotherapy, it is entirely possible that this dialogue represents the moment at which the very notion of psychotherapy was born in the Western philosophical tradition. Note that this term occurs for the first time in the context of a discussion of courage, in a conversation in which two fathers express a deep concern for the education and training of their adolescent sons. I think that this dialogue, with all its ironies and ambiguities, absurdities and pathos, has a great deal to do with the very notion of psychotherapy, particularly psychotherapy for adolescents.

The recurrent pairs of contrasting figures in the *Laches* suggest to me something of the equivocal character of courage itself. Always, from antiquity to the present, courage or valor, manliness, intestinal fortitude—however one wants to name it—has been a strange virtue and one that is always problematic. Courage seems to require (in its most conventional form) war and killing in order for it to be realized. No matter what one's attitude toward war might be, there always remains the uneasy sense that the price of Achilles' distinction and excellence as a warrior was the death of Hector, one of the few genuinely lovable people in Homer's *Iliad*. What can we make of such a virtue? There are those— perhaps like Socrates—who would like to extend the range of courage so that it can be realized not only in the martial arena but in practically any area of life. But if Achilles and Hector display courage in their fight to the death, each knowing that the other is a deadly fighter of enormous skill and power, what are we to say of the person on a diet who resists the temptation to have a hot fudge sundae? Can we really compare *that* to the behavior of men who risk their lives in defense of their cities and families or to avenge the death of a friend?

All of my friends with whom I have discussed courage in recent months have wanted to talk about it in terms of risk taking. But the risk that someone takes when he actually puts his life on the line by going into military combat seems to me very different from the risk that one takes in getting a new job, getting married, or leaving home and going off to college—not to speak of the small risks that we all take every day of our lives as we pursue our daily affairs. The scope of courage, then, remains profoundly ambiguous. Are we, like Aristotle, to restrict it simply to those situations in which we literally risk our lives? Or can it in fact extend to the whole of life?

If courage is a virtue, it is a strange, morally ambiguous virtue. What are we to make, for example, of those SS troops, those dedicated Nazis, who fought resolutely and well in the last days of World War II when their cause was lost and they knew it? Are they, the murderers of Auschwitz and Buchenwald, to be called courageous, virtuous? We feel much better when what seems to be courage occurs in service of an unambiguously good end. But, after all, those who fight in the name of other values— even bad ones—may also fight well and risk just as much. Is courage, then, a morally neutral virtue? This is a puzzling and disturbing possibility.

If the contrasting pairs of figures around which the *Laches* is structured suggest something of the problematic character of courage, those same dualities also suggest that each member of a pair has something defective about it, something that is at least in some degree corrected by the other member of the pair. Thus, if Lysimachus says more than he should, Melesias says too little and is too easily silent. This suggestion is particularly interesting if we think about it in relation to the views of Nicias and Laches, because it suggests that the problem with each general lies in the partiality of his views, a partiality that can be corrected by incorporating the views of the other. Thus Laches, with his notion of courage as brute endurance, may rightly emphasize the way in which courage is rooted in character, but he may seriously underestimate the role of intelligence and choice. Nicias, with his notion of courage as a kind of knowledge, may in turn underestimate the significance of character.

If this approach is valid, then the problem with Laches' and Nicias's divergent views of courage is not that each of them is wrong but that each is only partially right. The truth about courage would thus be found neither by rejecting both views nor by accepting one or the other but by finding a way to synthesize the two views into a coherent whole. These two views, however, are presented by their spokesmen as being diametrically opposed to each other. Each general sees the other's view as an account not of courage but of a vice to which courage is ordinarily contrasted. Nicias thinks of Laches' conception of courage as *rashness*. Laches thinks of Nicias's notion of courage as *cowardice*. It is Aristotle—as always the most thoughtful and moderate of thinkers—who locates courage as the mean between the two extremes of rashness and cowardice. Should we, then, with Aristotle, think of courage as a state of character that enables us to endure in the face of fearful things? This permits us to use our reason to discover what is the good thing to do in a given situation without being moved more than we should by the possible fearful consequences of our choice. This kind of courage has two things to be said in its favor. First, it very nicely resolves the inconclusive character of the *Laches* by producing a unified understanding of courage; second, the view of courage that emerges conforms very closely to the view of courage presented by Aristotle in Book 3 of his *Ethics*—and any conception that can claim to be close to Aristotle's view of things has a lot to be said for it.

Unfortunately, this solution will not work precisely because it begs the question that the dialogue so startlingly raises about courage; regardless of whether courage is endurance, wisdom, or a synthesis of the two, must we not know what is truly fearful and what is truly hopeful? But is this not exactly what we do not know—or, to express the situation better, what we wrongly believe that we know? And is it not precisely the role of Socrates to bring home to us that comprehensive and fundamental ignorance that we so desperately attempt to deny or ignore? And is it not this ignorance that renders futile the efforts and careers of Aristides and Thucydides in founding the empire, of Lysimachus and Melesias in their concern for their sons; of Nicias and Laches in their martial eminence. Is it not precisely the basic ignorance of all these pairs that renders the dialogue so pathetic and ironic? We, of course, with the wonderful hindsight of history, can look on these men with an amused superiority. But are we not, in fact, in our own lives, in our relations to our careers and families and each other, in exactly the same predicament? Faced with the world in which we live, courage is exactly the virtue that we all need and exactly the one that none of us seems to be able to achieve. But in saying this I think I have gone too far. I think that I have turned the Socratic ignorance into a counsel of despair. Let us pause for a moment and back up.

In her essay on *The Human Condition* (1958), Hannah Arendt proposes a distinction between "behavior" and "action," a distinction that she thinks is rooted in the classical thought of Plato and Aristotle but has been almost lost in the modern world. Most of the time in the ordinary course of our lives, she says, we are engaged in behavior; the things we do are predictable and in character. But once in a while, Arendt thinks, we stop behaving and begin to act. From the point of view of the neutral observer or the objective scientist, the difference may be hard to see. However, to those of us who undertake to act, the difference is clear. We act when we cease to be determined by the past, when the past no longer serves either as the sole key to what we are doing in the present or as the reliable basis for predicting what we will do in the future. We act, Arendt thinks, when we initiate something; when we break the chain of causation that binds the present and future to the past; when we start a new line of causation, a new situation that is, in its very existence, inherently unpredictable. Behavior is fundamentally repetitive; action, by contrast, is original, unique, and individual. Animals behave; humans can act. Action, the occasion of creating something new, always carries with it the possibility of greatness. And that is why it is actions that we celebrate in song and story, that we record in history—not the everyday behavior of people who do today and will do tomorrow what they have already done yesterday but those unique, initiating events that will somehow or other make the world different.

Conclusions

Courage, I propose, is the specific human excellence that makes action possible. For how, without courage, could we ever bring ourselves to take the overwhelming risks involved in acting? Courage is indeed a problematic, ambiguous virtue, because action itself is always problematic and ambiguous. To act, to start a chain of events the outcome of which is unknown and in principle unknowable, is to admit one's fundamental ignorance and not to deny it. To act is to risk failure, real failure. The only way to avoid failure is never to act but always to behave in predictable patterns, never to initiate anything new. Since there can be no action without courage, so in turn, I think, there can be no philosophy without action. I am thinking of philosophy not in the sense of a body of doctrine but rather in its root, Socratic sense, as being the love of and the search for wisdom. The Socratic career, the philosophical endeavor, the active search for wisdom, requires as its first step the acceptance of our fundamental ignorance. The discovery of our own ignorance—the realization that we do not know what we so desperately want and need to know—is, furthermore, not just the first step of philosophy; it is not a temporary stage along the way that will be overcome as we gather wisdom. The Socratic ignorance that is so beautifully illustrated by the failure of the *Laches* to come up with an answer to the question of what is courage and what those two boys should be taught in order that their souls may be properly cared for—this ignorance and this failure are what make it possible for us to achieve and to maintain our excellence and our virtue as human beings.

I am arguing that philosophy—the love of and the search for wisdom—is a kind of action and that, as such, it is impossible without courage. I am arguing that philosophy and courage are linked by the unique human capacity to act. The Socratic search for wisdom, moreover, is not just one action among many but perhaps the most daring of all, because it requires that we be willing to risk everything, that we be prepared to fail at what we care about most.

Nicias and Laches, with their ignorant self-assurance, each believes that, because he possesses the skill of a general, he has a kind of guarantee against failure. Lysimachus and Melesias, on the other hand, have no such guarantee; they know that they lack the competence that they need to educate their boys rightly. From their own experience they know all too well—or so they think—that their boys might turn out like them—that is, badly. Perhaps the deepest irony of the *Laches* is that the question that so concerns the two old gentlemen—What shall we do about our boys' education, and how shall we care for their souls?—has already been confronted before the dialogue begins. Both boys have already made the acquaintance of that master psychotherapist, Socrates. And we know from the two generals that he would not teach the boys anything. He is no Stesilaus who would train the boys in some particular skill that may or may not prove to be useful. From their acquaintance with Socrates, the two boys, if they listen and talk seriously, may learn to confront their own fundamental ignorance. They may learn that it is possible for them to act, to start something new and not to be the mere passive victims of their own pasts. Through their acquaintance with Socrates, the two boys may experience the joy and the terror of thinking for themselves and taking responsibility for their own lives. That experience may or may not lead to an eminent public career, but it is the necessary first step in the life of an excellent human being. In truth, psychotherapy and courage have a fair beginning here.

NOTE

The Joel Handler Memorial Lecture. Presented to the Chicago Society for Adolescent Psychiatry, October 17, 1984.

REFERENCE

Arendt, H. 1958. *The Human Condition*. Chicago: University of Chicago Press.

4 GIFTEDNESS AND CREATIVITY IN CHILDREN AND ADOLESCENTS

AARON H. ESMAN

The study of gifted and creative children has been of interest in psychology since the latter's emergence as a field of independent scientific investigation. Psychiatrists, and particularly psychoanalysts, have also from time to time ventured into this area in less systematic ways. Papers by Fisher (1981), Gedo (1983), Greenacre (1957, 1958), and others have explored developmental aspects of creativity, but the bulk of the literature in the field has appeared in journals of developmental and cognitive psychology, where clinicians are unlikely to explore it. As a result, most clinicians have at best a limited acquaintance with current knowledge and speculation in the realm of giftedness and creativity studies.

The limitations of our understanding of exceptionally gifted children are vast. We do not know what produces them or how best to educate them, or the relationship between such unusual capacities and psychopathology, or the long-term outcome of such children's development. Some have attributed this ignorance to the egalitarian bias of American society and its educational arm. Though there is some merit in this point, I am not aware that any less egalitarian society has anything more to tell us about these matters. A fair case can be made for the very rarity of exceptionally gifted children as a major source of our lack of knowledge, and Feldman (personal communication, 1984) has suggested that they can elicit in others a sense of the uncanny. Few clinicians can claim any extensive experience with them. It is my purpose in this chapter, therefore, to bring some of the literature in this area to an audience of clinicians who may, from their experience, be able to add to the store of knowledge and to reduce to some degree the scope of speculation.

The history of scientific interest in giftedness goes back at least to the early days of intelligence testing. The early psychometricians, such as Terman (1926), believed that giftedness is synonymous with high IQ and is a hereditary given. Further, giftedness (or high IQ) was assumed to be equivalent to creativity. As Cox (1926), one of Terman's associates, stated: "the extraordinary genius who achieves the highest eminence is also the gifted individual whom intelligence tests may discover in childhood" (pp. 215 ff). Or, as Feldman (1982) put it, "to be labeled 'gifted' or 'creative' in the psychometric manner . . . was to be given a promissory note" (p. 32). These early views of an inevitable linkage among high IQ, giftedness, and creativity were, however, not borne out by experience. Terman's (1926, 1947) classic sample of 1,000 California children with IQs over 140 yielded, on twenty-five-year follow-up, a group of successful achievers in conventional fields such as medicine, law, university teaching, and business, but few of them demonstrated exceptional creativity in adult life. Even an unusually high IQ (over 180) does not appear to predict originality of thought or creative achievement.

These failures did not, however, dampen the ardor of the psychometricians or diminish their zeal to develop ways of identifying and nurturing the potentially creative person. A new generation of tests was evolved specifically designed to measure and predict "creativity." Rather than measure intelligence, they sought to assess cognitive styles or approaches to problem solving. Guilford (1967) devised a set of measures to assess what he termed "convergent" and "divergent" production styles. In his view, "divergent" production, characterized by factors he defined as "fluency" and "flexibility," was conceived as being related to, and perhaps predictive of, future creativity. Strikingly, it proved to be poorly correlated with IQ and thus seemed to offer a wholly new dimension for appraising potential creativity. This work led, therefore, to a proliferation of efforts to assess this new factor and to devise new psychometric instruments toward that end.

Getzels and Jackson (1962) essentially confirmed Guilford's findings. They developed a battery of so-called creativity measures, including tests of word association, "uses of things," "hidden shapes," and others, and applied them to a group of intellectually gifted, that is, high-IQ, secondary school students. They factored two groupings—"creatives" and noncreative "high IQs" based on performance on these tests. Students in both groups did equally well academically, though "creatives" had somewhat lower measured IQs. The "high IQ's"—that is, the low "creatives"—appeared to be stereotyped, nonhumorous, and conventional in their thinking, while the "creatives" were somewhat deviant, valued humor, and were nonconformists. Thus their "creatives" resembled Guilford's "divergent" thinkers, while the "high IQs" were like Guilford's "convergent" type.

Strikingly, Getzels and Jackson found significant differences in family environment between their groups. The "high IQs'" parents were mostly academics, valued conformity, and were socially insecure. Many had had impoverished childhoods and pushed their children to perform. The parents of "creatives" were most likely to be in business, were more tolerant of risk and deviation, were more widely read, and were more concerned about their children's ethical values than with their academic performance.

At about the same time, Hudson (1966) in England was also engaged in pursuing the same issues. He, too, studied a group of bright adolescent boys in a private school. Using similar test measures, Hudson confirmed the existence of the "convergent" and "divergent" styles of thinking. And, like Getzels and Jackson, he found that the "convergents" were likely to have higher scores on standard IQ tests. He also confirmed Getzels and Jackson's observation that the parents of the "convergers" encouraged conformity and the development of practical skills, while those of the "divergers" were more concerned with personal relations, discouraging the acquisition of practical skills. Hudson found, however, that "creativity" was no more likely with one style than with the other; the "convergers" tended to find their way into science and mathematics, while the "divergers" moved into the arts and humanities.

Operating from a broader conceptual base than the previously mentioned American workers, however, Hudson saw "creativity" not so much as a matter of cognition but as a matter of "risk taking." "Intellectual discovery," he says, "is a personal business, not a purely intellectual one." The creative person "abandons himself, and finds once the crisis has passed that he has survived intact . . . the longing to be engulfed totally by someone else" (p. 115). That is, the creative process is akin to a merger experience or a loss of self-definition boundaries. Only those who can risk this transient loss of self-definition are likely to achieve creative work. This view is akin to Kris's (1952) concept of "regression in the service of the ego."

It will occur to some that these findings of distinct styles of cognitive processing and production might have some relationship to the well-

AARON H. ESMAN

known work of Witkin and Goodenough (1981) on field-dependent and field-independent cognitive styles. They suggest that a parallel may indeed exist between "field independence" and "convergent" thinking, but they do not develop this theme, nor do they at any time suggest a correlation between the cognitive styles they defined and either intelligence or creativity.

Indeed, the early enthusiasm for such correlations has waned considerably in recent years. All such testing and assessment procedures were founded on the premise that some special intrinsic factor of a cognitive nature must underlie and be demonstrably correlated with creative potential; further, that this presumably innate characteristic could be psychometrically demonstrated in childhood before any actual creative achievement had become evident. Even if not identical with "giftedness" or high IQ, it must still be there as a deviation from the conventional and could serve as a predictor. Today, however, none of those factors that psychometricians have proposed has stood the empirical test, and the psychometric approach to creativity studies has, therefore, fallen into desuetude.

Psychoanalytic investigators from Freud on have, as noted earlier, been interested in creativity. The literature they have generated on the so-called creative process is vast, if not always illuminating. Many speculations have been proposed about the possible influence of childhood traumata on later creative effort, but remarkably little has been written on actual creative achievement in the preadult years.

In the heady psychoanalytic era of the 1950s, the New York Psychoanalytic Institute, under the guiding aegis of Ernst Kris, undertook a project designed to study psychoanalytically a group of so-called gifted adolescents (Loomie, Rosen, and Stein 1958). Little, however, emerged from this project; few of the patients studied were in fact adolescents, and, apart from a recognition of the critical role of identification in their development, nothing specifically bearing on their supposed "giftedness" or their creative functioning appears to have emerged.

Greenacre (1957, 1958) contributed two penetrating essays that have become landmarks in the field of creativity study and continue to offer valuable insights. In "The Childhood of the Artist" she proposed that the potentially creative child (1) is innately endowed with greater sensitivity to sensory stimulation, (2) has an unusual capacity for awareness of relations among a wide range of stimuli, (3) has a predisposition to a wider than usual range of empathy, and (4) has an intactness of sensorimotor equipment sufficient to allow for the buildup of motor discharge for expressive purposes. She spoke of an unusually close relationship with the mother in early childhood followed by an intense identification with the father or father figure. "Fortunate is such a child if the own father fulfills the need for the model with which then to identify" (p. 62). The creative child experiences a particularly intense "love affair with the world" during what Mahler (1972) came to call the practicing period of separation/individuation, and the ultimate artistic product can often be seen as a love gift to the world and unconsciously to the parent figures. Greenacre also postulated particularly intense "family romance" fantasies in the potentially creative child caused by his sense of "difference" and consequent loneliness.

Greenacre's is a model of variant but essentially normal development in a child with exceptional endowment but not necessarily extraordinary IQ. Robbins (1969), on the other hand, conceived of artistic creativity along the lines of a pathological model using as his text the psychology of a psychotic adolescent who, he assures us, was before his treatment a gifted draftsman but who, after his "cure," lost interest in creative activities. Robbins speaks of such characteristics as "primitive perceptual orientation" as a necessary component of the creative personality. His view seems to be rooted in the Romantic equation of madness and genius that has been left behind by most contemporary students in the field.

Winnicott (1953) proposed a theory of the origins of creativity that has gained wide currency, a theory rooted in his concept of "transitional phenomena." He spoke of the "transitional space" between mother and infant bridging the gap between the sense of oneness and that of separation, affording the child the illusion of omnipotent control that his environment leaves, for a time, unchallenged. It is this illusion, Winnicott suggests, that is the root of later creative activity, and it is in this metaphorical transitional psychic space that creative work occurs. Premature closure of this "transitional space" by an unempathic intrusive mother or failure to develop this presymbolic capacity owing to severe deprivation or maternal inconsistency will stifle the emergence of creative potential. Winnicott is concerned here with what Rose (1980) has called "the creativity of everyday life" as well as with the capacity to create works of artistic or cultural significance.

More recently, Gedo (1983), in his penetrating essays on the creative personality, has sketched his own picture of the "childhood of the artist." He, like Greenacre, emphasizes the atypical qualities of the potential creator, exemplified by his greater sensitivity to sensory experience or his exceptional innate graphic or mathematical talents, to which the child has tended to respond both with anxiety and with grandiose fantasies of unlimited future possibilities. The fate of these exceptional gifts—often appearing in the context of otherwise unexceptional intelligence—depends, Gedo suggests, in large measure on the response of parents. Customarily, he says, the parents react to their child's unusual qualities with fear and envy; they are threatened by the possibility that the child may be "different" and endeavor to "normalize" him or her by discouraging the expression of exceptional gifts. It is only, Gedo proposes, in those rare situations in which parents respond with appreciation and encouragement to their child's extraordinary talents that these are likely to flower early and without crippling conflict.

Slaff (1981) offers one of the rare clinical descriptions of a multi-talented, potentially creative child and, like Greenacre and Gedo, emphasizes the feeling of "difference" and isolation such children experience with relation to their "normal" peers. He compares creative states with psychopathological conditions but, at the same time, distinguishes them: "The despair followed by happiness at the successful confrontation with a creative challenge is a function of the creative process at work. It is not a psychopathological experience" (p. 84).

Gruber (1982) suggested that one appropriate strategy for investigating giftedness and creativity is the retrospective study of the lives of established creative geniuses. He has conducted such studies of the lives of Darwin and Piaget. In conformity with my particular interest in adolescence, I have attempted to review the biographies of a small number of creative geniuses in the arts whose exceptional gifts revealed themselves during—or, with Mozart, before—adolescence through the creation of work of master quality. It is of interest that they are most prominent in the field of music, which is perhaps the closest of all the arts to mathematics, are less prevalent in the plastic arts, and rare indeed in literature.

Some Specific Case Examples

Unique, of course, is the case of Wolfgang Amadeus Mozart, whose unparalleled genius revealed itself early in childhood. At four he was playing the clavier and by six was performing publicly and had begun to compose. By age twelve he was already an established composer with five symphonies, two operas, and a variety of other instrumental and vocal works in his catalog. For him adolescence led to a deepening and enrichment of his art rather than its emergence; the work of the seventeen-year-old Mozart is clearly that of a defined autonomous and inimitable genius, while the early compositions, though on at least a par with most of what was being written in his time, lacked the individual stamp that came with his maturity.

Mozart was born into a musical family. His father was a moderately successful court musician and violin teacher; his mother was musically accomplished as well. He was a somewhat pampered child who, as a result of his precocity as a clavier performer, was exhibited and fussed over by crowned heads and nobility all over Europe from the time he was four years old. His father was his only teacher in all areas except for a brief informal tutelage at age nine by Johann Christian Bach in London. From the accounts of his extraordinary achievements it is evident that he was gifted constitutionally with remarkable powers of memory and melodic inventiveness which, together with the adulation they yielded him, contributed to a high level of self-esteem that at times seemed to have bordered on grandiosity and arrogance.

Illustrations of his extraordinary cognitive gifts abound. One of the most dramatic is the story of the prelude and fugue he sent his sister as a gift from one of his early travels. He apologized for the unusually untidy appearance of the manuscript of the prelude; he had, he wrote, written it down while he was simultaneously thinking out the fugue. This capacity for managing two trains of thought simultaneously seems to be related to, if not identical with, those cognitive qualities that Rothenberg (1979) has called "Janusian" and "homospatial" thinking. Later Mozart went through a phase-appropriate though somewhat belated process of adolescent rebelliousness—displaced in part from his pedantic and authoritarian father to the archbishop of Salzburg, who employed him. He finally left both at the age of twenty-five to make his fortune in Vienna. Regrettably, he failed to do so, dying at thirty-five and leaving that priceless legacy of incomparable music with which we are all familiar.

The second example is that of Franz Schubert. His father was a schoolmaster and a competent amateur musician, who, though he overtly discouraged his son from pursuing a musical career, recognized his talent quite early and began when the boy was five to teach him the piano, and, when he was eight, the violin. In his own words, "I proceeded far enough with him to enable him to play duets fairly well. Then I sent him for singing lessons." His teacher said, "Whenever I set out to teaching him something new I find that he knows it already" (presumably having learned it from his father). Young Schubert was sent to the Vienna Choir Boys' Academy at eleven and began composing at thirteen. By fifteen he had written the first of his endless profusion of great songs, "The Erlking," and at sixteen "Gretchen at the Spinning Wheel," in which he demonstrated a preternatural musical grasp of the experience of a young woman driven mad by disappointed love. Like Mozart, he composed with great speed and inexhaustible melodic inventiveness. At sixteen he had also written his first symphony, and by seventeen he had composed two quartets, a mass, and more great songs. He died, his work, like his eighth symphony, unfinished, at thirty-one.

The third musical prodigy, and certainly the most flamboyant adolescent genius of the eighteenth century, was Felix Mendelssohn. In his latency years he was regarded as a "second Mozart," the prototypic child prodigy who dazzled Europe with his extraordinary piano performances. At age twelve he was introduced to Goethe, whom he succeeded in charming. His training in composition began when he was nine, and at seventeen his genius was revealed to the public in the now familiar and properly admired "Midsummer Night's Dream" overture. Less familiar but equally dazzling was the masterpiece he created at sixteen, the Octet for Strings.

Mendelssohn was born to wealth and power, the son of a prosperous Jewish banker who had converted to Christianity for political and social reasons. His father was deeply concerned with Felix's development and strongly encouraged his devotion to music. He was a stern, demanding paterfamilias who was capable of writing to his son when the boy was eight in this vein: "Mind my maxim—'true and obedient'—you cannot be anything better if you follow it . . . your letters have given me pleasure but in the second I found some traces of carelessness . . . you must endeavor to speak better, then you will also write better. . . ." Also, when Felix was eight his father placed him under the tutelage of a music master and composer, named Carl Friedrich Zelter, who was the boy's constant companion, teacher, and career manager throughout his adolescence. After a brilliant career as composer, conductor, and virtuoso, Mendelssohn died at thirty-eight.

Now let us shift to another medium, that of the plastic arts. It is striking that of the three instances I have discovered that qualify for this discussion all are in fact among giants in the history of art. The first, Raffaelo

Santi, was born in the Umbrian city of Urbino in 1483, the son of a moderately successful painter, Giovanni Santi, with a significant local reputation. Typically, the boy showed talent for draftsmanship early and his father undertook his tutelage until, by age fourteen, he was technically accomplished. Giovanni then followed the common practice of the time and sent his son to serve as an apprentice to one of the masters of the era, Pietro Perugino. Raffaelo served as studio assistant to Perugino for about four years, but already at seventeen was receiving and executing independent commissions. The first of these, *The Coronation of St. Nicholas de Tolentino*, no longer exists, but the preparatory drawings such as this (fig. 1) demonstrate Raphael's total mastery of the medium. By age nineteen he was himself an acknowledged master, as demonstrated by the great altarpiece, *The Assumption of the Virgin*, today one of the glories of the Vatican Museum. A preparatory drawing for this work (fig. 2) achieves the highest level of Renaissance draftsmanship. He died at thirty-seven still growing and recognized along with Michelangelo as the supreme master of his time.

The second instance is that of the Baroque sculptor Gianlorenzo Bernini, born in Naples in 1598. His father was a sculptor of moderate talent who took his family to Rome a few years later to make his fortune. He was his son's only teacher; Gianlorenzo revealed his unusual talent at an early age and under his father's tutelage was carving competent portrait busts at ten. He worked with his father until his early adolescence but by sixteen was operating as an independent artist. A testament to his precocity is the marble group *The Goat Amalthea, the Infant Jupiter, and the Faun* (fig. 3), carved about 1614 at age sixteen, regarded for many years by art historians of later periods as a masterwork of classical antiquity. At eighteen he created a *Saint Sebastian* and a *Martyrdom of St. Lawrence* under the strong influence of Michelangelo. Bernini lived a long, productive, and immensely remunerative life, dying in 1680 at the age of eighty-two. Modern Rome is virtually a monument to his ceaseless creativity in sculpture and architecture.

The third of the adolescent masters was, of course, Pablo Picasso, who not incidentally compared himself with Raphael as a draftsman. He was born in Málaga, Spain, in 1881. His father, Don Jose Ruiz, was a moderately successful academic painter whose favorite subject appeared to be pigeons (note Picasso's fondness for painting doves). Picasso (his mother's surname) began to draw and paint as soon as he could hold the necessary implements and, by eight or nine, was doing respectable pic-

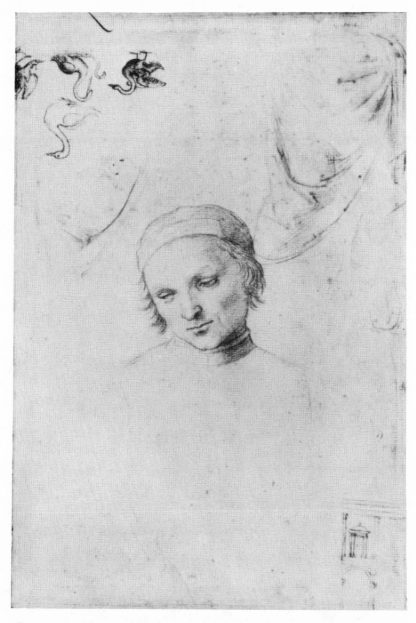

Fig. 1.—*The Coronation of St. Nicholas de Tolentino*. Courtesy of Art Resources, New York.

tures of bullfights. His father was his only teacher until at eleven he entered the local academy in which his father taught. Picasso always maintained that his father was the only effective teacher he ever had. According to a recent biographer, Mary Gedo (1980), Picasso experienced severe anxiety when separated from his father until his late adolescence. One assumes that he dropped his father's surname as a

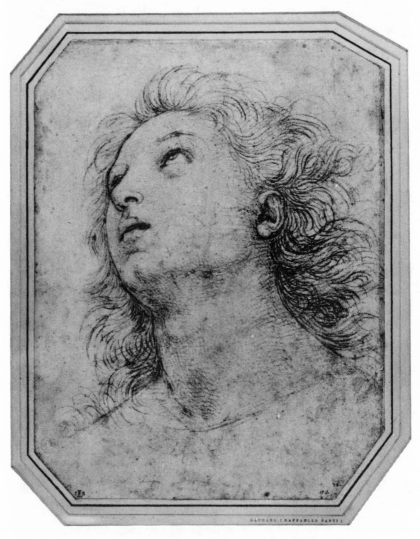

FIG. 2—*The Assumption of the Virgin*. London, British Museum.

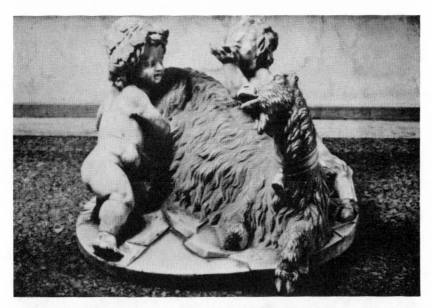

FIG. 3.—*The Goat Amalthea, the Infant Jupiter, and the Faun.* Courtesy of Art Resources, New York.

late-adolescent gesture of individuation. At fifteen he produced this portrait of his mother (fig. 4) and a major painting, *Science and Charity,* in which his father posed for the figure of the doctor (fig. 5). Though hardly preparing us for what was to come, this painting was already the work of a totally accomplished craftsman, and it won him awards in at least two important competitions in Spain. At eighteen, his future direction became more clearly stated in his early masterpiece, *Le Moulin de la Galette* (fig. 6). Picasso's close friend and biographer Jaime Sabartes called Picasso "not only Don Jose's child but his finest work." Like Bernini, but unlike all the others we are discussing, Picasso lived a long and prosperous life, painting to the end at ninety-three.

We move now to literature, where the cases are few. Indeed, the only instance I have found of major adolescent literary achievement in the English language is that of the bizarre genius Thomas Chatterton, who did not survive his eighteenth year. Though his father, again a schoolmaster, died three months before Thomas's birth in 1752, the boy was fostered and educated by his father's brother, a churchman. Indeed, it was while rummaging in his uncle's church that Chatterton, a lonely, depressive boy, discovered documents that fanned his already obsessive

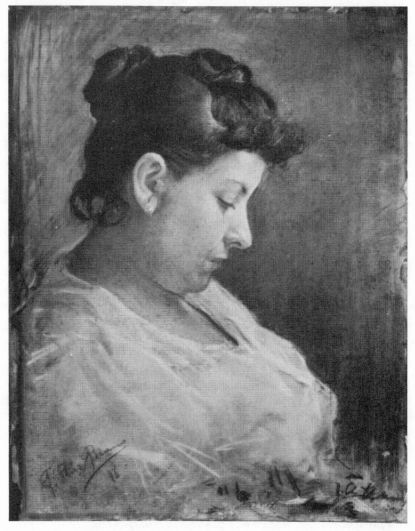

FIG. 4.—*Portrait of the Artist's Mother.* Courtesy of the Museo Picasso, Barcelona.

preoccupation with medievalism and provided matter for his inspired forgeries of medieval epic poems. He began inventing these at twelve, and created, as their putative author, a fifteenth-century monk, Thomas Rowley, perhaps a replacement father figure who incorporated also the clerical lineaments of his uncle and foster father (Greenacre 1958). When at seventeen he descended on London to make his fortune, his financial prosperity did not match the critical enthusiasm that had originally greeted his (or "Rowley's") works (which at that time were still regarded by many as authentic discoveries), and after two months he fell into despair and committed suicide. He was possibly an early-onset manic-depressive. His work, however, continues to be regarded as the most brilliant body of literary fraud ever perpetrated in the English language. As Dr. Johnson said, "This is the most extraordinary young man that has encountered my knowledge. It is wonderful how the whelp has written such things" (Boswell 1791, p. 31).

What then are we able to say about creative genius in adolescence? We have first the fact that, in adolescence, certain generic and universal developmental conditions obtain that are associated with the emergence of artistic and other sorts of creative potentiality. Among those are the simple mastery of technical skills through practice, rote learning, increasing muscular coordination, and control. But of crucial importance, I believe, is the emergence during early adolescence (between twelve and fifteen), at least among the educated classes in developed societies, of the capacity for formal operational thought as described by Piaget. This capacity allows, for the first time in the course of development, for conceptual thinking, the play of abstract ideas, and the conceptualization of previously unexperienced and even unimagined possibilities—including the anticipation of the future. This enrichment and expansion of the cognitive world is certainly the developmental precondition for the well-known emergence of mathematical genius in adolescence. I believe it to be similarly a precondition for the appearance of truly original creative work in the arts as well. What else is art about, after all, than the experiencing of previously unimagined possibilities? Or, as Edelson (1978) says, "Imagination is the capacity or power to entertain or contemplate not only what is, but what may be—to entertain, contemplate, or construct symbolic forms designating states of affairs that are neither necessarily existent or immediate" (p. 110). Flavell (1963), in comparing, from the Piagetian point of view, the adolescent with the preschool and latency child, says, "The adolescent has something of both: the 7–11 year old's zeal for order and the pattern coupled with a much more sophisticated version of the younger child's conceptual daring and uninhibitedness. Unlike the concrete-operational child, he can soar; but also unlike the preoperational child, it is a controlled and planned soaring, solidly grounded in a bed-rock of careful analysis and painstaking accommoda-

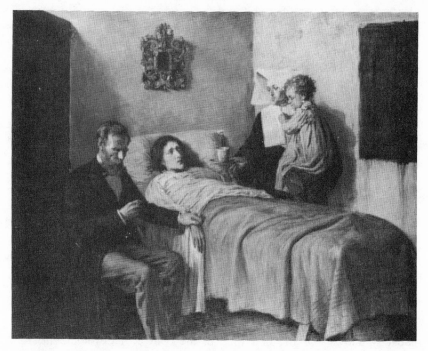

Fig. 5.—*Science and Charity.* Courtesy of the Museo Picasso, Barcelona.

tion to detail" (p. 211). I can think of no better description of the cognitive foundation for creative effort than this one.

I believe, too, that the predominance of musical wunderkinder can also be understood developmentally. Unlike the complexities and richness of verbal language, music is a language with a limited number of elements that are structured—or at least that were during the premodern era—by a system of clear and defined syntactic rules. It is not difficult for any intelligent child to learn the elements; the combinatory and organizing rules can also, with somewhat more difficulty, be learned as the rules of games are learned by latency-age children. Little in the way of the life experience required by the literary artist is needed for this; the abstract principles of music can be learned like those of mathematics. One can see this in Mozart's early work; the very first compositions are the imitative efforts of a child who is learning the basic vocabulary of the language, usually by copying and varying the work of an older master. Somewhat later, during his preadolescent years, he was able to demonstrate his

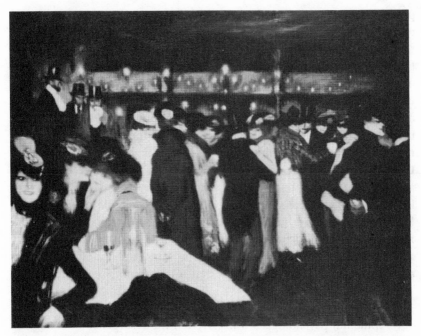

Fig. 6.—*Le Moulin de la Galette.* The Solomon R. Guggenheim Museum, New York. Gift of Justin K. Thannauser.

mastery of the rules of the game with work of superior technical skill. It is only in his adolescent years that the stamp of true originality appeared in his works in which he dared to challenge the rules, to play with the combination of elements in ways previously unheard of, much as the mathematical genius can, in adolescence, see new solutions to old problems or, like the current computer wizards, to new problems as well.

But beyond these maturational universals, what else do we have? We have a group of some half-dozen geniuses, all of whose histories seem to bear out the formulations offered years ago by Greenacre—boys of innate talent and unusual intelligence whose gifts were recognized early and fostered by fathers or father surrogates, many of them artists themselves, who served as teachers and as role models. It is true, of course, that one can find, if one looks into the histories of creative persons, data to support virtually any thesis one sets up to account for their creativity. Niederland (1976) has found a high incidence of physical handicap and defect in creative people—a sort of Adlerian focus in which the creative process is seen as a means of compensating for and mastering the sense of defectiveness such handicaps induce. A number of students, especially the Kleinians from one perspective (Brink 1977; Lee 1959) and Pollock (1978) from another, have considered early object loss as a crucial genetic determinant of creativity, with the work of art or the creative process itself serving to reconstitute the lost object in fantasy. Neither these nor any other unitary construct seems adequate, however, to deal with the infinite variety of individuals and their life histories that make up the roster of creative personalities over the span of time. In any case, none of these theories focuses specifically on the early appearance of creative achievement. About this, it would seem thus far that we can, at the very least, say that the early flowering of creative genius in adolescence is favored by an intense supportive relationship and identification with the father figure—that such a relationship may be a necessary, though hardly a sufficient, condition. And for those who wonder about adolescent girl artistic geniuses, I can only report that, to date, none has come to my attention.

This formulation seems to be consistent with those of the cognitive and developmental psychologists who have led the resurgence of studies of giftedness and creativity in recent years (Bloom 1985; Feldman, personal communication; Gardner 1982; Gruber 1982). There seems to be virtually universal agreement among them on the following points: "Intelligence" is not a universal but a multidimensional function involving a wide range of "realms" or "domains" of cognitive activity; "giftedness" in one area or "domain" does not necessarily correlate with "giftedness" in others, an extreme example being the "idiot savant"; development in one "domain" need not be consistent with that of others; for example, Mozart's total mastery of the keyboard at six was not matched by equal verbal or mathematical skills. This is consistent with Anna Freud's (1963) concept of "developmental lines." Timing and sociocultural context are crucial; for example, the case of the Indian Ramanujan, cited by Gardner, who had possibly the most gifted mathematical mind of the twentieth century "but was introduced to formal mathematics too late to make major contributions" (Feldman 1982, p. 35). Had Mozart been born in the Australian outback rather than in the musically overheated culture of central Europe, it is unlikely that he would have become a composer, though a Bernini born into a West African tribe might well have been a sculptor. In other words, there must be what Feldman calls "coincidence" among innate gift, opportunity, and sociocultural support. "Extraordinary mastery of the field is the result of prolonged systematic and guided interaction with specific environmental forces such as teachers, peers, educational materials, technologies, competitions, and performances" (Feldman 1982, p. 34). Bloom (1985) has particularly emphasized the crucial role of parents—especially fathers—in the early nurturance of children's talents: "No matter what the innate characteristics (or gifts) of the individual, unless there is a long and intensive process of encouragement, nurturance, education, and training, the individuals will not attain extreme levels of capability." "Discovery depends," as Perkins (1981) says, "not on special processes but on special purposes. Creating occurs when ordinary mental processes in an able person are marshalled by creative or appropriately 'unreasonable' intentions" (p. 101). These intentions are, to a large degree, guided by crucial identifications.

Discussion

Are there any clinical implications that we can derive from such work as I have presented here? I believe that there are, especially for child and adolescent psychiatrists. In this increasingly professionalized age, we are more and more likely to be consulted by the parents of unusually gifted children who seek advice, either out of concern that their child may be or become deviant in some way, or in the search for guidance toward optimal education for their child or the enrichment of his special talents. As to the latter—especially for the child with multiple domains of special competence—the usual educational facilities in most communities are likely to be quite inadequate. For the former, the gifted child is, as Gedo and others have pointed out, often a lonely child who is not understood by his peers or does not share their interests. The parents of such children are at times obliged, perforce, to make special, makeshift arrangements to provide tutors and mentors for their offspring. I am not certain that these may not be appropriate for such children. Certainly the creative development of Mozart, Schubert, Picasso, Raphael, and Bernini does not seem to have suffered from such informal and (by current standards) unconventional arrangements.

The problem is, of course, to provide concurrent social experience, and that is more difficult, given the paucity in the usual community of intellectual peers. And in fact such children, and others even less gifted, do grow up somewhat lonely, more accustomed to relating to adults than to agemates. Schubert was fortunate in that he was placed in the Vienna

Choir Boys Academy at eleven, where he had the benefit of superior teaching and a group of peers with similar interests, if not similar talents. But even he, notoriously gregarious as he was, was considered socially inept and awkward. Mozart was, of course, even more so, and suffered all his life from having, as Sitwell (1932) said, "been far too long in leading strings" (p. 138). For the less gifted but still unusually bright or talented child, socialization through elementary and even secondary schools is often difficult; true peers may not be found until these children get into high-status colleges and universities where they may, for the first time, find people who share their interests and style of thinking.

This is one of those situations that may lead to the "pathologizing" of the behavior of these children—the assumption, on the part of well-meaning adults including mental health professionals, that their deviations from the standard American model of outgoing, athletic immersion in the normative peer culture denotes psychopathology and requires some form of "therapy." The child and adolescent psychiatrist has a role to play here in challenging such judgments and placing the gifted child's developmental concerns in a wider and more helpful perspective.

Parents may also need help in avoiding premature display of their gifted children. We know too many cases, from Mozart on, in which children's talents are exploited by their parents for their own advantage— usually to the disadvantage of the child's emotional and social development. This is particularly important in the light of what we know, or believe we know, about the cognitive changes that occur in early and midadolescence. Bamberger (1982), in her study of musical prodigies, has suggested that a transition occurs at this time between two types of musical "intelligence"—a "figural" style characteristic of musically naive adults and preadolescent musicians and a "formal" style characteristic of mature, trained musicians. It is her hypothesis that the careers of early prodigies often founder on the mid-adolescent transition between these styles of cognition—a transition that seems congruent with that from concrete to formal operational thinking in other realms. If she is right, it would seem prudent to ascertain with reasonable certainty that this critical transition is assured, at least with the field of special competence, before launching a young musician prematurely on what may prove an abortive and disappointing career.

In this connection, another observation comes to mind. I have had occasion to interview a number of young physicians and medical students, applicants for residency positions, who in childhood had shown unusual talent and were trained and groomed for careers as performing artists. In each case, at some point in mid to late adolescence these young people undertook a reassessment of their career goals and arrived at one of two conclusions—either that the discipline required by a musical career entailed the sacrifice of too many other aspects of life, or that they were not destined, however good they were, to attain the very top levels of professional success in the intensely competitive musical world. In either case, they concluded that a change in career direction was in order.

It seems to me that this process of self- and reality assessment is a clear manifestation of that phase-specific aspect of late adolescence that Erikson (1950) has called "identity formation" and Blos (1968) has designated as "consolidation of character." It entails a painstaking and often painful self-examination that will, in many instances, lead the young person to seek professional guidance and support; indeed, many of the older adolescents we see come to us in just such a crisis. It is incumbent on us to help such multitalented youths in the evaluation of their gifts and to assist them in their choice of that "domain" in which they are likely to achieve greatest personal fulfillment. We must, however, be wary of our own narcissistic counteridentifications with such exceptional young people. As Fisher (1981) has said, "The therapist has to resist his grandiose impulse to unleash a patient's unusual talent. What we can unleash in our patients is only the power to make an authentic choice" (p. 538).

Conclusions

Slaff (1981) speaks of creativity as both a "blessing" and a "burden" for the child or adolescent endowed with such capacities. It seems to be an appropriate aim for mental health professionals to assist parents and educators so that the blessing of giftedness and creativity can be enhanced and the burdens minimized. Study of the life course of gifted children and of the intrinsic and environmental forces that promote or stifle the expression of their gifts represents a major item on the agenda for future developmental research.

NOTE

Presented as the Peter Blos Biennial Lecture of the Jewish Board of Family and Children's Services, New York, December 1985.

REFERENCES

Bamberger, J. 1982. Growing up prodigies: the mid-life crisis. In D. Feldman, ed. *New Directions in Child Development: Developmental Approaches to Giftedness and Creativity.* San Francisco: Jossey-Bass.

Bloom, B. 1985. Quoted in *New York Times,* February 12.

Blos, P. 1968. Character formation in adolescence. *Psychoanalytic Study of the Child* 23:245–263.

Boswell, J. 1791. *The Life of Samuel Johnson, LLD.* London: Routledge.

Brink, A. 1977. *Loss and Symbolic Repair.* Hamilton, Ont.: Cromlech.

Cox, C. 1926. *Genetic Studies of Genius.* Vol. 2, *The Early Mental Traits of 300 Geniuses.* Stanford, Calif.: Stanford University Press.

Edelson, M. 1978. What is the psychoanalyst talking about? In J. Smith, ed. *Psychiatry and the Humanities,* Vol. 3. New Haven, Conn.: Yale University Press.

Erikson, E. 1950. The problem of ego identity. In *Identity and the Life Cycle.* New York: International Universities Press, 1959.

Feldman, D. 1982. A developmental framework for research with gifted children. In D. Feldman, ed. *New Directions in Child Development: Developmental Approaches to Giftedness and Creativity.* San Francisco: Jossey-Bass.

Fisher, S. 1981. Some observations on psychotherapy and creativity. *Adolescent Psychiatry* 9:528–538.

Flavell, J. 1963. *The Developmental Psychology of Jean Piaget.* Princeton, N.J.: Van Nostrand.

Freud, A. 1963. The concept of developmental lines. *Psychoanalytic Study of the Child* 18:245–265.

Gardner, H. 1982. Giftedness: speculations from a biological perspective. In D. Feldman, ed. *New Directions in Child Development: Developmental Approaches to Giftedness and Creativity.* San Francisco: Jossey-Bass.

Gedo, J. 1983. *Portraits of the Artist.* New York: Guilford.

Gedo, M. 1980. *Picasso: Art as Autobiography.* Chicago: University of Chicago Press.

Getzels, J., and Jackson, P. 1962. *Creativity and Intelligence: Explorations with Gifted Students.* New York: Wiley.

Greenacre, P. 1957. The childhood of the artist. *Psychoanalytic Study of the Child* 12:47–72.

Greenacre, P. 1958. The family romance of the artist. *Psychoanalytic Study of the Child* 13:9–43.

Gruber, H. 1982. On the hypothesized relationship between giftedness and creativity. In D. Feldman, ed. *New Directions in Child Development: Developmental Approaches to Giftedness and Creativity.* San Francisco: Jossey-Bass.

Guilford, J. 1967. *The Nature of Human Intelligence.* New York: McGraw-Hill.

Hudson, L. 1966. *Contrary Imaginations: A Psychological Study of the Young Student.* New York: Schocken.

Kris, E. 1952. *Psychoanalytic Explorations in Art.* New York: International Universities Press.

Lee, H. B. 1959. The creative imagination. *Psychoanalytic Quarterly* 18:301–360.

Loomie, L.; Rosen, V.; and Stein, M. 1958. Ernst Kris and the gifted adolescent project. *Psychoanalytic Study of the Child* 13:44–57.

Mahler, M. 1972. On the first three subphases of the separation-individuation process. *International Journal of Psycho-Analysis* 53:333–338.

Niederland, W. 1976. Psychoanalytic approaches to artistic creativity. *Psychoanalytic Quarterly* 45:185–212.

Perkins, D. 1981. *The Mind's Best Work.* Cambridge, Mass.: Harvard University Press.

Pollock, G. 1978. Process and affect: mourning and grief. *International Journal of Psycho-Analysis* 59:255–276.

Robbins, M. 1969. On the psychology of artistic creativity. *Psychoanalytic Study of the Child* 24:227–251.

Rose, G. 1980. *The Power of Form.* New York: International Universities Press.

Rothenberg, A. 1979. *The Emerging Goddess.* Chicago: University of Chicago Press.

Sitwell, S. 1932. *Mozart.* New York: Appleton.

Slaff, B. 1981. Creativity: blessing or burden? *Adolescent Psychiatry* 9:78–87.

Terman, L. 1926. *Genetic Studies of Genius.* Vol. 1, *Mental and Physical Traits of 1000 Gifted Children.* Stanford: Stanford University Press.

Terman, L. 1947. *The Gifted Grows Up.* Stanford: Stanford University Press.

Winnicott, D. 1953. Transitional objects and transitional phenomena. In *Collected Papers*. New York: Basic, 1958.

Witkin, H., and Goodenough, D. 1981. *Cognitive Styles: Essence and Origins*. New York: International Universities Press.

5   SOME FORMS OF NARCISSISM IN ADOLESCENTS AND YOUNG ADULTS

RICHARD L. MUNICH

The self-consciousness of adolescents and young adults that accompanies the consolidation of identity or the concept of self illustrates many elements of pathological narcissism. Graphically represented by prolonged gazing in a mirror, this self-consciousness is often a painful consequence of normal development. Sometimes, however, it borders on and is indistinguishable from a diffusion of identity, a fragmentation of the self, or even a frank paranoia. Usually it is somewhere between these extremes, inextricably bound to the turmoil we come to expect of this phase of life.

Many authors, including Blos (1962), Deutsch (1944), Jacobson (1964), and Malmquist (1968), have written about the increase in manifestations of narcissism during adolescence. Commenting on the young person's absorption with growth, discovery, and pain, Spacks (1981) states that "compound nouns beginning with self almost all apply readily to adolescents, immersed in a life stage of heightened narcissism." In fact, all young adolescents must cope with substantial physical and endocrinological changes that focus attention on their bodies. Late adolescents and young adults, burdened with the consuming psychological challenges of separation from home, are breaking intensified libidinal ties with cherished objects and involving themselves in new relationships that require extensive experimentation with and commitment to physical and psychological intimacy. All of this physical and psychological activity requires both an underlying stability and a flexibility of the self. A modicum of narcissism in the most general sense, that is, an increased

85

investment in the self, is required to negotiate these changes and endeavors. Both patients that I will discuss, for example, sustained the first major exacerbation of their difficulties when they left home—one for preparatory school at age fourteen, the second a few weeks after entering college at age eighteen.

Self-consciousness has been of interest throughout history. Its vicissitudes are recorded in Ovid's account of the myth of Narcissus; while in the fairy tale, Snow White's mother asks, "Mirror, mirror on the wall, who's the fairest of them all?" Carly Simon's modern lines proclaim, "You're so vain, I bet you think this song is about you . . . ." Listen to John Milton's Eve in Book IV of *Paradise Lost* (1674):

> . . . I thither went
> With unexperienc't thought, and laid me down
> On the green bank, to look into the clear
> Smooth Lake, that to me seem'd another sky.
> As I bent down to look, just opposite,
> A shape within the wat'ry gleam appear'd
> Bending to look on me, I started back
> It started back, but pleas'd I soon return'd
> Pleas'd it return'd as soon with answering looks
> Of sympathy and love; there I had fixt
> Mine eyes till now, and pin'd with vain desire,
> Had not a voice thus warned me, what thou seest,
> What there thou seest fair Creature is thyself,
> With thee it came and goes.

Certainly one reason for our interest in the developmental stage of adolescence and young adulthood resides in its intense focus on self-consciousness, almost as if that stage were the prime aperture for exposing our own narcissistic concerns.

Mirrors have always played a critical role in self-consciousness and in this process of the consolidation of the self. Winnicott's (1965) notion was that the infant's first view of him- or herself is the reflection of what he or she sees in the mother's eyes. In this case, the mother, acting like a mirror, reflects the first distinguishable qualities of the inchoate self back to the infant.

Lacan (1936) writes about the mirror phase during infancy, in which the infant symbolizes in an "aha"-like manner the mental permanence of the I or subjective self. The mirror image, representing a far more coherent picture than the uncoordinated and even fragmented infant him- or herself experiences, is at the threshold of the visible world and serves to establish a relation of the organism to its reality. Lacan continues, ". . . the mirror phase is a drama whose internal impulse rushes from insufficiency to anticipation and which manufactures for the subject . . . the armour of an alienating identity, which will stamp with the rigidity of its structure the whole of the subject's mental development."

For Lacan, the unconscious is revealed in misrecognitions stemming from this mirror phase. A way of thinking about distortions becomes clear if we extend the notion of a mirror beyond that of a simple reflecting surface. All of us are aware of and extremely curious about the occasional discrepancy between our self-concept and what we might see on a videotape representation of ourselves, hear on an audio reproduction of our voices, or experience when we view our photographs. It is most troublesome, however, when the image of ourselves comes back from other people in a discordant and unexpected form, when it does not coincide with what we feel ourselves to be, or when it is incongruent with what we have sent out to them.

Erikson (1950) formulated the notion of identity as consisting of two major factors. The first involves what we think of ourselves; the second, what others in various ways let us know they think about us. The healthy human organism is most often able to bring into and keep these two factors in harmony with each other. The mirror can be used to practice this task of integration, and this practice is the hidden agenda for adolescents spending hours viewing themselves. Of course they are also watching themselves change physically, making themselves look just right, correcting defects, and practicing poses. But underneath, they are adjusting representations of themselves. It is impossible to look through a high school or college literary magazine without seeing this at work. For example, an eighteen-year-old wrote this passage in a story about a fight with his girlfriend: "It was a night flight and he had beaten his sister to the window seat. Paul looked into the window at his reflection. Because of the plane's two-layered window he saw two faces. The first one looked sharp. He admired himself, fixed his hair, squeezed a pimple. The second face was unclear and distant. Somehow his features were distorted; his nose and mouth were large, his eyes were mere blurred, tiny slits" (E.M., *Day Star*, Hopkins Grammar School).

This excursion through poetry and literature brings us to the first technical point. When, under the strain of his angry feelings, our eighteen-year-old author looks into the double window, he is led to two perceptions. One is a clear, sharp reflection of himself that, with only minor adjustments, he can admire. In self-psychology terminology, this is his ideal self. The other image, however, is distorted; the mouth and nose are large, the eyes are slits. This is referred to as an unacceptable self. We now have three entities: the actual self who is looking in the mirror, the ideal self, and the unacceptable self. All three concepts are associated with thoughts, feelings, and impulses, most of which are primarily unconscious and, when integrated, form a coherent self-representation.

We turn now to the internal object and find parallel notions. *E.T., The Extra-Terrestrial* (1982), although primarily about a latency-age child, Elliot, graphically illustrates the components of object representation. The internal object we are interested in here is Elliot's father, who has separated from his wife, leaving his son alone and alienated from his siblings and friends. The movie documents Elliot's efforts to reconstruct, mourn for, and finally separate from a coherent object representation of his lost father. The abandoned extra-terrestrial, E.T., is portrayed as a benevolent, healing creature who longs for the return to a safe home. Although its sex is ambiguous, the E.T. is the external representation of Elliot's ideal paternal object. The scientists pursuing the E.T., whom Elliot fears will do horrible things like lobotomize the E.T., who turn Elliot's living room into a modern intensive care unit, and with whom Elliot must do battle to save the E.T. are the external representation of his unacceptable paternal object. It is as Loewald (1949) wrote, that "reality . . . is represented by the father who is an alien, hostile, jealous force and interferes with the intimate ties between mother and child . . . ."

A footnote to the notion of the E.T. as ideal object is that he or she cannot survive in this world, even with all that modern science can provide. This was also true of more typical adolescent and young-adult ideal objects, such as John F. Kennedy, Martin Luther King, Jr., Mahatma Gandhi, Elvis Presley, or John Lennon. While very few ideal objects have actually survived, nonetheless, the intensity with which adolescents identify with such figures and their respective causes is well known and might be viewed as a slightly more grown-up version of the kind of externalized object representation that the E.T. is for Elliot. Often these figures serve only as extensions of various projected omnipotent and godlike narcissistic configurations of adolescents themselves. Of course, adolescence is also known for the intensity of its hatred toward various objects who do not measure up, even in very minor ways. The cruelty and exclusiveness of peer-group cliques is one painful example of this.

To continue, however, it is necessary to define yet another term that we will need later, that of self-object, a term prevalent in self-psychological theory. Again, I want to use the movie *E.T.* to illustrate in a concrete way what is meant by this perplexing term. First of all, notice the first and last letters of Elliot's name—E.T. Next, remember the strange sequence in the movie when Elliot is in school and the E.T. is raiding the refrigerator at home. The E.T. drinks beer from the family refrigerator, and Elliot, now at school, begins acting as if he were intoxicated. The E.T. bumps its head against a wall, and Elliot gets a headache. The E.T. yearns to be home, free from its new captivity, and Elliot leads a quiet revolution in the biology classroom by freeing all the frogs that are about to be anesthetized and dissected. And finally, the E.T. passes out, and Elliot slumps to the classroom floor unconscious. This parallel behavior is an external representation of a self-object, an internal, living reflection of a symbiotic attachment similar to that existing during the early months between mother and infant. Theoretically, this represents in ego psychology and object relations theory terms the projection and fusion of the omnipotent infantile self into and with the ideal maternal object.

One can now see that the internal object is quite parallel to the situation of the internal self-representation. That is, there is an actual object, an idealized object, and an unacceptable object, each with its constellation of thoughts, affects, and fantasies. Naturally, the developmental task parallel to construction of a coherent self-representation is the construction of coherent object representations. This leads us to the second technical point, the orderly differentiation of self- and object representations. We are accustomed to understanding, as a highlight of borderline-personality organization, major difficulties in this developmental task. Defensive refusion of self- and object representations, often under the threat of separation or rejection, leads to blurring of ego boundaries, faulty reality testing, and serious difficulties with impulses and identity. However, the narcissistic personality represents a particular form of this difficulty, one in which the ego boundaries have already become stable but in which the actual self, the ideal self, and the ideal object are fused to form what is referred to as the pathological grandiose self. This grandiose self is what the narcissistic person is in love with and to what all the libidinal investment seems to accrue. This leaves the unacceptable self, the unacceptable object, and the actual object in the position of forming a worthless and devalued object, one that is subject to the intense negative affect we come to expect from our narcissistically disordered patients when we become, via their projection, the external object that they want to devalue and destroy. We will take up the role of the superego in this problem later.

The third edition of the Diagnostic and Statistical Manual (DSM-III) reflects these constellations of self- and object representations in its description of the narcissistic personality disorder. There are five categories of signs and symptoms that are required to make the diagnosis. The first two refer to self-representations and include a grandiose sense of self-importance or uniqueness and preoccupation with fantasies of unlimited success, power, brilliance, beauty, or ideal love. The last two elements needed for the diagnosis refer to object representations and include first of all a response to criticism, rejection, or defeat ranging from rage to either indifference or feelings of inferiority, shame, humiliation, or emptiness. The second is a sense of entitlement (the expectation of nonobligatory care, respect, and affection) and interpersonal exploitativeness, with relationships characterized by either overidealization or devaluation and, most especially, a lack of empathy; some people feel that envy should be added to this part of the list. Finally, a symptom that is in between those representing self-representations and object representations, perhaps representing a kind of mirror between the two, is an exhibitionism by means of which the narcissistic personality seeks to meet its requirement for constant attention and admiration.

Before all my readers assume that they fall irrevocably into this diagnostic entity, I should delineate several levels of narcissism: at the lowest level, one might have narcissistic traits or defenses—and all of us do; next, there is a narcissistic character, which some of us have and with which all of us are familiar and to which many are attracted; most pathological is a narcissistic personality disorder per se. The differentiation of these levels of organization in the evaluation of adolescents is difficult and important.

For example, a prevalent and therefore normal symptom of adolescence and young adult life is depersonalization, often but not always accompanied by derealization. In this symptom, the person feels detached from while at the same time looking at himself. It is as if the person had taken his self-representation and made it into an object that the self, using an internal mirror, then views. The episodes are usually brief and benign and may include alterations in the sense of time. Although it is also a function of superego pathology, group pressure, and feelings of emptiness, much experimental drug taking in adolescence and young adult life seems calculated to produce this depersonalized and derealized state. It can be a temporarily effective means of relieving anxiety, even though its etiology certainly derives from anxiety (Munich 1977).

Sometimes, however, depersonalized states can be more troublesome. An attractive, frightened sixteen-year-old adolescent was admitted for long-term hospitalization after several moderately serious suicide gestures. She described rather lengthy episodes of depersonalization that had occurred over a period of two years. Previous unsuccessful treatment had included phenothiazines, antidepressants, a course of twenty ECTs, lithium carbonate, and brief psychotherapy. Her self-consciousness had become fixed in a way that had her permanently in her own mirror. Otherwise, the patient presented as a perfect young woman. She dressed appropriately, was well mannered, and deferential. On the other hand, her smile was somewhat fixed, and she had very little to say for herself. The patient's dissociated state seemed intensified and was complicated by an extreme anxiety that precluded any meaningful verbal contact. At times the patient's agony seemed unbearable to both of us. Once, after several months of treatment, in the mutual desperation that comes with these painful states, I asked the patient to take walks with me, during which the gargoyles on university buildings were of special interest to her. Very gradually a story of nightly harassments by her older brothers began to emerge. The brothers' persecution included episodes when her parents were out and the boys made noises outside her bedroom door and window. Such events led to her sleeping with kitchen knives and experimenting with taking various household poisons as far back as age eight. Preoccupation with suicide and death had been prominent since that time. We were finally able to establish that her first episode of depersonalization had occurred at age fourteen following the wedding of one of her brother's friends. The symptom became more frequent (at times lasting several days) during a family ski trip, after she had lost control during a downhill race with one of her brothers. The patient was able to identify as a fairly reliable precipitant a rejection of any sort. She was able to recall feelings of emptiness and even detachment, especially when father was away from home.

Although this case example must be formally diagnosed as an atypical

affective disorder or depersonalization neurosis, the presence of hysterical and narcissistic features and the role of a narcissistic character structure cannot be overestimated, particularly since this patient received two
years of inappropriate treatment. Some of this treatment made
psychotherapy more difficult to begin and sustain, since the patient
feared I might at any moment respond with a recommendation for ECT.
More serious, however, were the problems that occurred when the
patient found herself in a difficult situation with or aware of negative
feelings toward her mother. In fact, her only substantial affective expressions occurred during mother's visits, when she would fly into rages and
then seal silently over.

Here is where we pick up the superego thread I alluded to earlier. In
narcissistic disturbances, the superego is not well integrated into the
personality structure. It is not hard to see how little room there might be
in a grandiose self-representation for delegates from the outside world.
This accounts for the oftimes exploitative, manipulative, and even antisocial tendencies of these patients. Superego precursors are primarily
associated with the devalued, unacceptable object representations who
become threatening and aggressive figures against whom one must be
defended. Guilt itself becomes a dreaded and terrifying complex of
feelings, to be given lip service to protect the grandiose self but mainly to
be used as fuel in the frequent rage reactions such patients experience
when they do not get what they want or when there is a challenge to the
integrity of the grandiose self.

So when our patient experienced an identification with and negative
feelings toward her mother, she attempted to avoid them—and the
ensuing guilt about them—by withdrawing from the unpleasant stimuli.
In this case, the withdrawal was from the condensed unacceptable self,
unacceptable object, and actual object into a pathological grandiose self.
It stimulated the wish to be reunited with an idealized picture of the
father to whom she had felt so close—and who had, by the way, jumped
to his death from her window during an earlier hospitalization. For
example, after these blowups with mother, she would vigorously refuse
any contact with nurses or other female patients (or would become
clinically worse while with them) and would only sit with me, albeit in
virtual silence. At these times, when asked what was happening, she
might reply that she was thinking of dying or that she had the "old
feeling" of looking at herself again. The self she attempted to present at

these times was the accomplished, athletic, attractive, appropriate upper-class and blamelessly perfect daddy's little girl who could do no wrong and whom everyone misunderstood.

At this point the psychoanalytic clinician might legitimately comment that a discussion of many critical issues is missing from this account. To name but a few such issues, there are envy of and competition with the taunting male siblings, conflicts over incestuous impulses for father, and intrapsychic details about the obviously ambivalent relationship with her intrusive and controlling mother. Is not this just a slightly more compli-cated example of oedipal trends at work? Major questions might also be raised about the treatment, including transference and countertrans-ference issues, especially concerning the meaning of the scanty verbal contact and its apparent change as a result of my taking walks with the patient at one point during the treatment. But the narcissistic defenses, in combination with previous treatment, made getting to these more tradi-tional themes in traditional ways virtually impossible.

This brings us to the third technical point, the difference between the content of a psychoanalytic therapy and its conditions. When psychoanalysis shifted its focus of inquiry from conflicts to defenses against those conflicts, from explication of the id to elaboration of the ego, from investigation of impulses to analysis of resistances, it began on its path to the current controversy about the relationship between the transference and the therapeutic alliance. Many of the major theoretical disputes in our field have revolved around disciples' efforts to return to the original path. Abraham, Klein, and Lacan are good examples of the effort to keep or return psychoanalysis to a more consistent focus on Freud's original formulations of psychosexual conflict. Freud himself, his daughter Anna (*The Ego and Mechanisms of Defense*), Hartmann, and Jacobson pushed ahead on the modern ego-psychological road. Object-relations theorists form a special tributary of that road, viewing sig-nificant early figures in the individual's life as the first and most important reality with which the ego must deal. To put it most boldly, internal ego development and self-representation cannot proceed without corre-sponding object input from the external world. When, at the end of the book, the analyst in Phillip Roth's *Portnoy's Complaint* (1967) tells his impulse- and conflict-ridden patient that "now, perhaps, we are ready to begin," he is reminding his narcissistically disordered patient first of all that there is another person in the room. But more important, he is telling his patient that in modern psychoanalysis the discourse is carried on at another level, an important aspect of which is the patient's efforts to act as if that other person were not there.

Modern theorists such as Kohut and Kernberg have written extensively about this issue, particularly with respect to the development and treatment of self-pathology in narcissistic and borderline patients. Both analysts are particularly interested in the framework and conditions of the treatment situation and therapeutic alliance. With adolescents and young adults this focus is especially important, since the inner content of mental activity is still in the process of being consolidated with rapidly shifting identifications and strong dependent and rebellious needs. The main issue for patients with narcissistic psychopathology is the tenuous quality of or lack of connection with significant objects or therapists in their life; so the combination of adolescent turmoil and its disorganizing effect on functioning with a narcissistic configuration is difficult to treat at best. One often feels impelled to construct an empathic net around such a patient; yet an equally good case can be made for confronting the patient head-on.

A twenty-year-old man was referred for intensive psychotherapy following his discharge from inpatient treatment of two years. He had been admitted three weeks after leaving home to start college and following a dramatic suicide attempt in one of the bathrooms of his dormitory. Strikingly handsome and earnest, he had an outstanding academic record in high school, where he had also been the lead actor in many dramatic productions. It appeared that this patient felt most kindly toward himself only when getting A's or starring in plays. Otherwise, he was plagued by obsessional ruminations about life's mundane details and the ways in which he was falling short of brilliance and stardom. His suicide attempt was related, at least on the manifest level, to his inability to complete his first paper assignment in a way acceptable to the very high standards he held for himself. His parents had been divorced when he was thirteen years old. His heterosexual relationships and experiences were quite limited, but during his two-year hospitalization he formed a symbiotic, sibling-like relationship with another patient who was three years older. The patient had many acquaintances but almost no genuinely close friends. Most significant was the patient's excellent capacity for surface adjustment and making a good impression; underneath, however, he felt either empty and shallow or deeply tormented. Whatever his Axis I diagnosis, this patient most certainly demonstrated a narcissistic personality disorder. In many ways he reminded one of a man in mid-life who has just come to the realization that he has lived on a very superficial and meaningless level. The well-known poem by Edwin Arlington Robinson (1916), "Richard Cory," reflects this kind of crisis. Richard Cory glittered when he walked and was admirably schooled in every grace. But, as the last stanza goes,

So on we worked, and waited for the light,
And went without the meat and cursed the bread;
And Richard Cory, one calm summer night,
Went home and put a bullet through his head.

The patient's behavior in therapy for the first several months was compliant, endlessly and entertainingly verbal, and quickly and positively responsive to my interventions. It was as if the therapeutic alliance was fueled by the implicit understanding that the most responsive and articulate patient was responding to the most insightful and empathic analyst. This therapeutic bliss was rarely challenged. He found an appropriate job and even terminated the relationship with his girlfriend in the service of, among other things, "really getting down to things" in the therapy. Even vacations and occasional missed sessions were sustained with unusual equanimity. One day, several months into the treatment, he casually asked at the end of the hour if I would mind writing a letter to the dean recommending his return to school as a special student. I paused and he immediately remarked that it looked to him as if I really did not want to do it. Again even before I could respond, he continued, saying that he of course understood and would have the matter taken care of himself. From that day on, the treatment had a very different character. Although he returned to college successfully, the patient's superficial adjustment outside the treatment hours diminished markedly, and the quality of the sessions become more difficult—so much more difficult, in fact, that what appeared to be a severe narcissistic personality disorder now appeared to be a defensive response to something more serious. Instead of a humorous, literate, and elegant verbal mode of communication, the patient rambled and ruminated about failing his courses and being asked to leave school, thus disappointing those very few people left who cared about him. He felt certain that he was wasting the hours and that I was angry with him and occasionally had thought blocking with the intrusion of violent imagery and suicidal ideation. He complained bitterly of loneliness and emptiness. Life seemed to have no meaning. He was at the same time desperately pleading for help, insisting that he was receiving none, and ignoring all of my interpretive efforts. From his point of view the worst sin I had committed had been to allow him to return to school before he was ready. Even though he realized that he had neither really asked for my advice nor explored his decision, it was still my responsibility to have known how unprepared he was and put a stop to his crazy acting out. It appeared that the transference was subsequently devalued to the same extent that it had been idealized during the first several months. Most remarkably, although each test and each paper was a major crisis, he continued to receive A's in his academic work.

Here the narrative account ends, and we return to what in retrospect was a critical moment in the therapy—the requested letter. To formulate the situation in Kohut's (1971) terms, that is, the idealizing transference and the mirror transference, the first several months were characterized by the patient's view of me as a self-object or a partial object that existed only as an extension of the patient's ideal self. Unlike a positive neurotic transference, this idealized transference was not a substitute for a loved or loving object. Rather it was a replacement of something the patient perceived as missing in his psychological structure, something closely related to the empty and shallow infrastructure of his personality that he complained about. To the extent that the patient was capable of identifying with me then, the first months also involved a substantial amount of mirroring. I had become the grandiose self that the patient wanted so much for himself, bound to reflect back to him his narcissistic demands for exhibitionism and recognition. In this context, my obvious unwillingness to write the required letter was an empathic failure—the mirror did not work right, and immediate restitutional work had to be done. But the damage had been done, and the patient struggled for the next several months to find or reconsolidate the fragmented self-object he had worked on so carefully during the first months of treatment.

Kernberg would see things somewhat differently. He would see the requested letter as representing the patient's efforts to exploit the situation and manipulate the therapist into supporting the pathological grandiose self. Quite the opposite of the conception of the therapist as being a mirror, in this context the therapist is a devalued, unacceptable object representation that the patient must destroy to maintain his internal status quo. The subsequent reaction is predictable narcissistic rage consequent to a misperceived rejection; in other words, he projected onto me his grandiose self and saw my rejection as deprecatory. In either case, the projection should be pointed out and interpreted sooner rather than later. Rather than accept Kohut's explanation of the patient's subjective experience of emptiness as being caused by something actually missing in the psychological structure, Kernberg (1975) postulates that the normal relations between integrated self and integrated internal objects are replaced by the pathological grandiose self. In this circumstance, he continues, the internal object representations deteriorate—perhaps as a result of attack by the unintegrated superego—and the experience of emptiness is intense. For Kernberg, this emptiness "represents the hope for reestablishment of significant object relations on the one hand and the (effort) to refuse all good self and object images on the other."

When my patient's pathological grandiosity was challenged by the therapist-mirror's sending back an incongruent or discrepant image, the patient experienced, because of the projective identification described above, a traumatic sense of humiliation bordering on defeat. In the instance of the letter, however, the patient was able to compensate and maintain his self-esteem for the time being. On actually returning to school, however, he was confronted with the same challenges to his grandiose self that he experienced on first starting school and that led to his suicide attempt and hospitalization. The patient was unable to maintain the grandiose self and decompensated into a prolonged, rageful temper tantrum that had the effect of threatening his reality testing, impulse control, and object tie to his therapist. Under these conditions feelings of loneliness and emptiness take over and death seems preferable.

By my reading of things, both Kohut's and Kernberg's theoretical positions are useful ways of thinking about the material. For example, with the letter, Kohut might have said, "your anxiety about getting back into school and what I would think of that must have made it difficult for you to bring this up so that we could discuss it in our regular way." Following Kernberg, though, one might have said, "since you know we are here to discuss things, you must be quite angry to bring this up at the last minute when it is impossible for us to discuss it." Kohut capitalizes on the mirror; Kernberg takes the initiative in shaping its reflection. An important issue that neither Kohut nor Kernberg takes up is that of timing. Each seems to argue for his particular intervention irrespective of the temporal vicissitudes of the treatment alliance. Sometimes it might be better to mirror; sometimes to confront.

Timing depends on the patient, the therapist's style, and the phase of treatment. In the moment the letter was requested, this therapist was paralyzed. Several weeks later, when the general situation had become worse, I began addressing the contradiction between the patient's good grades as registered and his poor performance as reported. I also kept the focus on the interactive aspects of this communication and on how hard the patient was attempting to bolster his self-esteem by angrily denigrating his therapist and that therapist's efforts. Perhaps at this later time we were both more prepared to deal with these critical transference issues, because important genetic material concerning the mother's alternately depriving and stimulating behavior subsequently surfaced.

There are risks associated with both approaches. With Kohut, the risk is that of conveying to the patient that the therapist cannot tolerate anger; and with Kernberg that one cannot tolerate idealization. One could lose a patient under both conditions. As a last but extremely important point: as much as the narcissistic personality may want to distance himself from and even destroy the devalued object, he also fears his capacity to achieve this and needs the object—hated though it is—to bolster his self-esteem. In this way, the narcissistic personality begins to look similar to the borderline-personality disorder and organization.

Conclusions

The developmental tasks of adolescence and young adult life, particularly those concerned with a consolidation of the self-concept and sense of identity, are both facilitated and complicated by a normal and necessary increase in narcissism. Although mirrors and mirroring experiences promote development from the individual's earliest days, reflections from outside are critical adjuncts during this necessarily turbulent phase after childhood and before adult life. By posing an essentially unanswerable question—when is looking in the mirror too much?—and by choosing two examples of adolescents in severe turmoil, I have attempted to demonstrate several points: (1) the mechanism whereby a pathological grandiose self develops, and how that mechanism relates to accepted diagnostic criteria; (2) some forms of pathological narcissism that might easily pass for, be obfuscated by, or be confused with other forms of psychopathology; and (3) how a focus on the therapeutic alliance and its management may be far more important for dealing with narcissism and especially its adolescent and young-adult manifestations than is concern with the psychodynamics that have produced the manifest difficulty.

NOTE

Portions of this manuscript were presented at the Symposium on Clinical Aspects of Narcissism, New Haven, Connecticut, April 1983, sponsored by The Western New England Institute of Psychoanalysis.

REFERENCES

Blos, P. 1962. *On Adolescence*. New York: Free Press.
Deutsch, H. 1944. *Psychology of Women*. Vol. 1, *Girlhood*. New York: Grune & Stratton.
Erickson, E. 1950. *Childhood and Society*. New York: Norton.
Jacobson, E. 1964. *The Self and Object World*. New York: International Universities Press.
Kernberg, O. 1975. *Borderline Conditions and Pathological Narcissism*. New York: Jason Aronson.
Kohut, H. 1971. *The Analysis of the Self*. New York: International Universities Press.
Lacan, J. 1936. *Ecrits: A Selection*. London: Travistock, 1977.
Loewald, H. 1949. Ego and reality. In *Papers on Psychoanalysis*. New Haven: Yale University, 1980.
Malmquist, C. 1978. *Handbook of Adolescence*. New York: Jason Aronson.
Milton, J. 1674. *Paradise Lost*. Book 4. In M. Y. Hughes, ed. *Complete Poems and Major Prose*. New York: Odyssey, 1957.
Munich, R. 1977. Depersonalization in a female adolescent. *International Journal of Psychoanalytic Psychotherapy* 9:187–198.
Robinson, E. A. 1916. "Richard Cory." In *Collected Poems*. New York: Macmillan.
Roth, P. 1967. *Portnoy's Complaint*. New York: Random House.
Spacks, P. 1981. *The Adolescent Idea*. New York: Basic.
Spielberg, S., and Kennedy, K. (producers). 1982. *E.T., The Extra-Terrestial*. Universal Pictures.
Winnicott, D. W. 1965. *The Maturational Process and the Facilitating Environment*. New York: International Universities Press.

6 FACTORS COMPLICATING THE PSYCHIATRIC DIAGNOSIS OF ADOLESCENTS

ELISA G. SANCHEZ

If the diagnosis of psychiatric patients in general is a difficult task, suffering from great deficiencies and involving innumerable contradictory opinions (Feinstein 1977; Garza-Guerrero 1980; Grinker 1977; Stoller 1977; Wing 1977), then the diagnosis of the adolescent patient is an even more complex undertaking. Adolescence is a stage in life that implies growth, change, and intricate adaptive processes. The difficulties in understanding these processes have led to the formation of many myths (Adelson 1964; Blos 1971; Elkin and Westley 1955; Jahoda and Warren 1965; Rutter, Graham, Chadwick, and Yule 1976; Weiner 1971) that obscure the true diagnosis of adolescent patients.

Is the adolescent's experience due to age? Is the problem transitory? Is the conduct an attempt to obtain peer approval, or does it represent an effort to adapt to sociocultural environment? In search of an answer to these questions, I reviewed the pertinent literature on adolescent diagnosis and found that there are differing opinions about evaluation (Kernberg 1978; Meeks 1973; Offer, Ostrov, and Howard 1981; Offer and Sabshin 1963; Wilson 1971) and systems of classification of mental disorders in adolescents (Masterson, Tucker, and Berk 1963, 1966; Spitzer 1980; Spitzer, Sheehy, and Endicott 1977; Weiner 1980). These reflect a lack of conceptual consistency in the field of adolescent diagnosis.

Because of the difficulties that beset nosology and classification, these problems will undoubtedly persist. The focus of this work is, therefore, limited to the consideration of those factors that complicate the diagnostic process itself. Although these factors overlap, they will be delineated in the following categories: characteristics of adolescence; personal characteristics and conceptual framework of the therapist; sociocultural factors; familial factors.

Characteristics of Adolescence

During adolescence, growth and development take place in the biological, intrapsychic, and social spheres. Among the developmental tasks to be resolved are: (1) detachment from the parents through achievement of autonomy; (2) attainment of the genital stage of psychosexual development with the resulting capacity to engage in heterosexual relationships; (3) integration of identity; (4) predominance of the secondary thought process; and, as a result of the resolution of these tasks; (5) achievement of a stable and nonconflictual relationship between the intrapsychic structures (Blos 1979; Blotcky and Looney 1980; Josselson 1980; Laufer 1965; Offer and Offer 1971; Spiegel 1958).

The completion of these tasks is a difficult endeavor but one that adolescents can successfully accomplish through the adaptive abilities and defensive mechanisms that lend distinctive features to this stage of life. Consequently, adolescents must be understood in their own developmental context, thus avoiding the potential misinterpretation of normal clinical manifestations as psychopathological in nature. The following clinical manifestations are a result of normal adolescent development:

1. The changes in corporal sensations and increased sexual drives overload the ego and its defense mechanisms and produce conflicts between instinctive urges and internal prohibitions. The results are feelings of guilt, shame, and inferiority. These feelings can also originate from the opposing self-images that the adolescent has, what he wants to be, and what he really is (Jacobson 1961). The fluctuation in the adolescent's identity and self-esteem is also related to the devaluation that he makes not only of his parents but also of the parents' attitudes and behavior that had previously served him as a model for his own value system. In the devaluation of his superego parental introjects, the adolescent loses the protective and gratifying function of the introjects. He then seeks a substitute for this loss of gratification by narcissistically centering on himself. The results will be feelings of superiority that alternate with periods of self-devaluation and a hypersensitivity to the physical and

psychological modifications that he is experiencing (Geleerd 1961; Jacobson 1961; Josselson 1980; Josselyn 1954; Marcia 1980; Spiegel 1951).

2. Another source of conflict and ambivalence for the adolescent is the process of detachment from parents. Though the adolescent experiences growth and a drive for independence, he at the same time does not feel prepared to face them either emotionally or economically. He is afraid of losing the love of the persons who up to this time have been predominant in his life. The adolescent's dependency-independency conflict is evidenced by the establishment of a "negative dependency" (Offer and Offer 1971). By this mechanism, the adolescent adopts opposite attitudes over daily issues that irritate his parents in order to feel independent from them. Since the adolescent's range of activity is now more ample, he begins to seek relationships out of his home with his peer group. The peer group provides an ally in his battle for autonomy and in his search for identity (Adelson and Doherman 1980; Coleman 1980).

3. Obviously, the conflicts that the adolescent is undergoing will affect directly his emotions. In this regard, Jacobson (1961) has described changing moods as the inevitable handmaidens of adolescence. However, Grinker, Grinker, and Timberlake (1962), Masterson and Washburne (1966), Offer (1967), and Rutter et al. (1976), among other authors, do not agree with the statement that changing moods are present in all adolescents, including the "normal" adolescents studied by them. They found a variety of symptoms, most commonly anxiety and depression, that were generally moderate and transitory. The depression manifested itself in feelings of guilt and self-depreciation.

These characteristics of adolescence can complicate the diagnosis of the adolescent patient in several ways:

1. Because of the adolescent's difficulties in maintaining his self-esteem, he is very sensitive to outside opinion and easily feels criticized and devaluated. In an effort to avoid these feelings, he frequently chooses not to inform the therapist of his emotions. His mistrust is also related to his negativism, which grows out of his desire to become independent, since trust may be experienced as dependence (Geleerd 1961). This obstructs the gathering of information needed to make a good diagnosis, and some aspects, in particular the sexual ones, must await revelation until a good relationship has developed.

2. The accentuation of narcissistic traits that occurs during the adolescent period can cause the therapist to wonder whether he is dealing with a

narcissistic personality disorder. In order to make a differential diagnosis, it is essential to determine whether or not the following signs, never present in pathological narcissistic structures, are present in the adolescent patient: (1) the capacity for feeling depressive guilt, (2) the ability to establish lasting, nonexploitative relationships, and (3) the aptitude for having his own value system (Kernberg 1978).

3. The adolescent's attempt to acquire independence can produce behavior that is sometimes difficult to differentiate from pathology. The therapist can avoid that mistake by keeping in mind two important points: even when the adolescent devaluates his parents, he should have the capacity to appreciate their positive aspects; the more conspicuous the clinical manifestations are, the more difficult the resolution of the separation process (Marohn 1980). This indicates that serious delinquent behavior or open rebelliousness should not be considered a part of the normal separation process. Their presence necessitates an exhaustive diagnostic evaluation with the thought in mind of serious psychopathology.

4. The affective symptoms that almost inevitably affect the adolescent may, if they are present with a certain intensity, require a differential diagnosis from those that pertain to well-established psychopathology. This need is more important with depressive symptoms, because of their frequency in adolescence.

This case example illustrates some of the characteristics of adolescence and their influence during the diagnostic process.

CASE EXAMPLE 1

The patient is a single, middle-class, nineteen-year-old male patient, in college. His academic performance had been satisfactory until he experienced a fainting sensation that prevented him from completing an exam. This happened several months prior to his seeking psychiatric help and has continued intermittently since then. At times this sensation is so intense that he does not step outside of his home. In the first evaluation interviews, it was difficult to get the patient to search within himself for the origin of his difficulties. He was under the constant impression that he suffered from an organic disease, and he paid inordinate attention to every physical complaint that he felt. This situation continued even in the face of the negative findings of the physical and laboratory examinations.

During the evaluation interview, the therapist took note of the glowing manner in which the patient described himself.

> P: I'm a very kind, agreeable and polite person. I have my good moments as well as my bad ones, but I'm sincere and intelligent. I like helping other people a lot and I have good social relationships.
>
> T: I notice you describe yourself very favorably.
>
> P: That's how I feel and everyone who knows me thinks the same way.
>
> T: Is there something about you that you do not like?
>
> P: Well, like most people, I occasionally have some bad moods. For example, my father and my friends bother me when they don't understand that I am right about something but when they see their mistake, I'm not annoyed any more.
>
> T: And you're usually right?
>
> P: Well, it doesn't happen often but logically I'm usually right, like when I want my sister to do something for me and she doesn't do it immediately.

At this point the therapist could not resist feeling antipathy toward the patient for his self-centered attitude. However, this antipathy yielded to the need to accept the patient on his own terms. The therapist recognized this attitude as a device to protect the patient's self-esteem, which had been threatened by increasing pressures at school, anxieties about the propriety of masturbation, and doubts about his sexual attractiveness. His oedipal conflict was now reawakened and he was experiencing more intense rivalry and ambivalence toward his father. Despite these anxieties the therapist could perceive the patient's concern for others and his ability to empathize, which extended to his sister—whom he loved and respected in spite of the quarrels between them. The patient had a well-integrated, though rigid, superego, demonstrated by his capacity to feel reparatory guilt and by his autonomous value system that governed him without many contradictions.

The Therapist's Conceptual Framework

The therapist's conceptual framework determines his definition of normality and pathology and the selection of criteria used for evaluation.

In reviewing the literature on adolescence, one finds two predominant trends that define "normality" during adolescence: psychoanalytical writings and empirical investigation studies (Mitchell 1980). Until recently, the works of the classical psychoanalysts (Bernfeld 1938; Blos 1962, 1967; Erikson 1968; Fountain 1961; Freud 1958; Geleerd 1961; Josselyn 1954; Lindemann 1964; Spiegel 1951; Winnicott 1971) served as the basis for evaluating adolescents. But a heterogeneous group of investigators who recently have conducted investigations on a greater number of adolescents, patients, and nonpatients have mounted a challenge to traditional concepts (Douvan and Adelson 1966; Grinker et al. 1962; Masterson 1967; Masterson and Washburne 1966; Offer et al. 1981; Rutter et al. 1976). These authors think that classical psychoanalytic theory on adolescence was the product of unsupportable generalizations and that the classical authors did not clarify whether they were talking about their findings in patients or about their theories on adolescence in general.

Under the classical point of view, adolescence is considered a chaotic condition triggered by the new feelings and emotions that accompany physical development. The new sexual drives are so menacing that the adolescent tries to manage them by adopting one of two opposing postures: asceticism or sexual promiscuity. The principal threat of the sexual drives is that they are accompanied by the reappearance of oedipal desires that compel the adolescent to reject his parents. The adolescent looks for refuge and identity in his peer group, which finally takes the parents' place in giving rules and principles. The clash of the adolescent's increased aggressiveness with his efforts to achieve independence frequently gives rise to open rebelliousness, delinquency, and drug addiction. Classical analytical authors also theorize that adolescent moods are oscillatory, which makes planning for his future a confusing and difficult task. In summation, classically, adolescence is a turbulent state where anything can occur and where equilibrium is an abnormality. These authors' opinion on adolescent psychopathology is that clinical entities are badly defined, very unstable, and transient. This makes the diagnosis an almost impossible undertaking because it is difficult to determine whether the symptoms are due to "the age crisis" and are likely to disappear without a trace.

In opposition to the classical viewpoint, recent researchers depict the adolescent as capable of adequately managing the tension produced by his physical and emotional changes without significant modification in his personality. They label the adolescent's conduct as judicious, consistent, and oriented toward the implementation of future plans. His moods are stable, and he is capable of sublimating his aggressions through sports, hobbies, or long talks with a friend. His sexual attitude is conservative, and he is conscious of the responsibilities that sexuality entails. In addition, he is respectful of his parents and shares many of their moral standards (Feather 1980). These authors view the so-called turmoil of adolescence as overrated and stereotyped in the literature. The only signs of turmoil they found were isolated, moderate, and transitory symptoms.

The conclusions reached by these researchers regarding adolescent psychopathology were: (1) the symptoms remain unchanged through time (Rutter el al. 1976); (2) the difference in the stability of diagnosis between adolescents and adults is not very marked, for example, 54 versus 76.7 percent, respectively (Weiner and del Gaudio 1976); (3) the adolescent psychopathology tends to progress into an adult disorder (Masterson 1967); (4) good adjustment during adolescence indicates stability in adulthood (Peskin and Livson 1972; Vaillant 1978); (5) the problem in diagnosing an adolescent does not lie in distinguishing between psychopathology and a veritable adolescent turmoil but, rather, in correctly diagnosing the former (Masterson 1967).

Although there is a significant contrast between the two reference frameworks described, both contain very helpful principles for the understanding of adolescent patients, particularly if clinicians are able to integrate them adequately. The risks of an uncritical and dogmatic adherence to either of these frameworks would be: (1) A prejudicial proclivity toward a "traditional classic" point of view may lead the clinician to consider psychopathological manifestations as normal adolescence vicissitudes. He may take an expectant position with the inherent danger of delaying treatment; (2) the uncritical assumption that adolescence is an untroubled age may cause the clinician to exaggerate the importance of adaptive symptoms and behaviors and thereby diagnose them as "illness." The clinician may thus ignore psychoanalytic theory, which furnishes sound psychodynamic explanations for such clinical manifestations.

The Personality of the Therapist

As traditionally assumed, the personality of the therapist affects his understanding of the patient's behavior and feelings. Clinicians who have experienced a very conflictive adolescence or who have had children with the same problem tend to have a distorted view of the adolescent. Mistakes in diagnosing can also be made by therapists who feel uncomfortable and threatened by the nonconformance of adolescents (Kernberg 1976; Oldham 1978).

The foregoing difficulties may cause the clinician: (1) to diagnose a nonexisting pathology if he exaggerates clinical observations that clash with his personal values; and (2) to fail in diagnosing pathology if he underestimates clinical manifestations that suit his personal needs.

This clinical example illustrates how both the conceptual reference framework and the personality of the therapist can affect the diagnosis.

CASE EXAMPLE 2

The patient is a sixteen-year-old, single, male, upper-class high school student. The parents sought psychiatric treatment for him because of his frequent quarrels, aloofness from family activities, and addiction to drugs. He had undergone prior psychiatric treatment, so the new therapist obtained a clinical opinion from the former therapist, who felt the patient's problems were part of the adolescent turmoil as well as the result of environmental influences. For instance, he believed that the social status of his former patient, which was higher than his own, was the cause of the patient's drug addiction and that some of the patient's symptoms corresponded to the "poor rich child" syndrome with the attendant lack of love and attention from his socially involved parents. In order to compensate for this deficiency, the original therapist undertook the role of a parental surrogate. The treatment ended in a great friendship between them but obviously brought about little beneficial change.

The new therapist's evaluation differed considerably from that of his colleague. He saw the patient's psychopathology in his inability to achieve stable and lasting interpersonal relationships. His identity was diffuse to the extent that he had engaged in both homosexual and heterosexual relationships. He had poor impulse control and an unsoundly structured superego, which was corroborated by his inability to possess his own value system or to respect that of others. These defects had led him to commit delinquent acts. The final diagnosis was borderline personality disorder.

Sociocultural Factors

Because sociocultural factors have a pervasive influence on adolescent behavior, most authors on this subject agree that adolescents should never be evaluated without taking into account the social and cultural medium in which they develop (Saltzman 1974). Adolescence is the phase of development where the individual's field of action expands outside his family, which until then had been the principal provider and supporter. In the wider field of his community the adolescent confronts the difficult task of finding his own place, a process that helps him consolidate his identity. This can be achieved only if society responds to the adolescent's needs by providing support and by assigning a position and a function (Erikson 1968). These needs are very difficult to fulfill because of the numerous changes in our society. For instance, in our industrial society the young do not have the essential role in the economy of the country that they had in preindustrial times when their role was predetermined. Scientific and technological advances have multiplied vocational options and lengthened academic training, causing greater difficulty in career choice and prolonging dependence on parents (Giovacchini 1980).

Because of rapid cultural change, society is now more tolerant of mental illness and deviant behavior, sending a confusing message to the adolescent that may complicate healthy identity consolidation and have a deleterious effect on his behavior.

The demands and expectations that society has for adolescents are another influential factor in their conduct (Miller and Simon 1980; Offer and Offer 1971). Every society, in different epochs, has formed an image that it expects the adolescent to fit. The present images have been shaped by myths and generalizations from psychopathological behavior, which because of its visibility has attracted greater attention (Adelson 1964; Jahoda and Warren 1965). There is a risk that adolescents may end up by accepting these descriptions and forming a deviated self-image (Anthony 1969).

The problems caused by the interplay between adolescents and society may cause the therapist to make errors in diagnosis: (1) Behavior may be qualified as pathological when the therapist fails to consider the sociocultural context in which it occurs. The behavior may be the product of adaptive mechanisms or of attempts to fulfill the expectations of society. (2) Behavior that is frankly pathological may be diagnosed as normal and adaptive. (3) The therapist may respond primarily to societal stereotypes rather than to the individual patient. (4) The therapist may be influenced by societal attitudes toward mental illness. (5) The therapist may not be able to differentiate between behavior influenced by fads and that caused by authentic cultural changes (Kernberg 1976).

Familial Factors

As described by Lidz, the family is the first teacher of social interaction and emotional reactivity. It provides identification and self-esteem and exposes the children to the parents' interpretations of reality and forms of communication (Lidz, Cornelison, Carlson, and Fleck 1971). Consequently, the family influence is decisive in the formation of the children's behavior. This influence takes on more importance during adolescence when the teenager begins to acquire independence and practice in society what he has learned in his family circle. This process places a great amount of stress on both adolescent and family and tests their capacity to cope with change. The result may be maladaptive mechanisms reflected in adolescent behavior. Ackerman (1962) thinks that many times the adolescent's irrational behavior in extrafamilial situations is simply the adolescent's carrying out his familial conflicts. For example, parents may use the adolescent as the scapegoat of the family's pathology or may impede his independence to maintain the family's emotional equilibrium (Arnstein 1980). The parents may also encourage certain behavior in their adolescent children in order to gratify their own unacceptable desires (Johnson 1972; Shapiro 1969).

The participation of parents is an important part of the evaluation process to furnish helpful information and to give the therapist an opportunity to appreciate the family's dynamics (Kaplan 1971). The parents' information may show a tendency to underestimate or to exaggerate their children's problems. There are numerous reasons that may cause the parents to misinterpret the behavior of their adolescent children: (1) their difficulties in keeping abreast of rapid cultural changes and evaluating their adolescent children's behavior in the context of these changes (Offer et al. 1981); (2) the reactivation in the parents of their own adolescent conflicts (Benedek 1959; Estrada Inda 1982); (3) the reawakening of parents' unsatisfied dreams and the accompanying envy toward their adolescent children at a time when the parents are passing through the middle-age crisis (Lidz 1969).

The interplay of these circumstances could lead the therapist to make the following mistakes in the diagnosis of adolescents: (1) the therapist may be overinfluenced by the parents' interpretation of the adolescent's problems; (2) the therapist may be incapable of understanding the adolescent's problems as they relate to the dynamics of the family; and on the other hand, (3) the clinician could exaggerate the impact of family dysfunction on the adolescent's clinical manifestations to the point of ignoring individual psychopathology and its contribution to family dysfunction.

This clinical vignette demonstrates sociocultural and familial factors and the manner in which they affect the diagnostic evaluation.

CASE EXAMPLE 3

The patient is a seventeen-year-old, single, male college student who comes from an upper-middle-class family. He was coerced into seeking psychiatric consultation by his mother and sister because he was suspected of using marijuana. Drug abuse was totally unacceptable to this conservative family. The family physician, also a man of conservative values, previously saw the patient and angrily identified him as a drug addict.

During the psychiatric evaluation, the psychiatrist learned the following about the patient: He had smoked marijuana two or three times over a few months to obtain peer-group acceptance, but he had stopped when the novelty passed. He was a studious individual and had received acceptable grades in school. He had significant friendships and was respectful of others and loyal to his peer values. The patient had the capacity for falling in love and maintaining nonexploitive heterosexual relationships. He was developing his own value system that allowed him to appreciate the values of others, including those of his parents, whom he loved and respected.

During a joint interview of the patient and his parents, the therapist discovered that the mother was excessively infantile and very possessive. The son had explained to his mother that his use of marijuana had been a short and transitory occurrence, but she ignored him and insisted on psychiatric counseling in order to continue exploiting the situation. Although she complained to her husband that his neglect and irresponsibility toward the family had brought about the son's use of marijuana, she was actually conveying her own disappointment in feeling neglected by her husband. At the end of the evaluation, the clinician recommended marital therapy as the treatment of choice, with the possibility of including the son in some of the sessions.

Conclusions

The diagnosis of adolescent patients is multifaceted and involves therapist-patient, social, and familial systems. It is necessary to evaluate the adolescent as a whole and to understand his behavior and symptomatology in the context in which they occur, that is, age, conflicts inherent in the adolescent stage, and the familial, sociocultural, and economic environments.

Furthermore, the diagnostic task with the adolescent is directly related to the therapist-patient interaction. It is important to evaluate adolescent behavior in terms consistent with the patient's underlying motivations and intrapsychic meanings. In doing this, the therapist injects his own personal traits and his training background.

The cases reported exemplified how the diagnosis procedure may be complicated and even impeded if the therapist fails to take into consideration all the factors described throughout this chapter.

NOTE

The American Society for Adolescent Psychiatry Research Fund Award Address, presented at the annual meeting, Dallas, Texas, May 1985. This award is supported by a grant from the Gralnick Foundation, Port Chester, New York.

REFERENCES

Ackerman, N. 1976. *Grupoterapia de la familia.* Buenos Aires: Horme.
Adelson, J. 1964. The mystique of adolescence. *Psychiatry* 27:1–5.
Adelson, J., and Doherman, M. J. 1980. The psychodynamic approach to adolescence. In J. Adelson, ed. *Handbook of Adolescent Psychology.* New York: Wiley.
Anthony, E. J. 1969. The reactions of adults to adolescents and their behavior. In A. H. Esman, ed. *The Psychology of Adolescence.* New York: International Universities Press, 1975.
Arnstein, R. L. 1980. The student, the family, the university, and transition to adulthood. *Adolescent Psychiatry* 8:173–183.

Benedek, T. 1959. Parenthood as a developmental phase: a contribution to the libido theory. *Journal of the American Psychoanalytic Association* 7:386–417.

Bernfeld, S. 1938. Types of adolescence. *Psychoanalytic Quarterly* 7:243–253.

Blos, P. 1962. *On Adolescence: A Psychoanalytic Interpretation.* New York: Free Press.

Blos, P. 1967. The second individuation process of adolescence. *Psychoanalytic Study of the Child* 22:162–186.

Blos, P. 1971. The generation gap: fact and fiction. *Adolescent Psychiatry* 1:5–13.

Blos, P. 1979. *The Adolescent Passage: Developmental Issues.* New York: International Universities Press.

Blotcky, M. J., and Looney, J. G. 1980. Normal female and male adolescent psychological development: an overview of theory and research. *Adolescent Psychiatry* 8:184–199.

Coleman, J. C. 1980. Friendship and the peer group in adolescence. In J. Adelson, ed. *Handbook of Adolescent Psychology.* New York: Wiley.

Diagnostic and Statistical Manual of Mental Disorders III, 3d ed. (*DSM-III*). 1980. Washington, D.C.: American Psychiatric Association.

Douvan, E., and Adelson, J. 1966. *The Adolescent Experience.* New York: Wiley.

Elkin, F., and Westley, W. A. 1955. The myth of adolescent culture. *American Sociological Review* 20:680–684.

Erikson, E. H. 1968. *Identity: Youth and Crisis.* New York: Norton.

Estrada Inda, L. 1982. *El Ciclo vital de la familia.* Mexico, D. F.: Xochitl.

Feather, N. T. 1980. Values in adolescence. In J. Adelson, ed. *Handbook of Adolescent Psychology.* New York: Wiley.

Feinstein, A. R. 1977. A critical overview of diagnosis in psychiatry. In V. M. Rakoff, H. C. Stancer, and H. B. Kedward, eds. *Psychiatric Diagnosis.* New York: Brunner/Mazel.

Fountain, G. 1961. Adolescent into adult: an inquiry. *Journal of the American Psychoanalytic Association* 9:417–433.

Freud, A. 1958. Adolescence. *Psychoanalytic Study of the Child* 13:225–278.

Garza-Guerrero, A. C. 1980. Una revisión crítica sobre diagnóstico en psiquiatría y psicoanálisis. Trabajo presentado en el Depto. de Psiquiatría, Hospital Universitario, Universidad Autónoma de Nuevo Leon, México.

Geleerd, E. R. 1961. Some aspects of ego vicissitudes in adolescence. *Journal of the American Psychoanalytic Association* 9:394–405.

Giovacchini, P. P. 1980. Sociocultural factors, life-style, and adolescent psychopathology. *Adolescent Psychiatry* 8:65–84.

Grinker, R. R., Sr. 1977. The inadequacies of contemporary psychiatric diagnosis. In V. M. Rakoff, H. C. Stancer, and H. B. Kedward, eds. *Psychiatric Diagnosis.* New York: Brunner/Mazel.

Grinker, R. R., Sr.; Grinker, R. R., Jr.; and Timberlake, J. 1962. "Mentally healthy" young males: homoclites. *Archives of General Psychiatry* 6:405–453.

Jacobson, E. 1961. Adolescents' moods and the remodeling of psychic structure in adolescence. *Psychoanalytic Study of the Child* 16:164–183.

Jahoda, M., and Warren, N. 1965. The myths of youth. *Social Education* 38:138–149.

Johnson, A. M. 1972. Sanctions for superego lacunae of adolescents. In S. I. Harrison and J. F. McDermott, eds. *Childhood Psychopathology and Anthology of Basic Readings.* New York: International Universities Press.

Josselson, R. 1980. Ego development in adolescence. In J. Adelson, ed. *Handbook of Adolescent Psychology.* New York: Wiley.

Josselyn, I. 1954. The ego in adolescence. *American Journal of Orthopsychiatry* 24:223–237.

Kaplan, A. H. 1971. Entrevistas conjuntas de padres como parametro en el psicoanalisis de los adolescentes. *Cuaderno de la Sappia* 2:17–32.

Kernberg, O. 1976. Cultural impact and intrapsychic change. *Adolescent Psychiatry* 4:37–45.

Kernberg, O. 1978. The diagnosis of borderline conditions in adolescence. *Adolescent Psychiatry* 6:298–319.

Laufer, M. 1965. Assessment of adolescent disturbances: the application of Anna Freud's diagnostic profile. *Psychoanalytic Study of the Child,* pp. 99–123.

Lidz, T. 1969. *El Adolescente y su familia.* Buenos Aires: Horme.

Lidz, T.; Cornelison, A. R.; Carlson, D. T.; and Fleck, S. 1971. *Interaccion familiar. Aportes fundamentales sobre teoria y tecnica.* Buenos Aires: Tiempo Contemporaneo.

Lindemann, E. 1964. Adolescent behavior as a community concern. *American Journal of Psychotherapy* 18:405–417.

Marcia, J. E. 1980. Identity in adolescence. In J. Adelson, ed. *Handbook of Adolescent Psychology*. New York: Wiley.

Marohn, R. C. 1980. Adolescent rebellion and the task of separation. *Adolescent Psychiatry* 8:173–183.

Masterson, J., Jr. 1967. The symptomatic adolescent five years later: he didn't grow out of it. *American Journal of Psychiatry* 123:1338–1345.

Masterson, J., Jr.; Tucker, K.; and Berk, G. 1963. Psychopathology in adolescence: clinic and dynamic characteristics. *American Journal of Psychiatry* 120:351–365.

Masterson, J. Jr.; Tucker, K.; and Berk, G. 1966. The symptomatic adolescent: delineation of psychiatric syndromes. *Comprehensive Psychiatry* 7:166–174.

Masterson, J., Jr., and Washburne, A. 1966. The psychiatric significance of adolescent turmoil. *American Journal of Psychiatry* 124:1549–1554.

Meeks, J. E. 1973. Nosology in adolescent psychiatry: an enigma wrapped in a whirlwind. In J. C. Scholar, ed. *Current Issues in Adolescent Psychiatry*. New York: Brunner/Mazel.

Miller, P., and Simon W. 1980. The development of sexuality in adolescence. In J. Adelson, ed. *Handbook of Adolescent Psychology*. New York: Wiley.

Mitchell, J. R. 1980. Normality in adolescence. *Adolescent Psychiatry* 8:200–213.

Offer, D. 1967. Normal adolescents: interview strategy and selected results. *Archives of General Psychiatry* 17:285–290.

Offer, D., and Offer, J. L. 1971. Four issues in the developmental psychology of adolescents. In J. G. Howees, ed. *Modern Perspectives in Adolescent Psychiatry*. New York: Brunner/Mazel.

Offer, D.; Ostrov, E.; and Howard, K. I. 1981. *The Adolescent: A Psychological Self-Portrait*. New York: Basic.

Offer, D., and Sabshin, M. 1963. The psychiatrist and the normal adolescent. *Archives of General Psychiatry* 9:427–432.

Oldham, D. 1978. Adolescent turmoil: a myth revisited. *Adolescent Psychiatry* 6:267–279.

Peskin, H., and Livson, N. 1972. Pre- and post-pubertal personality and adult psychologic functioning. *Seminars in Psychiatry* 4:343–353.

Rutter, M.; Graham, P.; Chadwick, O.; and Yule, W. 1976. Adolescent turmoil: fact or fiction. *Journal of Child Psychology and Psychiatry and Allied Disciplines* 17:35–36.

Salzman, L. 1974. Adolescence: epoch or disease. *Adolescent Psychiatry* 3:128–139.

Shapiro, R. L. 1969. *El Adolescente y su familia*. Buenos Aires: Horme.

Spiegel, L. A. 1951. A review of contributions to a psychoanalytic theory of adolescence. *Psychoanalytic Study of the Child* 6:375–393.

Spiegel, L. A. 1958. Comments on the psychoanalytic psychology of adolescence. *Psychoanalytic Study of the Child* 13:296–308.

Spiegel, L. A. 1961. Disorder and consolidation in adolescence. *Journal of the American Psychoanalytic Association* 9:406–416.

Spitzer, R. L.; Sheehy, M.; and Endicott, J. 1977. DSM III: guiding principles. In V. M. Rakoff, H. C. Stancer, and H. B. Kedward, eds. *Psychiatric Diagnosis*. New York: Brunner/Mazel.

Stoller, R. J. 1977. Psychoanalytic diagnosis. In V. M. Rakoff, H. C. Stancer, and H. B. Kedward, eds. *Psychiatric Diagnosis*. New York: Brunner/Mazel.

Vaillant, G. 1978. The natural history of male psychological health. *American Journal of Psychiatry* 135:653–659.

Weiner, I., and del Gaudio, A. 1976. Psychopathology in adolescence. *Archives of General Psychiatry* 33:187–193.

Weiner, J. B. 1971. The generation gap: fact and fancy. *Adolescence* 6:155–166.

Weiner, J. B. 1980. Psychopathology in adolescence. In J. Adelson, ed. *Handbook of Adolescent Psychology*. New York: Wiley.

Wilson, M. R. Jr. 1971. A proposed diagnostic classification for adolescent psychiatric cases. *Adolescent Psychiatry* 1:275–295.

Wing, J. K. 1977. The limits of standardization. In V. M. Rakoff, H. C. Stancer, and H. B. Kedward, eds. *Psychiatric Diagnosis*. New York: Brunner/Mazel.

Winnicott, D. W. 1971. Adolescence: struggling through the doldrums. *Adolescent Psychiatry* 1:40–50.

PART II

PSYCHOTHERAPEUTIC ISSUES IN ADOLESCENT PSYCHIATRY

EDITORS' INTRODUCTION

The psychotherapy of adolescents requires of the therapist the highest degree of flexibility and self-awareness. Not only must he respond to the shifting developmental patterns of his patient, but he must be continuously vigilant regarding his countertransferential responses and prepared to adapt his technical approaches to the vagaries of adolescent mores. In particular, he must accommodate himself to the fact that many troubled adolescents are, at best, reluctant patients, at least at first, and that they are often enmeshed in families that lend less than optimal support to therapeutic endeavors.

Daniel Offer, Eric Ostrov, and Kenneth I. Howard report their study of emotional disturbance, juvenile delinquency, and mental health resource utilization among normal adolescents. They found that a substantial percentage were psychologically disturbed, performed delinquent acts, but had never been seen by a mental health professional or come to the attention of school authorities or other adults as needing help. Offer, Ostrov, and Howard conclude that, while only a minority of adolescents are disturbed, this represents a very large number, and at least half have not received mental health care. The authors speculate that both nonrecognition by adults and parents and the inability of adolescents to initiate and carry through help-seeking behavior explain the low level of service.

David Dean Brockman discusses psychoanalytic approaches in college students when time restraints and developmental considerations require abbreviation of the therapeutic work. He believes that these externally imposed time factors and internally imposed developmental issues need not lead to compromises in analytic procedures. He recommends that a therapist should follow standard techniques, and his experiences are that

119

a meaningful transference neurosis will develop with progress manifested by removal of symptoms, development of insight, and expansion of ego boundaries.

Frank S. Williams writes that most seriously disturbed adolescents who undertake psychotherapy suffer from developmental defects. Therapists must address these issues, and the analytic treatment of the adolescent frequently requires parenting, education, and guidance in addition to genetic reconstruction and interpretation. Adolescents have reality resistances to analysis that are not resistances to the developing transference. When the family is not providing necessary parenting, family therapy intervention may be helpful. Williams concludes that in treatment of adolescents guidance can be a pathway to insight and growth.

John L. Schimel discusses the art of interpretation—particularly during psychotherapy with adolescents. Therapy with adolescents contributes additional challenges beyond usual analytic transactions: problems in communicating with the young; the special psychodynamics of adolescence; transference-countertransference issues; confrontational experiences; and a note of playfulness reminiscent of parent-child relationships. The author emphasizes the different roles the developing adolescent is playing as well as the multiple positions the therapist assumes—the many people in the room—and warns of the introduction of premature interpretations that may have a devastating effect. Schimel concludes that, particularly with adolescents, the development of a working relationship depends on the groundwork performed using creative approaches through interpretation.

Kenneth M. Schwartz reviews the meaning of charismatic religious groups or cults to late adolescent development. He discusses clinical management of cult members who present voluntarily for treatment, particularly with regard to conflicts around leaving a group and reintegrating into society. The author concludes that some adolescents use cult membership to help deal with normal adolescent issues. Other, more seriously disturbed, use the cult as a retreat.

Loretta R. Loeb discusses the psychoanalytic treatment of an early adolescent with an obsessive-compulsive neurosis. She reviews sexual and object development and concludes that an obsessive-compulsive neurosis is formed when an individual is unable to resolve and deal with early conflicts and regresses back to using the defenses of isolation, reaction formation, and undoing.

120

7 SELF-IMAGE, DELINQUENCY, AND HELP-SEEKING BEHAVIOR AMONG NORMAL ADOLESCENTS

DANIEL OFFER, ERIC OSTROV, AND KENNETH I. HOWARD

The purpose of this chapter is to describe the extent of emotional stress perceived by adolescents, the amount of delinquency performed by them, and how many of those who have emotional problems seek and obtain mental health care in their community.

It is a commonly held notion that adolescence is, by nature, a period of emotional turmoil. Adolescents, it is held, resolve their inner problems by acting out, behaving unpredictably, rebelling against their parents, and having mood swings. Even mental health professionals who work with adolescents tend to think that normal teenagers are as disturbed and as unhappy as hospitalized, psychiatrically ill teenagers actually are (Offer, Ostrov, and Howard 1981a).

Review of the Literature

Review of the empirical literature has shown that the vast majority of adolescents are not in great turmoil, are not in a state of rebellion in their relationships with other family members, and have relatively smooth transitions from childhood to adulthood (Csikszentmihalyi and Larson 1984; Douvan and Adelson 1966; Offer and Offer 1975; Offer, Ostrov, and Howard 1981b; Westley and Epstein 1969).

The empirical literature indicates that, tested at any one point in time, approximately 20 percent of adults attest to being psychiatrically ill to a clinically significant degree (Uhlenhuth, Balter, Mellinger, Cisin, and

Clinthorne 1983). There is almost no literature bearing on the specific kinds of psychiatric illness found among disturbed teenagers in the community. Similarly, almost no literature exists bearing on the prevalence or characteristics of disturbed adolescents who do not receive treatment or are not the subject of intervention efforts.

There is some evidence, though, that a large proportion of disturbed adolescents do not come to the attention of adults as needing or requiring help. An early epidemiological study was that of Krupinski, Baikie, Stoller, Graves, O'Day, and Polke (1967), which was conducted in the small Australian town of Heyfield. On the basis of this research, it was concluded that 16 percent of the male adolescents and 19 percent of the female adolescents in the town had psychiatrically diagnosable conditions. A Scandinavian study (Bjornsson 1974) reported a prevalence rate for moderate or severe disorder of 21 percent for boys and 14 percent for girls among the thirteen- to fourteen-year-old adolescents in an industrial town.

In a series of studies by Rutter and associates (Graham and Rutter 1973; Rutter, Graham, Chadwick, and Yale 1976), data collection was based on information obtained from individual interviews of the adolescents by psychiatrists and interviews with parents and teachers of the youths studied. According to the authors, "More than a fifth of the boys and girls reported that they felt miserable or depressed, and the same proportion reported great difficulty in sleeping and waking unnecessarily early in the morning" (Rutter et al. 1976, p. 42). Using parents' interviews as the source of information about adolescents, these investigators found that the prevalence of psychiatric disorder among fourteen-year-olds was 13 percent. On the basis of interviews with the adolescents themselves, it was concluded that 16 percent could be diagnosed as having psychiatric disorders. Based on data from multiple data sources, it was concluded that "the corrected prevalence rate for psychiatric disorder in fourteen- to fifteen-year-old children is 21 percent" (Graham and Rutter 1973).

In the United States, there have been very few studies either of the prevalence of emotional disturbance among adolescents or of the kinds of disturbance shown by those adolescents who are disturbed. This fact was emphasized by Locksley and Douvan (1979), who wrote, "Although national surveys of the incidence of psychopathology among adolescents have not been conducted as yet, this may be a direction for research ultimately as profitable as those directions heretofore pursued" (p. 73).

Langner, Gersten, and Eisenberg (1974) conducted one of the few studies of the epidemiology of psychiatric illness among U.S. adolescents. This study used a questionnaire administered to mothers regarding their children's behavior. The sample studied consisted of 1,034 children aged six to eighteen years who were randomly selected from a cross section in New York. Questionnaire results were rated by a psychiatrist for degree of impairment. Results showed that 17–20 percent of the black and Spanish children showed extreme impairment rates, while only 8–9 percent of the white children did. Unfortunately, the results were not reported separately for adolescents as distinguished from children in other age groups. In the Locksley and Douvan study cited earlier, sophomores, juniors, and seniors attending a Midwestern urban, lower-middle-class high school were studied using a self-report questionnaire. Longitudinal data were obtained by readministering the questionnaire to a subsample of the sophomores during their senior year. Locksley and Douvan (1979) reported that males had a significantly higher frequency of aggression and feelings of resentment than did females, while, on the average, females reported a significantly higher frequency of feelings of tension and psychosomatic symptoms. The sexes did not differ in reported feelings of depression. Unfortunately, the data provided by Locksley and Douvan did not include an estimate of the prevalence of psychiatric disorder among the adolescents studied.

Other studies in the literature conducted in the United States have concerned the incidence of depressive symptoms among adolescents and not the incidence of psychiatric illness generally. For example, Schoenbach, Kaplan, Wagner, Grimson, and Udry (1980) report on a study based on a self-reported depressive-symptom checklist administered to 384 junior high school students. Elevated symptom scores among blacks and low-socioeconomic-status whites were cited in this study. Prevalence rates of depression were not reported, but the authors state that, compared to adults studied with the same instruments, adolescents showed similar symptom "persistence," that is, they reported that they felt symptoms of depression most or all of the time during the preceding week at the same rate as did adults. Studying small samples of seventh and eighth graders from one parochial school in suburban Philadelphia and using the Beck Depression Inventory as a source of data, Albert and Beck (1975) concluded that 33.3 percent of their early adolescent sample fell into the moderate-to-severe depressive symptomatology range while only 2.2 percent fell into the severe range.

Kandel and Davies (1982) studied the epidemiology of depression among adolescents. They studied adolescents, fourteen to eighteen years

123

of age, representative of public high school students in New York State in 1971 through 1972. They found that adolescents from families with very low incomes were more depressed than were those from any other social economic status group. Girls were more depressed than were boys. The one prevalence rate cited in this study was that 20 percent of the adolescents reported "feeling sad or depressed in the past year."

Concerning the issue of what proportion of psychiatrically ill youths seek or obtain professional help, a review of the literature revealed only two studies relevant to help-seeking behavior among adolescents. One study (Leslie 1974) was conducted in Britain. It concluded that "the parents of 24 out of the 67 children with psychiatric disorder (or 36 percent) had not sought advice at any time; some did not perceive abnormality, but others did not know of anyone who would help with such problems" (Leslie 1974, p. 118). The other study, Kellam, Branch, Brown, and Russell (1981), presents even more dramatic results. According to these authors, an adolescent's acceptance of an offer of help through counseling was associated not with how disturbed the adolescent was but with the characteristics of the persons offering the help. The implication seems to be that many adolescents in need of help probably do not receive it, particularly when it is left up to them to initiate and carry through on help-seeking behavior.

The 1983 Epidemiological Study

The authors carried out this study, conducted in the Chicago area, to learn more about emotional disturbance, juvenile delinquency, and mental health resource utilization among adolescents. General findings are that about 20 percent of the adolescents studied were psychologically disturbed and/or performed delinquent acts. Many of these disturbed adolescents had neither ever been seen by a mental health professional nor come to the attention of school authorities or other adults as needing help.

SUBJECTS

As a first step in our study, the cooperation of the trustees of a Chicago suburban township was obtained to collect data from township adolescents. Students in the township high schools were studied. We randomly selected every fourteenth student in the entire high school. Since the school had a student body of 4,530, a list of 324 students was obtained. Among four cells—male freshmen/sophomores, male juniors/seniors, female freshmen/sophomores, and female juniors/seniors—the smallest was identified. This cell contained sixty-five students. Sixty-five students were then randomly drawn from each of the other cells, yielding a total of 260 students to be studied.

For these teenagers, questionnaires were mailed to their homes with a request that the teenagers fill them out and return them to the investigators. As an incentive for the teenagers to do so, those who cooperated with this research were promised (and given) a five-dollar gift certificate to be used for purchase of a record at a local store. Adolescents not responding to the mailed questionnaires were called by the investigators as a way of encouraging participation. To achieve a higher percentage of returns, the investigators hired a research assistant to go to the teenagers' homes to encourage them to fill out the questionnaires. As a result of these efforts, 87 percent of those students sampled from this suburban high school who were still resident in the areas when the research was being conducted completed the study.

Responses obtained from these students constitute the core of the data that were collected. To make the data base demographically more diverse, data were also collected from two Roman Catholic parochial high schools located in Chicago. One of these high schools is all male, all black, and located in a lower-class to lower-middle-class neighborhood in Chicago; the other parochial high school is almost entirely white, enrolls only girls, and is located in a lower-middle-class to upper-middle-class neighborhood in Chicago. In contrast, students from the suburban high school are almost all white, attend a coeducational school, and come from an upper-middle to lower-upper-class neighborhood in a Chicago suburb. In the parochial high schools, only juniors were studied because limited resources did not allow wider data collection. Juniors were chosen because follow-up after a year would be easier to obtain than it would be with seniors; conversely, it was thought their self-image would be more stable than that of freshmen or sophomores. Data were obtained from all present in school on the day of the testing.

INSTRUMENTS

Instruments given to the adolescents studied comprised the Offer Self-Image Questionnaire (OSIQ) (Offer et al. 1981b), the Delinquency

Check List (DCL) (Short and Nye 1957), a survey of mental health services utilized, and open-ended questions regarding problems and unmet needs for mental health services. A fact sheet requesting demographic data, including parents' marital status, also was included. Questionnaires were given anonymously, but the adolescents surveyed could write their names, addresses, and telephone numbers in a space provided for that purpose if they were willing to participate in future research.

OFFER SELF-IMAGE QUESTIONNAIRE (OSIQ)

The OSIQ contains 130 items that cover adjustment in eleven areas important to the psychological life of the adolescent. Adjustment in each area is measured by a scale score; the eleven scale scores, in turn, are clustered into five psychological selves. The different selves and corresponding scale scores are:

Psychological self—impulse control
Psychological self—mood
Psychological self—body image
Social self—social relations
Social self—morals
Social self—vocational and educational goals
Sexual self—sexual attitudes and behavior
Familial self—family relations
Coping self—mastery of the external world
Coping self—psychopathology
Coping self—superior adjustment (coping)

Scores for each scale are expressed as standard scores. In this metric, a score of 50 represents functioning in a given area equal to the mean of a like-age, same-sex, nationwide normative group. The standard scores are adjusted so that the standard deviation of the norming group is 15. In this metric, too, a higher score represents better adjustment in a particular area. OSIQ scale scores are internally consistent and moderately stable (Offer et al. 1981b). This questionnaire's value as a measure of adolescents' self-image and adjustment has been demonstrated in many studies (Offer, Ostrov, and Howard 1984).

In the data analysis, OSIQ data were scored using the standard-score format. As a result, OSIQ standard scores describing functioning in eleven areas relevant to adolescents were obtained for teenagers from

126

each community. These OSIQ scores were then used as a criterion of disturbance: if a student scored one standard deviation or more below the mean (a score of thirty-five or less in standard-score terms) on three or more OSIQ scales, that student was considered disturbed.

DELINQUENCY CHECK LIST (DCL)

The DCL is a self-report delinquency inventory based on the work of Short and Nye (1957). Short and Nye wrote items covering a wide range of delinquent behavior; items were responded to on a five-point scale ranging from "never" to "very often." In the DCL, all the Short and Nye items were retained except that the list of drug use items was expanded to reflect modern usage, for example, using cocaine. When Short and Nye factor-analyzed their instrument, they obtained four factors: rule-breaking behavior, defiance of parents, drug use, and assaultive behavior. With the exception of assaultive behavior, we retained these factors, placing new items into the appropriate factor. Factor scores are expressed as average responses to items in that factor. Consequently, the higher the factor score, the more the reported delinquency with respect to that factor. We have found this test to be helpful in our previous study of juvenile delinquents (Offer, Marohn, and Ostrov 1979). In this paper, an adolescent was considered "delinquent" if he or she attested to having been either apprehended by the police for any offense, put on suspension by a court, or held in a juvenile detention center or other correctional facility. A delinquent was also defined as an adolescent who had engaged in a pattern of serious delinquent offenses.

Results

SELF-IMAGE AND DELINQUENCY

Table 1 shows the percentage of disturbed and delinquent male and disturbed and delinquent female adolescents in the three communities combined.

The OSIQ scale score means for boys and girls from the three communities studied are well within the range of the normal. These results imply that the teenagers tested in this study and those tested as part of the national norming group (Offer et al. 1981b) were, on the average, very similar in self-image.

In order to better understand the relationship between self-image and

127

TABLE 1

PERCENTAGE OF MALE AND FEMALE ADOLESCENTS IN
THREE CHICAGO COMMUNITY HIGH SCHOOLS WHO
WERE DISTURBED AND DELINQUENT

	% Disturbed	% Delinquent
Male ($N = 156$)................	17	36
Female ($N = 170$)..............	21	27

NOTE.—Disturbed is defined in terms of an adolescent's being one standard deviation or more lower than the norming group average on three or more of eleven Offer Self-Image Questionnaire (OSIQ) scales. All other adolescents were considered normal. Delinquent is defined as someone who has been either apprehended by the police for any offense, put on suspension by a court, or held in a juvenile detention center or other correctional facility. A delinquent is also defined as an adolescent who has engaged in a pattern of serious delinquent offenses. (The numbers of subjects differ slightly among the tables because of problems with missing data.)

delinquency, we correlated the three main factors of the DCL test with the eleven scales of the OSIQ. The delinquency factors used in this chapter are: rule-breaking behavior, drug use, and defiance of parents. The factors and the items can be found in Appendix A.

As can be seen from the results, the general findings are that the more delinquent the adolescent, the poorer his or her self-image. Gender stands out in the sense that girls act out more in sexual terms and boys act out more with respect to issues that have to do with rules and regulations. Specifically, in table 2 we see that adolescents who are more rule breaking tend to have familial problems and a poor sense of what they want to do.

Rule-breaking males have very deviant self-images but feel that they have the support of their peers. Both male and female rule-breaking adolescents tend to have quite liberal sexual attitudes.

As table 3 shows, among the adolescents who use drugs, both males and females have a low sense of direction and low ethical standards. Female drug users are very liberal sexually. They attest to relatively good peer relationships. Male drug users acknowledge having poor impulse control. They also attest to poorer family relations, poorer general adjustment, and more overt psychopathology than do non–drug users. Adolescents who have familial problems have by far the poorer psychological selves (see table 4). We are saying neither that poor family relationships cause the latter nor that the reverse (i.e., poor psychological self as a cause of poor family relations) is the case. What we have found is that the relationship between these two factors is very strong. To put it differently, a good relationship with one's parents makes one feel better

TABLE 2
OFFER SELF-IMAGE QUESTIONNAIRE (OSIQ)
SCALE CORRELATES OF DELINQUENCY:
RULE-BREAKING BEHAVIOR

	Teenage Boys (N = 166)	Teenage Girls (N = 130)
Psychological self (PS):		
PS-1 Impulse control	−.21*	−.12
PS-2 Emotional tone	−.06	−.03
PS-3 Body and self-image	−.14*	−.04
Social Self (SS):		
SS-1 Social relationships	.13*	.11
SS-2 Morals	−.23*	−.20*
SS-3 Vocational-educational goals	−.21*	−.21*
Sexual self—Sexual attitudes	.25*	.43*
Familial self—Family relationships	−.30*	−.17*
Coping Self (CS):		
CS-1 Mastery of the external world	−.15*	.05
CS-2 Psychopathology	−.17*	.05
CS-3 Superior adjustment	−.18*	.06

*P < .05.

TABLE 3
OFFER SELF-IMAGE QUESTIONNAIRE (OSIQ)
SCALE CORRELATES OF DELINQUENCY:
DRUG USE

	Teenage Boys (N = 166)	Teenage Girls (N = 130)
Psychological self (PS):		
PS-1 Impulse control	−.21*	−.12
PS-2 Emotional tone	−.09	.05
PS-3 Body and self-image	−.09	−.01
Social self (SS):		
SS-1 Social relationships	.12	.19*
SS-2 Morals	−.20*	−.24*
SS-3 Vocational-educational goals	−.18*	−.19*
Sexual self—Sexual attitudes	.09	.33*
Familial Self—Family relationships	−.27*	−.07
Coping self (CS):		
CS-1 Mastery of the external world	−.12	−.04
CS-2 Psychopathology	−.19*	.08
CS-3 Superior adjustment	−.18*	−.06

*P < .05.

TABLE 4
OFFER SELF-IMAGE QUESTIONNAIRE (OSIQ)
SCALE CORRELATES OF DELINQUENCY:
DEFIANCE OF PARENTS

	Teenage Boys ($N = 167$)	Teenage Girls ($N = 128$)
Psychological Self (PS):		
PS-1 Impulse control	$-.23*$	$-.20*$
PS-2 Emotional tone	$-.20*$	$-.15*$
PS-3 Body and self-image	$-.19*$	$-.18*$
Social self (SS):		
SS-1 Social relationships	$-.17*$	$.01$
SS-2 Morals	$-.07$	$-.13$
SS-3 Vocational-educational goals.............	$-.16*$	$-.06$
Sexual self—Sexual attitudes	$.03$	$.28*$
Familial Self—Family relationships	$-.40*$	$-.34*$
Coping Self (CS):		
CS-1 Mastery of the external world	$-.17*$	$-.08$
CS-2 Psychopathology	$-.19*$	$-.09$
CS-3 Superior adjustment	$-.19*$	$-.03$

$*P < .05.$

TABLE 5
PERCENTAGE OF MIDWEST SUBURBAN HIGH SCHOOL
NONDELINQUENT VERSUS DELINQUENT ADOLESCENTS
USING MENTAL HEALTH PROFESSIONALS

	% Nondelinquent ($N = 160$)	% Delinquent ($N = 59$)
Consulted mental health professionals more than once	13	27
Consulted mental health professionals excluding school counselor one time	22	20
Never consulted a mental health professional	65	53

TABLE 6
PERCENTAGE OF MIDWEST SUBURBAN HIGH SCHOOL
NONDISTURBED VERSUS DISTURBED ADOLESCENTS
USING MENTAL HEALTH PROFESSIONALS

	% Nondisturbed ($N = 167$)	% Disturbed ($N = 32$)
Consulted mental health professionals more than once........................	12	25
Consulted mental health professionals excluding school counselor one time	25	22
Never consulted a mental health professional..	63	53

about one's psychological self. The adolescent males who have problems with their families have poor peer relationships and poor coping abilities. The adolescent females who score high in this regard have liberal sexual attitudes.

MENTAL HEALTH UTILIZATION

In the suburban high school sample, specific data exist concerning the adolescents' mental health care utilization. Data presented in tables 5 and 6 show that although more delinquent and disturbed adolescents than normal adolescents used mental health care, a significant number of disturbed adolescents did not ever consult a mental health professional.

Figures 1 through 6 show that disturbed adolescents can be distinguished on the basis of how they utilize mental health services. In comparison to the normals (standard score of 50), they are considerably disturbed. Those adolescents (males and females) who see a mental health professional only once have a more disturbed self-image than do those who are in psychotherapy. The latter group seems to show areas in which they have improved. In comparison, those adolescents who never consulted a mental health professional are consistently below the norm. There are no areas in which they are similar to the normative group.

Discussion

As has been true whenever research has been conducted with representative groups of adolescents, these results also show that the vast majority of adolescents studied are happy and well adjusted. Consistent with the results of previous epidemiological studies, data gathered here indicate that about 20 percent of the adolescents studied are emotionally disturbed to a meaningful degree. Largely unknown until now has been the percentage of disturbed adolescents who do not manifest this disturbance either through antisocial behavior sufficient to warrant their being apprehended by the police more than once or through being seen by a mental health professional more than once. The data suggest that about one-third of boys and two-thirds of girls who are disturbed have not either received help or come to the attention of authorities. In the suburban high school, more than half of the disturbed or delinquent adolescents had never seen any mental health professional. It is of interest to note that if the OSIQs of teenagers identified as disturbed in these samples are compared with the OSIQs of youths who are hospital-

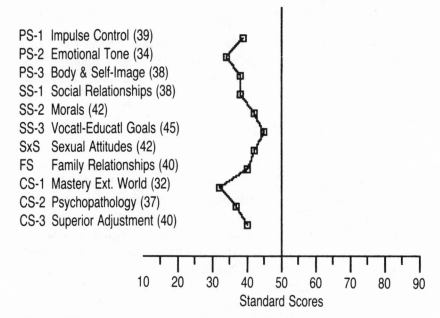

FIG. 1. Offer Self-Image Questionnaire standard score profile for twenty-three twelve- to nineteen-year-old disturbed female adolescents who had never used mental health services. Numbers in parentheses are standard score values for each scale. PS = psychological self; SS = social self; SxS = sexual self; FS = familial self; and CS = coping self.

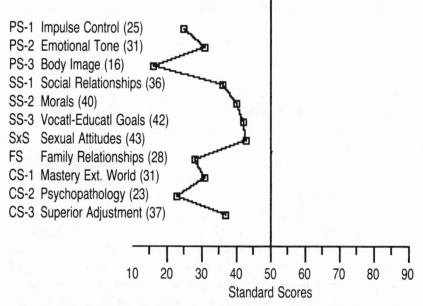

FIG. 2.—Offer Self-Image Questionnaire standard score profile for six twelve- to nineteen-year-old disturbed male adolescents who had used mental health services once. Numbers in parentheses and abbreviations are as in fig. 1.

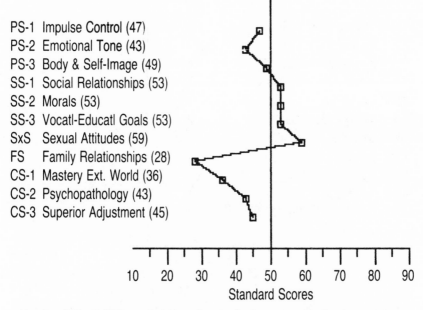

PS-1 Impulse Control (47)
PS-2 Emotional Tone (43)
PS-3 Body & Self-Image (49)
SS-1 Social Relationships (53)
SS-2 Morals (53)
SS-3 Vocatl-Educatl Goals (53)
SxS   Sexual Attitudes (59)
FS   Family Relationships (28)
CS-1 Mastery Ext. World (36)
CS-2 Psychopathology (43)
CS-3 Superior Adjustment (45)

Standard Scores

FIG. 3.—Offer Self-Image Questionnaire standard score profile for three twelve- to nineteen-year-old disturbed male adolescents who had used mental health services more than once. Numbers in parentheses and abbreviations are as in fig. 1.

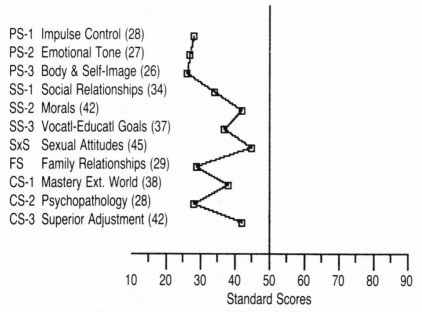

PS-1 Impulse Control (28)
PS-2 Emotional Tone (27)
PS-3 Body & Self-Image (26)
SS-1 Social Relationships (34)
SS-2 Morals (42)
SS-3 Vocatl-Educatl Goals (37)
SxS   Sexual Attitudes (45)
FS   Family Relationships (29)
CS-1 Mastery Ext. World (38)
CS-2 Psychopathology (28)
CS-3 Superior Adjustment (42)

Standard Scores

FIG. 4.—Offer Self-Image Questionnaire standard score profile for six twelve- to nineteen-year-old disturbed female adolescents who had used mental health services once. Numbers in parentheses and abbreviations are as in fig. 1.

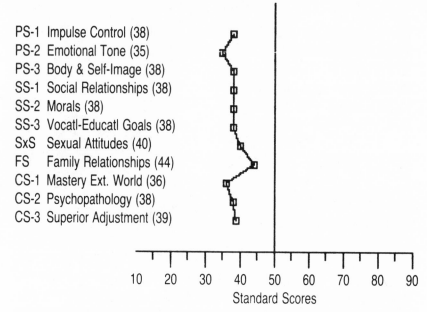

PS-1 Impulse Control (38)
PS-2 Emotional Tone (35)
PS-3 Body & Self-Image (38)
SS-1 Social Relationships (38)
SS-2 Morals (38)
SS-3 Vocatl-Educatl Goals (38)
SxS Sexual Attitudes (40)
FS Family Relationships (44)
CS-1 Mastery Ext. World (36)
CS-2 Psychopathology (38)
CS-3 Superior Adjustment (39)

Standard Scores

FIG. 5.—Offer Self-Image Questionnaire standard score profile for sixteen twelve- to nineteen-year-old disturbed male adolescents who had never used mental health services. Numbers in parentheses and abbreviations are as in fig. 1.

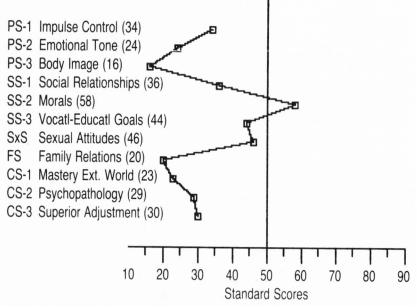

PS-1 Impulse Control (34)
PS-2 Emotional Tone (24)
PS-3 Body Image (16)
SS-1 Social Relationships (36)
SS-2 Morals (58)
SS-3 Vocatl-Educatl Goals (44)
SxS Sexual Attitudes (46)
FS Family Relations (20)
CS-1 Mastery Ext. World (23)
CS-2 Psychopathology (29)
CS-3 Superior Adjustment (30)

Standard Scores

FIG. 6.—Offer Self-Image Questionnaire standard score profile for six twelve- to nineteen-year-old disturbed female adolescents who had used mental health services more than once. Numbers in parentheses and abbreviations are as in fig. 1.

ized for psychiatric illness (see Koenig, Howard, Offer, and Cremerius 1984), it turns out that the profiles are very similar. This fact suggests that youths identified as disturbed in these samples are notably ill, even though almost none has been treated on an inpatient basis and even though many, particularly the girls, have not received any sustained professional help.

Among the boys in this sample who were identified as disturbed, those who are disturbed without acting out have relatively good impulse control and family relationships. But these disturbed boys have poor emotional tone, body image, and social relationships. Disturbed girls had very poor family relationships. For both adolescent boys and adolescent girls, it seems as if good family relations serve as an emotional inoculator that can ward off emotional stress that comes their way in their years of growing up to adulthood. Delinquents belong to many different subgroups. Our data have shown that adolescents with different problems relate differentially to their peers. Some cope fairly well with their emotional world, while others do not.

Conclusions

This study indicates that only a minority of adolescents are disturbed in the sense of feeling badly about themselves in a number of areas. Viewed nationally, though, that minority represents a very large number of teenagers. At this time, in the United States, there are approximately 18 million adolescents in high school. If 20 percent of those adolescents are disturbed, the implication is that nearly 3.6 million may require some kind of help or intervention. Our results suggest that of those 3.6 million, approximately 50 percent, or 1.8 million, have either not received any mental health care or have not been so overtly disturbed as to attract attention.

In the final paragraph of this chapter, we would like to focus on the help-seeking behavior of adolescents. It is incumbent on us to determine why so many disturbed adolescents do not seek or receive mental health care. Our next project is aimed at finding out what the attitudes of adolescents and their parents are toward the mental health professional. Only then can we improve the care that they receive.

NOTE

This work was supported in part by the Adolescent Research Fund: In Memory of Judith Offer.

Shioamay L. Young, David Parrella, and Tracy Thornberg have helped in the data processing and analysis.

REFERENCES

Albert, N., and Beck, A. T. 1975. Incidence of depression in early adolescence: a preliminary study. *Journal of Youth and Adolescence* 4:301–307.

Bjornsson, S. 1974. Epidemiological investigation of mental disorders of children in Reykjavik, Iceland. *Scandinavian Journal of Psychology* 15:244–254.

Csikszentmihalyi, M., and Larson, R. 1984. *Being Adolescent: Conflict and Turmoil in the Teenage Years.* New York: Basic.

Douvan, E., and Adelson, J. 1966. *The Adolescent Experience.* New York: Wiley.

Graham, P., and Rutter, M. 1973. Psychiatric disorder in the young adolescent: a follow-up study. *Proceedings of the Royal Society of Medicine* 66:58–61.

Kandel, D. B., and Davies, M. 1982. Epidemiology of depressive mood in adolescents. *Archives of General Psychiatry* 39:1205–1212.

Kellam, S. G.; Branch, J. D.; Brown, C. H.; and Russell, G. F. M. 1981. Why teenagers come for treatment: a ten-year prospective epidemiological study in Woodlawn. *Journal of the American Academy of Child Psychiatry* 20:477–495.

Koenig, L.; Howard, K. I.; Offer, D.; and Cremerius, M. 1984. Psychopathology and adolescent self-image. In D. Offer, E. Ostrov, and K. I. Howard, eds. *Patterns of Adolescent Self-Image: New Directions for Mental Health Services.* San Francisco: Jossey-Bass.

Krupinski, J.; Baikie, A. G.; Stoller, A.; Graves, J.; O'Day, D. M.; and Polke, P. 1967. A community health survey of Heyfield, Victoria. *The Medical Journal of Australia* 54:1204–1211.

Langner, T. S.; Gersten, J. C.; and Eisenberg, J. G. 1974. Approaches to measurement and definition in epidemiology of behavior disorders: ethnic background and child behavior. *International Journal of Health Services* 4:483–501.

Leslie, S. A. 1974. Psychiatric disorder in the young adolescents of an industrial town. *British Journal of Psychiatry* 125:113–124.

Locksley, A., and Douvan, E. 1979. Problem behavior in adolescents. In E. Gombera and V. Frank, eds. *Gender and Disordered Behavior.* New York: Brunner/Mazel.

Offer, D.; Marohn, R. C.; and Ostrov, E. 1979. *The Psychological World of the Juvenile Delinquent.* New York: Basic.

Offer, D., and Offer, J. B. 1975. *From Teenage to Young Manhood: A Psychological Study.* New York: Basic.

Offer, D.; Ostrov, E.; and Howard, K. I. 1981a. The mental health professional's concept of the normal adolescent. *Archives of General Psychiatry* 38:149–152.

Offer, D.; Ostrov., E.; and Howard, K. I. 1981b. *The Adolescent: A Psychological Self-Portrait.* New York: Basic.

Offer, D.; Ostrov, E.; and Howard, K. I., eds. 1984. *Patterns of Adolescent Self-Image: New Directions for Mental Health Services.* San Francisco: Jossey-Bass.

Rutter, M.; Graham, P.; Chadwick, D. F. D.; and Yale, W. 1976. Adolescent turmoil: fact or fiction. *Journal of Child Psychology and Psychiatry* 17:35–56.

Schoenbach, V. J.; Kaplan, B. H.; Wagner, B. H.; Grimson, R. C.; and Udry, J. R. 1980. Depressive symptoms in young adolescents. *Society for Epidemiologic Research Abstracts* 112:440.

Short, J. F., Jr., and Nye, F. I. 1957. Reported behavior as a criterion of deviant behavior. *Social Problems* 5:207–213.

Uhlenhuth, E. H.; Balter, M. B.; Mellinger, G. D.; Cisin, I. H.; and Clinthorne, J. 1983. Symptom checklist syndromes in the general population: correlations with psychotherapeutic drug use. *Archives of General Psychiatry* 40:1167–1173.

Westley, W. A., and Epstein, N. B. 1969. *The Silent Majority.* San Francisco: Jossey-Bass.

Appendix A: The Three Delinquency Check List (DCL) Factors and Their Items

RULE-BREAKING BEHAVIOR

Came to school late in the mornings.
Skipped school without a legitimate excuse.
Took part in a "gang fight."
Obtained liquor by having older friends buy it for you.
Bought or drank beer, wine, or liquor (include drinking at home).
Carried a switchblade or other weapon.
Used alcohol excessively.
Drank so much that you could not remember afterward some of the things you had done.
Went for a ride in a car you or someone else had taken without permission.
Had sexual intercourse with a person of the opposite sex.

DRUG USE

Smoked marijuana.
Sold drugs.
Used psychedelics (e.g., mescaline, PCP, LSD).
Used downers (e.g., barbiturates).
Used speed (e.g., amphetamines, cocaine).
Used inhalants or sniffed glue.
Used heroin.

DEFIANCE OF PARENTS

Went against your parents' wishes.
Defied your parents' authority (to their face).
Shouted at your mother or father.
Cursed at your mother or father.
Struck your mother or father.

8 FOCAL ANALYSIS OF A COLLEGE FRESHMAN

DAVID DEAN BROCKMAN

Analysis of college students as described here is a limited technical modification of usual psychoanalytic practice and can be invoked when time constraints and developmental considerations, such as realistic moves toward autonomy, require abbreviation of the therapeutic work. My thesis is that, in spite of these limiting factors, creditable psychoanalytic work can be done in selected cases. These externally imposed time factors and internally imposed developmental issues need not lead to unnecessary shortcuts, manipulation of the transferences, changes in the frequency of sessions, forcing preconceived notions about a nuclear conflict onto the patient, or attempting to produce a corrective emotional experience by acting in a contrived manner opposite to the pathogenic parental figures. In short, one need only follow standard technique in introducing the analytic process by means of interpretation of the initial transferences to produce a therapeutic alliance and interpreting, in the usual manner, subsequently appearing resistances and transferences. Dreams are used to facilitate the deepening of the analytic process and to elucidate the neurotic conflicts as they emerge in the transference. If this procedure is followed, a transference neurosis can be observed to develop.

There are obvious defects in this proposal, because all of the transferences cannot be dealt with in enough depth or with the thoroughness ordinarily accorded the working-through process, nor should they necessarily be, at this time. However, I will illustrate my thesis with data from a case from my clinical practice and then discuss some possible objections that might be raised.

Reprinted from D. D. Brockman. *Late Adolescence: Psychoanalytic Studies*.

The term "sector analysis" was introduced into the literature by Felix Deutsch (1949), who proposed a psychodynamic psychotherapy based on the associative anamnesis. The aim of his approach was to direct the patient's attention to a certain area and to link the presenting symptoms and complaints with underlying conflicts emanating from the patient's past experience. Therapeutic technique involved a persistent confrontational type of intervention designed to break up old associational chains and replace them with new ones using cue words or phrases taken from the patient's language. He used such terms as "the little one" (the person in the past) and "the big one" (the observing person in the present) who "becomes the observer together with the interviewer, who confronts the patient continually with the behavior of the 'little one' in the 'big one.'" Deutsch's aim was a "goal limited adjustment therapy" that in general terms was to "create the most favorable psychological conditions for the ego functioning." But, noble as that sounds, it still seems to me he was forcing something onto the patient. He admitted his technique was an active one, and, to his credit, it might well have special application with certain psychosomatic disorders. I am not using the term sector analysis here, although a more descriptive term might be "limited psychoanalytic therapy," but I wanted to convey a different meaning than brief psychotherapy. The patient's needs for help and growth were here calculatedly related. Instead of postponing major decisions until treatment had ended, the patient ended treatment to get on with his need for growth, development, and education as part of his normative late adolescent needs.

Many of the modern proponents of brief psychoanalytic psychotherapy, such as Balint, Ornstein, and Balint (1972), Davanloo (1980), Malan (1976), Mann (1973), Sifneos (1972, 1979, 1981), Socarides (1954), and Wolberg (1965), derive their research from the experiments of Alexander and French (1946) and Ferenczi (1920), as well as from Freud's work with late adolescent patients. This work was first reported with Breuer in *Studies on Hysteria* (Breuer and Freud 1893–1895) as the cases of Katharina, Elisabeth von R., and Rosalia, and then, independently, that of Dora (Freud 1905a). These modern writers emphasize strict selection criteria and the singling out of a focus or central conflict, usually oedipal, active and deep interpretation of the early transference reactions, and finally the linking up of these transferences with past and present in a "triangle of insight" (Menninger 1958). Of necessity, brief therapy is goal and time limited. As a matter of fact, Fenichel (1954) called it "the child of bitter necessity" (p. 243). In the 1960s and 1970s, clinic personnel were overtaxed by too many patients, and waiting lists grew so long that the patient population was underserved (Mann 1973). In the 1980s, necessity has taken the form of budget cuts and the consequent need to keep costs down. But whatever the reasons—numbers or economics—there has been a great deal of experimentation with the psychotherapeutic process: such a variety, in fact, that Mandel (1981) has annotated a bibliography on brief psychotherapy containing a total of 1,500 publications written by 1,000 workers in the field between 1920 and 1980. Of these, only fifty-two relate specifically to college youth. Various techniques for accomplishing the therapeutic aims of brief therapy are used, but some common denominators among them are manipulation of the frequency of interviews, active and early interpretations of transference, pedagogical tactics, anxiety-suppressing measures, and setting a limit on the length of treatment.

Frances and Perry (1983) recently identified three groups of researchers in the field of brief therapy, classifying them according to the point at which transference interpretations are recommended. The three groups are the conservatives, the radicals, and the skeptics. The conservatives (Berliner 1941; Deutsch 1949; Pumpian-Mindlin 1953) believe that, while transference interpretations are central to the psychoanalysis, they are inappropriate in brief psychotherapy. The radicals (Davanloo 1980; Malan 1976; Mann 1973; Sifneos 1972, 1979, 1981) advocate the use of transference interpretations actively early and, so it appears, quite forcibly, in an almost procrustean manner. The skeptics, Frank (1971) and Strupp (1975), regard transference interpretations as superfluous; in their opinion, the effective agent in brief therapy is nonspecific and interpersonal, that is, due to the relationship alone.

Frances and Perry (1983) follow standard technical criteria for the use of transference interpretations (p. 407): "1) Transference feelings have become the point of urgency and/or major resistance; 2) transference distortions have disrupted the therapeutic alliance and interpretations are necessary to strengthen the alliance; 3) conflicts revealed in the transference directly reflect conflicts responsible for the presenting problems or maladaptive character traits; 4) the patient has the psychological-mindedness to observe, understand, tolerate, and apply transference interpretations; and/or 5) the length of the remaining treatment will allow sufficient exploration of whatever transferences are made."

There are suitable cases among the college population for which the standard technique is the treatment of choice, using the basic principles of interpreting transferences and resistances and of permitting the transference neurosis to unfold without undue activity by the therapist (see also Basch 1980; Gedo and Goldberg 1973). According to Adatto (1980), the analysis of late adolescence is made difficult because the quality of the transference neurosis is "attenuated" or "sporadic" as compared with the experience with adults. The reason for this frequent failure to fully develop a consistent transference neurosis, he states, is that the as yet unconsolidated personality of the late adolescent is vulnerable to the threat of regression inherent in the psychoanalytic technique and process. In the case history to follow, I did not encounter this difficulty, as there was already a beginning consolidation of an adult personality. The patient, moreover, was highly motivated, receptive to self-exploration, and with an intact ego composed of a well-developed self-observing function. He enjoyed his parents' positive support, and he had been provided with a rich intellectual and cultural environment. He was a person with high intellectual capacities and verbal facility. Our personalities meshed in a positive way. I was able to create in the analytic situation an appropriately benign "container" which, together with therapeutic interventions, became linked with the natural strivings toward health inherent in this young man's personality. The treatment was successful in that he was restored to a high level of emotional and intellectual functioning, even though he interrupted the therapy to return to college at the end of six months of treatment.

Though psychoanalysis confined to a brief time span is a modification of usual practice, it was indicated in this case by the constraints imposed by the requirement of continuing the patient's college education (Isay 1980). It is important to keep in mind that only certain specially qualified persons have the psychological capacities to benefit from such abbreviated or focal analytic experiences.

Case History

Jeff was a high-achieving eighteen-year-old college freshman at a prestigious West Coast university. Even though he was not in academic trouble, he was unable to work at his usual high level and was struggling to keep his mental equilibrium. His increasingly frequent use of drugs, particularly hallucinogens, compounded the regressive process of a latent neurosis. The regressive swings he experienced were characterized by

142

excessive sleeping, fears about his sexual identity, a depression bordering on despair, and panic levels of anxiety. Above all, he did not know what was happening, nor could he stem the progressive and enveloping tide of these acute symptoms. It was in this state of acute distress that he returned home to seek consultation.

A casual observer would have been shocked by his physical appearance. He looked like a wild man. His thick, curly black hair stood out in all directions, and his face was obscured by an equally bushy beard. But I was reassured by his eyes, which sparkled with warmth and sincerity. Furthermore, he was clean and neat, and he gave a coherent, organized, and concise account of his recent experiences at school. In other words, his bizarre appearance was a superficial manifestation of a variety of underlying motivations, among which was an obscuration of his genuine interest in and high motivation for treatment as well as his exhibitionistic self-assertiveness.

Reluctantly, he had resumed the second semester only to discover that he was overwhelmed with inner turmoil. All excitement and joy had gone out of his personal life and academic pursuits. In the diagnostic interviews he reported a pair of dreams, the first of which was about carefree fun and games and innocence, while the other dealt with ancient Rome, Roman soldiers, and castrated slaves. He felt directionless, in contrast with his brilliant high school record of high grades, tutoring disadvantaged children and other social service projects, and popularity with his classmates. He realized soon after arriving at college that he was not the only student with an outstanding record and the promise of a brilliant career. What distressed him the most, though, was that he could not carry on an intelligent conversation with his father or senior persons. Invariably, he capitulated to his father's point of view early on in their discussions, which usually ended by his retreating to his room. There, as he seethed inside, he would be reduced to angry and frustrated tears. He had fantasies of demolishing his father's argument point by point that escalated to fantasies of physically beating up his father. He had discovered he could get some relief from anxiety by self-administered hallucinogenic drugs, specifically LSD and mescaline, eventually escaping into a stupor. Another solution was to accumulate as many sexual conquests as possible. During his first semester, he had engaged in long, intensely stimulating discussions on a wide variety of topics with his roommates, friends, and instructors. He was excited by the exchange of new ideas, but he became frightened by thoughts that he was certainly homosexual because he found these new relationships stirring and stimulating. Even though he had never acted on these friendly impulses in terms of overt homosexual behavior, his fears grew in intensity.

In response to his question about employment, I said that anything he could do on his own to help stabilize himself would be helpful and constructive. We were able to arrange an analytic appointment schedule that was mutually satisfactory. Thus we began.

In the first hour he reported a dream with triadic and primal scene meaning. He and some other friends watched while a male friend made out with a girlfriend. He became so angry he threw everyone out of his house except a second girl. He associated to feeling guilty about his actual relationship with the latter girl. In the second session he recalled an event from kindergarten days. He had bitten another boy in a tussle to get the boy's pineapple juice. When he skipped fourth grade, the bigger boys on the playground unexpectedly accepted him as one of them instead of picking on him because they liked his aggressive, bullying behavior. He tried very hard to be first and best in everything, including his schoolwork. He associated that now he really wanted to be liked by others and not be intimidating, as he remembered himself in grade school and as he perceived his father. I commented that he must be wondering if I would like him in spite of his antisocial behavior. He reported a small victory over his father in an argument about his clothes and style of dressing.

In the following session he reported a dream about a vicious argument with his father, who was making fun of him, calling him a fag, and mimicking him with a lisp. The patient threw a rock that smashed a vase behind father's head. Again he escaped to his room, but he felt better that he had at least got in touch with his rage in the dream. I commented that I could understand his worry about always taking flight from arguments and that he must be wondering whether the same conflict would turn up in the relationship with me.

The next dream was about feeling trapped in a forest surrounded by poisonous snakes (see Discussion); this reminded him of a recurrent nightmare from age three or four in which snakes covered the landscape. There was no place to step that was free of snakes. He was paralyzed with fear, but at the same time he was fascinated by them.

When his father insisted on talking with him about what was going on with him, and his parents requested a report from me, he became fearful of being found out and grew mistrustful of me. He felt like a sitting duck, helpless and angry. I commented that he was appealing to me for protection and understanding. In response, he described how lonely and unsupported he had felt, and he spoke again of his confusion about his sexual identity.

In the beginning phase of the therapy there was an idealized father transference. He saw his parents as such modern liberals that he could not figure out what they stood for; they were so permissive they let him do whatever he wanted. Only when he grew an outrageous Afro and bushy beard, used illegal drugs, and engaged in some public demonstrations was he able to provoke some kind of limit setting from them. In those rare instances, he was surprised that they cared enough to insist on certain canons of behavior. On the other hand, he generally shied away from confrontations with his parents over these or other issues. He reported that his brother's solution to the generational conflict was to avoid confrontations. He had fantasies of arguments with a girlfriend's parents about sleeping with her, and he tentatively argued with his father about students' occupying college administration buildings. As his neurotic regression worsened, new symptoms appeared—guilt about his sexual behavior, premature ejaculation, and, as if to confirm his need for punishment, a dream of being hit by a poisoned dart.

When his father offered a brief trip to London and Paris for the two of them, his first reaction was fear that he was being bribed into submission. When he wondered whether it was time to get a haircut, I warned him that agreeing too soon to give up his efforts to be his own person might be a premature closure. What I actually said was that accepting the trip was one thing and giving in was another. The patient responded to this intervention with a dream about seeing his girlfriend in somebody else's arms, and somebody commented about a person who was lost in a homosexual life-style. The premature ejaculation symptom strangely disappeared. In a second dream he swam nude in the purifying river Ganges and later walked along a country road in France with a macho movie character. When his father playfully approached him with trimming shears, Jeff clearly understood it as a thinly disguised enforcing of his father's will as well as an unconsciously communicated castration threat.

When Jeff returned from his trip he reported he was anxious and uneasy most of the time except when he was alone. Sleep came only with sedatives, and in spite of medication he had nightmares. One was of a ménage-à-trois with a Mrs. Robinson type and her hippie lover. His father appeared in the dream in a rage, yelling he would kill Jeff. The patient woke up protesting and telling himself maybe he should not be involved in this sexual situation in the first place. He reported he felt a great sense of relief—even though it turned him into a little boy—being in bed with both a man and a woman. I said he must have felt he had no other choice but to turn himself into a little boy who had little chance in a contest with his father *or* me.

It was clear that he had formed a firm positive attachment and therapeutic alliance with me; when he dreamed of being back at school, he wondered how he could be there and continue his sessions with me. He continued the dream with an open defiance of his father in a sexual scene and provocatively gave him the finger gesture.

He decided to be open and honest about being in therapy in his application for a job. When he comforted his girlfriend he was gratified to discover tenderness within himself because he had always seen himself as totally self-centered. I interpreted this as behaving like me, as a helping person. When he was forced to work late and learned the job had been misrepresented to him, he protested that his employer's business practices were unethical and quit. However, he was able to get another job right away. He more openly accepted his self-assertiveness and reported that the relationship with his parents had become a little easier.

In the transference he regressively retreated to a comforting mother figure, which was reflected in a dream in which he was drafted into the Union Army only to desert and run away with a girlfriend, Barbara. I suggested that he was afraid of a warring conflict with me as a Southerner and that he was now transferring his old conflict with his father onto the relationship with me. He acted out the escape through drugs, rationalizing it as proof to himself that he would not necessarily freak out. The premature ejaculation symptom returned as an expression of the dynamic transference relationship with me—taking drugs was equated with engaging in sexual behavior and defiance of me.

In his real relationship with his father, he attempted to make peace by giving him a birthday card and a present. At about the same time his maternal grandfather died, and he felt tenderly toward his mother in her loss. He saw his girlfriend Barbara as a maternal type who could comfort him as a kid, but he was at a loss to understand what role his mother or Barbara played in the overall picture of his conflicts. He then associated to feeling guilty. I commented that his premature ejaculation symptom and his guilt feelings in the relationship with Barbara were somehow connected to his tender feelings toward women, particularly his mother.

In the very next session Jeff reported that he still woke up every day with anxiety. He and a college friend decided together that their motivations to take drugs were not realistic and that they should avoid using them. He dreamed that the last fish had been killed (as though there had been a nuclear holocaust), while a hermit crab revived and grew bigger though seriously wounded. Help came but arrived too late. The patient was expressing how depressed and devastated he felt and was despairing of receiving help from therapy. I commented that externally his situation did not seem so serious as to be compared with a nuclear holocaust but that the conflicts he was struggling with internally were nonetheless very real to him. I added that our task was to see what solutions we could work out together.

Relief came almost too swiftly. He could not explain this, but it seems now to have been a transference improvement, only very short-lived. He dreamed that he was being sexually teased, first by his girlfriend; then he was tortured by his father's voice over a loudspeaker, laughing fiendishly and making the sky turn dark. In his associations he expressed his fear that other men, including his father, could steal his girlfriends. He felt tortured by women, too. He saw them as fickle with their love, and this made him feel even more insecure. In a dream, he escaped into his favorite restaurant. It was now clear that he was experiencing an intensification of the conflicted father transference that was prompting a regressive retreat to mother for comfort and food.

His anxiety attacks became much worse in the mornings (when he saw me), and his conflicts were all the more painful when he realized he could not escape them. He understood consciously that the conflict with his father was not experienced in the therapy with me. He recognized that he brought it on himself when he typically bowed out of competition. I suggested that the reason he bowed out of competitive situations was that he perceived them as dangerous and destructive, like activities back-alley toughs engage in (this figure was played back to him from one of his dreams). He experimented with this insight by engaging in a discussion about Huxley's *Brave New World* with his father, who happened to like what Jeff had to say. Though he felt complimented, he still felt hostile inside—ready to battle with his father—and answered curtly. As he struggled with his images of himself vis-à-vis his father and other men— me, peers—he began to perceive a possible difference in himself.

However, a threatened breakup of his relationship with his girlfriend added to his anxieties. He realized that he himself had started the breakup and that she was simply reacting. Again, I interpreted his actions as connected to the therapy and his bowing out of competition with me.

147

He was able to see that he had precipitated the breakup with Barbara "to get away from something else—you. I know what went wrong intellectually, but I'm not sure I am in control of it."

He noticed a change in his relationship with his parents. They saw how relaxed he was, and there was better communication with his father. Nevertheless, he noted that he felt "three times more anxious inside." He reported a dream about giving a Bar Mitzvah speech to a large audience—telling them off and setting fire to the place. In his associations he said he was disappointed he had never had a Bar Mitzvah. My comment was that leaving school was a disguised jab at his tradition-bound father who, it seemed to him, was selfishly interested in his son's success—and that in the dream he was attacking me as well. Jeff agreed that he saw me as part of a group that was trying to get him to do something for them.

In the next session, the patient announced that he had awakened that morning free of anxiety for the first time in a long while. He felt pretty well put together and understood more about himself. He reiterated his understanding from the previous session—that getting away from Barbara was like an escape from me.

In a dream he went to a bank to change rubles into American money, and the police were called to arrest him. He associated to not trusting me with his confidences, which I related to his fears of losing the support of the relationship with me and the fear during separations from me that he would not be able to sustain himself and the progress he had already made. He also wondered how lasting the effects of the therapy would be: were the insights permanent, or would his neurosis return some day? He experimented with his newfound freedom by discussing with his father his relationship with Barbara. Much to his surprise, he discovered he had less anxiety than before.

In the first session after a break, he said how glad he was to see me so he could report he was doing very well; he was eager to report the same to the school psychiatrist before being readmitted. That interview went well, and the projective tests (Rorschach, TAT, etc.) confirmed the clinical impression that he was making sufficient progress to return to school.

The school psychiatrist said Jeff "seemed to be functioning in an organized and optimistic manner." He went on:

I feel that this newfound organization is not simply the result of less stress but due to some real gains in maturity. His previous panic stemmed from the disintegration of his old self-image, and that was not of course readily replaced by a substitute. He has thought through a number of his relationships and styles of functioning with people, and seems, as a result of these insights, to have achieved a viable new self-image.

Most notably the conflicts with authority into which he was thrown when he began to question the "old Jeff" have subsided. His father now seems more like a person to him than simply an authority. He seems to approach college also with more humanized expectations. Generally, he seems more relaxed about himself, less competitive, and more open to emotionally expressive relationships with others.

In short, the degree of insight, maturity, and self-acceptance now observed would seem to suggest that his current high level of organization can continue in the face of the normal threats and anxieties he will encounter when he comes back to college.

He reported a dream of sleeping with his girlfriend in his parents' bedroom, only she confessed she had been sleeping with Bill, a mutual friend. He immediately recognized that Bill represented his father and Barbara his mother. The dream was filled with guilt, and he felt chased by tigers. "For the first time I woke up from that dream aware of what it meant, nor was I shocked by it. I realized it was partly my fault. The thing that struck me, though, was trying to put in on my father." He associated to cooling off on his relationship with Barbara and that he was resigned to that separation. "I'm not ready for marriage and I have other girls on my mind. I haven't done enough experimenting yet. That could lead to depressing things, too, but I think I can strike a balance." I again interpreted his separation from me with his plans to return to school.

In the next session, he continued to feel good and was free of anxiety. When he said goodbye to his friends, who were going off to other colleges, there was a sort of finality in terms of a conviction that "that circle should break up—we were held together only by the past. I'm less sure about the relationship with Barbara though. In a way, I don't want to lose her, nor am I sure I can pull off a good relationship with my father. I'm not hostile now toward him, and I still see a sharp line between us—competition yes, but not hostile. I'm not ready to make peace with him, but I want to."

He discussed with his mother his relationship with Barbara. He dreamed of going to the theater with the girlfriend. Even though they had reserved seats they somehow got separated. He resigned himself to being separated and to their cultural differences. In a second dream he was a gladiator assigned to fight a Vietnamese farmer. "There were mutilated bodies all around to psych you out. We fought to a complete tie—a rough and tumble fight. He was admitted to the Viet Cong and I was released. I got my freedom by fighting. We ended up by shaking hands." In a third dream he met a friend from school with whom he felt strong competition—for the biggest beard as well as in intellectual matters. "I saw a lot of my father in him, and reacted to him as though he were my father—he was sarcastic but bright and we had fun talking together." The patient made the connection among his friend, his father, and me. He saw, however, a subtle shift in his relationship with me and his father. For example, he no longer felt anxious in the sessions. He awakened from these three dreams understanding their meaning, which gave him confidence that he could analyze himself. "It is nothing so dramatic, but I've got to be careful I don't fool myself into thinking everything has changed. I could still get depressed or anxious. I can deal with my conflict with my father much better. I've reconciled with him, and I don't want to return to school being uptight." When he visited his buddies at their school, they had a big party with drugs, but the patient was relaxed and in control of himself. "I feel closer and closer with my parents. I want to talk with my father about a lot of things—my courses, getting into a small group seminar with Dr. A. C. [an internationally famous historian]. It's a relief to think about things other than myself. It takes the pressure off. I even praised my father to a friend. I told him how bright and unusual he is. I'm looking at him more objectively. Philosophers really offer no help, just word games, and tight logic, like a chess game." I commented that he must be feeling better about leaving me.

In the last session we reviewed what we had talked about and that he seemed back on the track of normal development. In a way, his neurosis forced his return home so that he could start over (Whitaker 1974). A neurotic view of destructive competition with other men—his peers, his father, and me—was at the center of his problem. I confided how much I had enjoyed working with him and understanding how his mind worked, and wished him the best of everything in his schoolwork, et cetera. I felt most confident about his future, which was well buttressed by his talents and intellectual skills. In a letter to me dated the following February he wrote:

The months since September have in some ways been as valuable a part of the analytic experience as the therapy itself. I don't feel articulate enough to give you a good written description of these months, except to say that they have comprised the first large segment of my life that I feel has been lived fully, excitingly, genuinely, honestly (as much as that is ever possible), and productively. Of course, it has been no utopia. I would never have it so, but something even better: the real world. There have been pains, anxieties, and depressions, but they have been dealt with and, even more important, *made use of*. There has been no paralysis in the face of torment, whether real or imagined; I have felt pretty much in constant control of my life.

In June, at the end of the school year, he returned for three follow-up sessions. He looked confident and was happy to report that he had finished the year with high grades. He had been able to sustain an analytic, self-observing posture and process. He left his drug friends behind and walked away from them and from Barbara, with whom he realized he had had a maternal relationship. In his associations, he talked about how much easier he felt about deciding to go into his father's profession, and that now he was dating a girl with whom he had a more adult relationship, which allowed both of them to be more free. She was also culturally and ethnically similar to him, which had not been true of previous girlfriends.

Discussion

The psychotherapeutic process in this young man began with him in a state of acute distress and panic. He knew that he had to return home for help to pull himself together, but it was there that his dimly appreciated conflict with authority was made worse. What I brought to this endeavor was an overall facilitating role and a benign therapeutic environment that, together with the interpretive work, aided him in reducing his panic and the actual neurotic aspect of his anxiety neurosis. I provided him a model for observing and processing his inner turmoil that he was able to identify with and employ in his own behalf. I was quite willing to wait for the unfolding of the process and the ensuing transferences. I did not actively intervene to pressure him prematurely. My patience was re-

warded when it became clear that Jeff's integrative capacities were basically intact and could restore his equilibrium and that the regressive
process was not deepening. Furthermore, the major elements of his
personality were not progressively disintegrating. He looked like a wild
man, but his appearance was deceptive. His motivations for his appearance and other aspects of his behavior were to enhance his self-regard,
but the main reasons involved an ambitious desire to be verbally, intellectually, and sexually competitive. His Afro and beard were like plumage.
He felt pushed from the inside in regard to these activities, but he was also
being driven from the outside, by his father's demands for achievement
and open aggressiveness. It is not unlikely that his father was vicariously
enjoying Jeff's efforts to solve the generational conflict. He was aware at
some level that he had failed to push his older son into being more
competitive, but this did not deter him from pursuing his ambitions for
Jeff.

I saw in this young man a neurotic process that was in the early stages of
formation. He was frightened by his dreams and fantasies of destructive
and murderous rage, which promoted regression to fantasies of passive
homosexual submission to men he perceived as all-powerful and castrat-
ing. In sum, it was a classic instance of an acute anxiety neurosis. The
patient's use of psychoactive drugs accentuated and accelerated the intrapsychic process of neurosogenesis. In keeping with this point of view,
one possible formulation was that the neurotic illness was a regressive
retreat from an oedipal conflict composed of competitiveness with other
males (peers and father) for the available (real or fantasied) female
(girlfriend, mother), who was perceived as the reassuring, giving, feeding, comforting source of refuge. In addition, he longed for his father's
benign love, respect, guidance, and direction. In the beginning transference reactions, Jeff wanted me to like him and help him in spite of his
hostile and murderous fantasies and dreams. His passive submissive
feminine identification combined with a perception of himself as a
homosexual partner to other men when he felt impotent, powerless, and
castrated. This interfered with his ability to think, feel, and act as an
equal to men in intellectual discourse, appearance, popularity, and sexual prowess. Repression of his fears of homosexual submission to his
father, in arguments with his friends, professors at school, and in the
developing transference with me, reappeared as mistrustfulness and a
suspiciousness in keeping with Freud's classical formulation of paranoid
thinking (1911). The premature ejaculation symptom, which came later,

could be viewed as a regressive self-castrating loss of his masculine power and avoidance of conflict with me as the feared father in the transference.

From another perspective, Jeff's neurosis could be formulated as a deficit in the self. The childhood history of fighting in grade school, biting a schoolmate to take away his pineapple juice, his inability to relate effectively with men, his use of drugs, and his selfish use of other people, particularly women, for what they could deliver to him in the way of immediate gratification, were in a way a caricature of what he perceived to be the masculine role exemplified by his father. There was a sense that he was special and unique, an exaggerated view of himself constructed out of his and his parents' grandiose expectations of his superior intellect, but based in part on his actual academic performance in the past. He was popular, and his classmates had liked him. His personal dream had been further inflated when he was accepted by the prestigious university of his choice. The bubble was pricked, however, when he arrived on campus to discover he was not the only student with promise of a bright future. Though this deficit formulation possesses a certain cogency, the evidence seems to point more clearly to a structured neurosis.

When his initial anxieties about beginning therapy were relieved, Jeff formed a sound and substantial therapeutic alliance. The father transference emerged pari passu as he expected me to object to his sexual and drug behaviors, which, in his mind, were equivalent. He already felt uncomfortable about his sexual behavior, and he could not reasonably expect me as a physician to be supportive of his experimenting with hallucinogenic drugs. Over the first two or three months he tested me to see whether I would intervene in a negative or demeaning way, as he expected in the father transference. He could see a friend's having irresponsibly wrecked a borrowed car as reprehensible, and he struggled with his sense of guilt about exploiting women sexually. He openly confronted his employer with what he thought were unfair, improper, and unethical business practices. The observable changes in his character—forthrightness, honesty, and a stable adherence to an elevated sense of values and rules of behavior—were substantial and seemed enduring. However, they more likely signified a new level of adaptation through a process of adopting what he perceived to be my standards as well as a reinforcement and consolidation of the parental standards already present in his personality.

Giving in to his father and to me in the transference was felt and interpreted as homosexual submission to me as the aggressor. He realized

153

from his nightmarish dreams and anxious nights on a trip with his father that such regressive solutions did not really deliver relief.

Regression to a maternal transference within the therapeutic relationship with me and with his girlfriend was a regular occurrence, but these regressive swings were temporary, reversible, and transitory. The reason for these regressive swings was castration anxiety precipitated by his back-alley view of the competitive battles between men. When he said it was like cutting off his nose to spite his own face, I responded "or cutting off something else." His view of competition as a fight to the death changed as a result of transference interpretations. In the gladiator dream his resolution of the battle with a Vietnamese farmer concluded with a handshake, and both combatants went their separate ways. In discussions with his parents and with me he felt freer to express his views without caving in or losing control. His recurrent snake dreams from childhood, in which he was surrounded on all sides by poisonous snakes, were understood as castration dreams. Snakes meant father, the feared and loved (fascinating) object.

Progress in a psychotherapeutic process can be evaluated according to several criteria—removal of symptoms, development of insight, or expansion of ego boundaries. Horowitz (1979) advocates a configurational analysis of mental or ego states, relationships with objects, and information processing. Jeff's therapy could be assessed in terms of the formation of the therapeutic alliance, the early transference reactions that were in time replaced by more stable, enduring, and interpretable transferences. His dreams were especially helpful in monitoring the therapeutic process and served to spotlight the most specific psychic intensities at any given moment, which were like a beacon guiding me in my therapeutic interventions. Jeff recovered from an acute anxiety neurosis, as revealed in his dreams, associations, and the school psychologist's evaluation. The follow-up sessions at the end of the school year confirmed our impression that he had been ready to return to school. He was able to maintain a self-analytic posture that sustained him when he felt internal pressure from the conflicts we talked about. The underlying oedipal conflict had reached a new phase in the process of resolution, and in my opinion he had reestablished connections with those natural processes of growth and strivings toward health that are at the center of development. Ideally, it would have been better for him to remain at home and continue the analysis, but to do so would have interfered with his natural growth processes of moving out of the parental home and getting on with his education.

In a letter written to me thirteen years later, Jeff described how his self-analytic work has endured through his use of free association and analysis of his dreams "to keep in touch with my unconscious." He has married and is working productively in an academic setting, making use of his intellectual skills.

For practical purposes, this case was what one might call an abbreviated analysis. He adopted an analytic-like style of observing himself and monitoring his dream life. The technique I adhered to was interpretation of unconscious meanings, when available to consciousness, particularly when resistances were manifest. His admission that he was still uncomfortable in expressing affectionate feelings to his parents indicates unfinished work. Furthermore, even though he has married, he does not describe his wife or his relationship with her. More important than this, though, is the fact that the mother transference was worked on only superficially. There were some separation feelings and mourning of the process but none of the usual termination features of recapitulation of the neurosis and the course of therapy. One might also say that there was insufficient repetition and working through of all the transferences. Naturally, working through demands more than six months to fully accomplish the task of uncovering all the antecedents of a neurosis.

My account of a brief six-month analysis raises many questions. First of all, was this treatment experience typical of analyses of college-age youth, and if not, in what way was it different? It was certainly not typical of most analyses of adults, in that analyses of character problems generally last much longer than six months, and in modern practice it is unusual to be consulted by a patient with a neurosis in the early stages of formation. Moreover, it is not typical for a person to be in an acute state of readiness and preparedness for analysis, as was my patient. The therapeutic split (Sterba 1934) and the therapeutic alliance were easily and rapidly established. Stated another way, the resistances were not so deeply entrenched as to make the beginning or "launching" phase so difficult, nor were the resistances so immutable. Therefore, in all these senses, there was something atypical and unusual that, in combination, made for an auspicious and serendipitous beginning.

Psychotherapy of college students is usually very brief—from one to twenty sessions—and often less than ten (Whittington 1962). Love and

Widen (1982) at Northwestern University's Student Health Service offer a "quarter or two" of therapy. However, the brief therapies or counseling (Hanfmann 1978) are usually limited to, or focused on, crises or otherwise circumscribed goals, which often take on the quality of educative experiences rather than the analysis of resistances. Hanfmann (1978) regards transferences in college students as episodic and not very important and feels that the active therapeutic agent is an "attitudinal factor" in the counselor, who must employ, as a real person, a positive, empathic, and communicative human relationship. The counselor's task was to uncover and promote the growth factors in the healthy self of the client. Cognitive development must be promoted, especially new capacities for thinking, communiciation, and problem solving.

Sifneos (1972, 1979) describes two kinds of short-term psychotherapy: one, crisis intervention, is anxiety suppressing; the other is anxiety provoking and more nearly approaches psychoanalysis. In the latter, the therapeutic alliance (positive transference) is manipulated to teach problem solving, and even though affects became the focus of some aspects of the therapy, Sifneos calls the changes effected a corrective emotional experience. Interpretations in the case material seem forced. Problems of oedipal conflict type are actively confronted with direct interpretations of drives and drive derivatives before resistance or defenses against the drives. Even though the therapeutic situation is termed "dyadic," preoedipal or narcissistic problems are avoided. Overt dislike of a patient is termed "countertransference."

Another type of brief therapy was described by Wedge (1958), in which an interpretive technique of surprise was used to loosen previously idiosyncratic adaptational patterns. This technique might have been effective in Jeff's case, but it seemed at the time of the diagnostic evaluation that analytic therapy was a more suitable approach.

A second question is, Was the result achieved a transference cure? Ordinarily speaking, a transference cure is silent in the sense that transferences and resistances are not made conscious through systematic interpretation. In severely narcissistic or borderline individuals, any attempt at interpretation of the transference is met with strong protests that what is expected is real parenting. Similarly, in parent loss or arrested development, patients who select the analyst to be the parent, the patients are actually seeking a transference cure. The replacement of the lost object actually interferes with the painful task of reliving and working through the mourning process or, for that matter, the restoration

156

of those developmental and growth processes that inevitably involve conflict. It is virtually impossible in some instances to overcome this formidable defense transference through application of a proper interpretive technique. Furthermore, the development of a utilizable and workable transference cannot occur, nor does the patient allow a deepening of the analytic process into a transference neurosis. The transference expectation is already conscious but is split off and disavowed.

By none of these criteria could my case be adequately explained as a transference cure. Another criterion involves use of the analyst as a new object rather than as a surrogate parent. Ritvo's discussion (1974) of this issue is very cogent. In the context of the transference situation, patients do make use of the analyst as a new object to facilitate growth and development, particularly when the transference-countertransference situation is maintained within appropriate boundaries of analytic abstinence. The use of the analyst as a real object seems to have more obvious meaning in child analysis (Sandler, Kennedy, and Tyson 1975). However, it is also evident in the analysis of adults who have lost a parent in childhood, especially when the mourning process has been worked through. "Frozen" development is unblocked and processes of growth are resumed. Ritvo's longitudinal studies point up the necessity of differentiating between interpretation of transference use of the new object and use of the analyst as a surrogate parent.

The evidence in my patient points to the conclusion that his was not a transference cure or a countertransference acting as a surrogate parent. More accurately, perhaps, he made use of me as a new object to facilitate further growth and development, freeing up an arrest in development (Mode IV in Gedo and Goldberg's [1973] formulations).

Sterba (1951) described Freud's suggestion treatment of Bruno Walter's psychogenic "rheumatic neuralgia" in his conducting arm—a veritable "professional neurosis." First Freud sent Walter to Sicily for a change of scenery. When he returned, Freud capitalized on the patient's confidence in him, encouraged the conductor to forget about his ailment, and urged him to overcome it. There is no question that this treatment, as recounted in Walter's autobiography (1946) and Sterba's formulations, amounts to suggestion therapy. Sterba speculated that Freud intuitively understood that Walter was suffering from a slight dynamic disequilibrium and that Walter's ego was "strong enough with some suggestive support to regain control over the muscular functions of which an unconscious inhibition had taken possession. . . . Freud used all the weight of his suggestive authority to press him out of his neurosis . . . by taking full responsibility that no failure would occur." Another instance was Freud's four-hour stroll in Leyden with Gustav Mahler, resulting in a cure of Mahler's impotence (Jones 1955).

As is easily seen from Sterba's description, there is no comparison to the clinical material of my case, in which the transferences were allowed to naturally unfold and were, as much as possible, systematically interpreted. Unconscious contents were made conscious, all the while using orthodox technique without parameters or deviations of expediency. It was not a cure by suggestion.

My critics might then raise the question, What of the possibility that it was all an intellectual-cognitive exercise like Sifneos's short-term anxiety-provoking therapy (1979), which could be regarded as another form of transference improvement through manipulation of the positive transference and a superficial consideration of already conscious or perhaps preconscious and only slightly conflictual mental contents? Against this, I would have to say, Jeff's affectively charged regressive transference represents a substantial argument.

Yet another critic might compare the account of Jeff's analysis to the experiments conducted by Alexander and French (1946). They advocated a deliberate experimentation with the therapeutic process to shorten the work or produce certain cathartic experiences they called, over all, "the corrective emotional experience." They also proposed that role playing was indicated to provide the patient a new experience opposite to or corrective of the childhood relationship to parents. Alexander (1965) frustrated the regressive dependency needs of his patients by changing the frequency of interviews or by planned interruptions of the therapy so as to shorten the therapy and, most of all, to tell the patient that the therapy should be completed as soon as possible (see also Love and Widen 1982; Whittington 1962). Alexander (1965) advocated that the therapist should actively counteract the patient's attempt to "parentify" him. He also compared therapy to education, using the concepts of learning theory (reward and punishment) to explain the therapeutic process and therapeutic technique. In fact, old behavior patterns were to be unlearned by engaging the patient's motivation for help. Fenichel (1945) said that transference improvements were based on educational measures. On the other hand, he pointed out (Fenichel 1954) that such efforts at manipulation may yield some success: "The nearer a given neurosis is to the traumatic end of this complementary series, the greater is the probability that external efforts to support the subject's spontaneous attempts at regaining mental equilibrium may be successful" (pp. 244–245). However, there was no traumatic precipitating factor in Jeff's case, and there was no artificial manipulation of the positive or other transferences. This was no corrective emotional experience therapy.

Phillips and Wiener (1960) openly and avowedly espouse a manipulative and educative psychotherapeutic technique to assist patients to structure their lives and solve problems. To them, Alexander and French did not go far enough.

Even though one can find references to the educative function of psychoanalytic therapy in Freud's writings—for example, "On Psychotherapy" (1905b)—I think he was referring to the overcoming of resistances; in the same paper, he stated that "analytic therapy . . . does not seek to add or introduce anything new, but to take away something, to bring out something; and to this end concerns itself with the genesis of the morbid symptoms and the psychical context of the pathogenic idea which it seeks to remove" (p. 261). Moreover, in his 1919 paper, "Lines of Advance in Psychoanalytic Therapy," Freud recognized the problems of applying analytic therapy to the population on a large scale. To do so would "compel us to alloy the pure gold of analysis freely with the copper of direct suggestion" (p. 168). He hastened to add, "But whatever form this psychotherapy for the people may take, whatever the elements out of which it is compounded, its most effective and most important ingredients will assuredly remain those honored from strict and untendentious psychoanalysis" (p. 168).

The corrective emotional experience has become such a pejorative term that it is no longer possible to speak of emotionally charged experiences in analysis without the specter of this old term being raised. Recently, Heinz Kohut said (quoted in Kirsner 1982) that the corrective emotional experience could be regarded as "being properly understood and properly explained to himself" through proper interpretation, something entirely different from what Alexander advocated (see also Tolpin 1983).

What of the possibility that my patient was suffering only from a temporary regression, one of a series of regressive-progressive swings observed in normal development, and specifically the phase-specific conflicts for the college-age youth? I think this unlikely, as the symptoms he presented were not transient and were moderately severe. Furthermore,

he was not sleeping well, was rapidly sinking into a more severe pathological process that was already affecting his capacity for work and for
affectionate relationships with men or women, and he was no longer
deriving pleasure from the intellectual activities of college. This was
clearly not a normal late adolescent crisis that could have been easily
managed by a telephone call home, a visit with his parents, or an
emergency consultation. In fact, all these measures had been attempted
and had failed to reverse the regressive process.

The patient made ample use of me as the participant–empathic observer who communicated understanding of the neurotic conflicts
through well-timed and well-placed interpretations.

Conclusions

Under the impact of the interpretive work done with the patient, his
symptoms gradually disappeared, reappeared, and disappeared again for
good. There was a clear strengthening (as objectively confirmed by the
school psychologist's tests) of the healthy defensive operations of the
patient's ego, along with a new level of mastery of unconscious conflict.
What I have described is a consolidation of the patient's personality
brought about in part by the therapy, which freed up an arrested adolescent development.

However, for a variety of reasons, late adolescents do interrupt their
analyses to continue their educational objectives or to concentrate on
establishing themselves in the real world. If there was a flight from this
therapy, it could be argued that Jeff ran away from facing the mother
transference. First of all, it might be said, the conflicts around the father
transference occupied most of our attention. Second, the mother transference emerged only toward the end of our work and in an abbreviated
fashion, and it was partially displaced onto his girlfriend. In retrospect, it
is now clear that, were he to resume analysis at some future date, the
issues pertaining to the mother transference would be a central part of the
new psychoanalytic work.

REFERENCES

Adatto, C. P. 1980. Late adolescence to early adulthood. In S. E.
Greenspan and G. H. Pollock, eds. *The Course of Life: Psychoanalytic*

Contributions Toward Understanding Personality Development. Vol. 2, *Latency, Adolescence, and Youth*. Washington, D.C.: National Institute of Mental Health.

Alexander, F. 1965. Psychoanalytic contributions to short-term psychotherapy. In L. R. Wolberg, ed. *Short-Term Psychotherapy*. New York: Grune & Stratton.

Alexander, F., and French, T. 1946. *Psychoanalytic Therapy*. New York: Ronald.

Balint, M.; Ornstein, P. H.; and Balint, E. 1972. *Focal Psychotherapy*. London: Tavistock.

Basch, M. F. 1980. *Doing Psychotherapy*. New York: Basic.

Berliner, B. 1941. Short psychoanalytic therapy: its possibilities and limitations. *Bulletin of the Menninger Clinic* 5:204–211.

Breuer, J. V., and Freud, S. 1893–95. Studies on hysteria. *Standard Edition*, vol. 2. London: Hogarth, 1956.

Davanloo, H. 1980. *Short Term Dynamic Psychotherapy*. New York: Aronson.

Deutsch, F. 1949. *Applied Psychoanalysis*. New York: Grune & Stratton.

Fenichel, O. 1945. *The Psychoanalytic Theory of Neurosis*. New York: Norton.

Fenichel, O. 1954. Brief psychotherapy. In *The Collected Papers*, 2d ser. New York: Norton.

Ferenczi, S. 1920. The further development of an active therapy in psychoanalysis. In *Theory and Technique of Psychoanalysis*, vol. 2. London: Hogarth, 1950.

Frances, A., and Perry, S. 1983. Transference interpretations in focal therapy. *American Journal of Psychiatry* 140:405–409.

Frank, J. D. 1971. Therapeutic factors in psychotherapy. *American Journal of Psychotherapy* 25:350–361.

Freud, S. 1905a. Fragment of an analysis of a case of hysteria. *Standard Edition* 7:7–122. London: Hogarth, 1953.

Freud, S. 1905b. On psychotherapy. *Standard Edition* 7:257–268. London: Hogarth, 1958.

Freud, S. 1911. Psycho-analytic notes on an autobiographical account of a case of paranoia. *Standard Edition* 12:9–79. London: Hogarth, 1958.

Freud, S. 1919. Lines of advance in psycho-analytic therapy. *Standard Edition* 17:159–168. London: Hogarth, 1955.

Gedo, J., and Goldberg, A. 1973. *Models of the Mind*. Chicago: University of Chicago Press.

Hanfmann, E. 1978. *Effective Therapy for College Students*. San Francisco: Jossey-Bass.

Horowitz, M. 1979. *States of Mind: Analysis of Change in Psychotherapy*. New York: Plenum.

Isay, R. A. 1980. Late adolescence: the second separation stage of adolescence. In S. E. Greenspan and G. H. Pollock, eds. *The Course of Life: Psychoanalytic Contributions toward Understanding Personality Development*. Vol. 2, *Latency, Adolescence, and Youth*. Washington, D.C.: National Institute of Mental Health.

Jones, E. 1955. *The Life and Work of Sigmund Freud*, vol. 2. New York: Basic.

Kirsner, D. 1982. Self psychology and the psychoanalytic movement: An interview with Dr. Heinz Kohut. *Psychoanalysis and Contemporary Thought* 5:483–493.

Love, R. L., and Widen, H. A. 1985. Short term dynamic psychotherapy: another kind of learning on campus. *Adolescent Psychiatry* 12:327–335.

Malan, D. H. 1976. *The Frontier of Brief Psychotherapy*. New York: Plenum.

Mandel, H. P. 1981. *Short-Term Psychotherapy and Brief Treatment Techniques: An Annotated Bibliography, 1920–1980*. New York: Plenum.

Mann, J. 1973. *Time-Limited Psychotherapy*. Cambridge, Mass.: Harvard University Press.

Menninger, K. A. 1958. *Theory of Psychoanalytic Technique*. New York: Basic.

Phillips, E. I., and Wiener, D. N. 1960. *Short-Term Psychotherapy and Structural Behavior Changes*. New York: McGraw-Hill.

Pumpian-Mindlin, E. 1953. Considerations in selection of patients for short-term therapy. *American Journal of Psychotherapy* 7:641–652.

Ritvo, S. 1974. The current status of the infantile neurosis: implications for diagnosis and technique. *The Psychoanalytic Study of the Child* 29:159–181.

Sandler, J.; Kennedy, H.; and Tyson, R. L. 1975. The treatment situation and technique in child psychoanalysis. *The Psychoanalytic Study of the Child* 30:409–441.

Sifneos, P. E. 1972. *Short Term Psychotherapy and Emotional Crisis*. Cambridge, Mass.: Harvard University Press.

Sifneos, P. E. 1979. *Short Term Dynamic Psychotherapy*. New York: Plenum.

Sifneos, P. E. 1981. Short-term dynamic psychotherapy: its history, its impact and its future. *Psychotherapy and Psychosomatics* 35:224–229.

Socarides, C. W. 1954. On the usefulness of extremely brief psychoanalytic contacts. *Psychoanalytic Review* 41:340–346.

Sterba, R. 1934. The fate of the ego in analytic therapy. *International Journal of Psycho-Analysis* 15:117–126.

Sterba, R. 1951. A case of brief psychotherapy by Sigmund Freud. *Psychoanalytic Review* 35:75–80.

Strupp, H. H. 1975. Psychoanalysis, "focal" psychotherapy, and the nature of the therapeutic influence. *Archives of General Psychiatry* 32:127–135.

Tolpin, M. 1983. Corrective emotional experience: a self psychological reevaluation. In A. Goldberg, ed. *The Future of Psychoanalysis*. New York: International Universities Press.

Walter, B. 1946. *Theme and Variations*. New York: Knopf.

Wedge, B. B. 1958. *Treatment of Idiosyncratic Adaptation in College Students: Psychosocial Problems of College Men*. New Haven, Conn.: Yale University Press.

Whitaker, C. 1974. The symptomatic adolescent—an AWOL family member. In M. Sugar, ed. *The Adolescent in Group and Family Therapy*. New York: Brunner/Mazel.

Whittington, H. G. 1962. Transference in brief psychotherapy: experience in a college psychiatric clinic. *Psychiatric Quarterly* 36:503–518.

Wolberg, L. R. 1965. *Short-Term Psychotherapy*. New York: Grune & Stratton.

9   THE PSYCHOANALYST AS BOTH
     PARENT AND INTERPRETER FOR
     ADOLESCENT PATIENTS

FRANK S. WILLIAMS

Most seriously disturbed adolescents who come or who are brought for psychotherapy often suffer from severe developmental deficits (Williams 1973). They may suffer from deficits in age-appropriate parent-child interactions. These interactions include the receiving of emotional nurturing and support, validation of their independent functioning and responsible actions, and validation of their individuating identities. They may suffer from deficits in their education around sexuality, adult responsibility, and intimacy. They frequently suffer from a lack of insight into what is behind their arrested passage from symbiotic family dependency to adulthood—as well as not recognizing a premature and often self-destructive passage into pseudoadulthood.

It is not a strategic accident that the therapist's functioning as a teacher and parent leads to insight. It is, rather, based on the very nature of the developmental processes of adolescence. In Mahler's (1968) terms, an infant moves from a normal autistic phase of development to a normal symbiotic phase in which there is a prologue to the later development of trust, empathy, intimacy, and a sense of self-value. The child then moves on through the phases of separation-individuation. We know that the passage in early years from symbiosis toward separation and individuation occurs most smoothly when a good deal of nurturing, support, and emotional caring is still available from the same parents who now encourage the child toward autonomous functioning and unique identity formation.

Blos (1962) described a second individuation in adolescence. Again, there is a passage from symbiotic family nuclear ties, which provide support and guidance, to a state of independent responsibility with an evolving distinct existential identity—separate and unique from the family identity. The adolescent must further develop trust in his own power, as well as the power of others around him—his friends, siblings, and parents—in order to develop a sense of intimacy and empathy. This second passage, during adolescence, is a more difficult and critical developmental passage than the original one during childhood.

A two- or three-year-old moving toward separation-individuation from symbiosis has little or no choice about extreme separation and self-autonomy; the young toddler cannot really leave home. Adolescents can and oftimes do leave home. They may run away to available peer groups to join others who have taken pseudoindependent action or who have been prematurely extruded from their symbiotic nuclear families and cut off. Unfortunately, adolescents and their parents are not forced to stick with each other to battle out and negotiate their problems and to define and clarify the intricate and difficult balance between needed symbiotic nurturing and needed independent responsibility and self-determination. There is very little control that a parent can assert if the adolescent really wants to leave. There is very little control that an adolescent can assert should his parents extrude him or be unable to take care of him.

Family Dynamics and the Role of Family Therapy

The adolescent's passage toward separation-individuation becomes a crisis for the parents as well as the young person in terms of mourning, depression, and anxiety that surround the loss of symbiotic parent-child bonds. Much in the literature has appropriately focused on the depression and mourning in adolescents moving toward individuation (Blos 1962; Erikson 1968). But little has been written about the parents' parallel normal mourning process, as their adolescent children—especially their last adolescent child—move on toward separation-individuation and young adulthood (Toews, Martin, and Prosen 1981).

Parental mourning and anxiety are induced by loss of the old symbiotic ties as well as the threat of loss of parental identity. With disturbed adolescents who have had deficient or overwhelming symbiotic attachments, we must involve the family in family diagnosis, even when the primary treatment modality may be individual psychoanalytic psy-

165

chotherapy for the adolescent. The parents need to work through enough of their mourning and anxiety, or the adolescent will remain confused about his or her next steps in life. Family therapy sessions also help during the ongoing treatment of an adolescent, particularly when the adolescent has severe intrapsychic problems around the symbiotic passage. The therapist can observe how the adolescent triggers anxieties in the parents in relation to readiness or unreadiness for adulthood. Unfortunately, the family field is not always receptive to helping an adolescent achieve the proper balance between accepting guidance and support while developing greater mastery, autonomy, and self-determination. The passage becomes very stormy and destructive when parents are too restrictive and controlling of an adolescent, or when an adolescent is too dependent on his parents. On the other hand, the passage can also be disruptive when parents are too carefree, not restrictive enough, and overencourage freedom on the adolescent's part. Such parents do not remain available enough on a day-to-day basis for support and guidance, and their adolescent children become too independent, not seeking out enough of their parents' guidance.

Clinical Example

A case that demonstrates such an adolescent crisis for parents and their sixteen-year-old is that of Joe. From the time Joe was thirteen, he was allowed too much adult responsibility, and he took too many pseudomature chances. Mother had been very close to Joe during his early years and through the pains of her divorce and separation. She suddenly seemed to abandon Joe in favor of her new husband when the boy was thirteen. Around the same time, Joe's father, an older man who had lost a financial empire and had become severely depressed, married a woman who could not tolerate Joe's drug using and rebellious behavior. Joe became a boy "without a family."

Joe's passage from adolescent family symbiosis to young adulthood was an especially stormy one, since his parents and Joe were confused about what was appropriate and inappropriate behavior for a sixteen-year-old. His parents were recommended for family therapy sessions to sort out their confusion over power, adolescent independence, and the generational boundaries. Unfortunately, the family therapy was limited by the parents' turmoil and chronic unavailability.

As a family's structure begins to collapse and stress continues, it becomes difficult to hold such parents in family therapy. Multifamily changes make the family therapy part of the treatment of an adolescent problematic, especially when divorce and remarriage occur at the same time that the adolescent is in treatment. When parents are not emotionally available, a great burden and responsibility fall on the therapist's shoulders. He must provide more of the parenting, more of the teaching, and more of the guidance. In many cases, the adolescent cannot wait for the parents to mobilize themselves to make the most of their family therapy.

The Analyst as Parent and Teacher

The case of Joe reflects the kind of parenting and teaching the adolescent requires from his therapist. From age thirteen to age sixteen, Joe had become a heavy drug user and a sexually acting-out Don Juan. He nearly killed himself in an auto accident while on drugs after beating up an older friend who made a homosexual overture toward him. During the course of treatment, the analyst provided reassurance; validation of Joe's uniqueness; validation of his strengths and accomplishments; verbal reinforcement of his developmental strides and mature judgment; and empathic human relatedness. The analyst guided him through certain age-appropriate tasks and discouraged tasks that were beyond Joe's level of responsibility. The analyst explored and responded to many real-life factors—the home environment, school life, teachers, peers, and employment matters, among others. Joe's acting out was viewed as a cry for such needed structure, guidance, and support.

Review of Case Background

Joe was adopted. His natural mother was a fifteen-year-old unmarried girl. His natural father was a seventeen-year-old boy who was killed, while drunk, in a motorcycle accident. His adoptive mother, Rose, and adoptive father, Jack, twenty years older than Rose, adored Joe and raised him as a "prince" during his early years. His mother was especially close to the boy through her separation and divorce and until her courtship and remarriage. Joe's adoptive father had always wanted Joe to be an obedient and charming little boy. During his infancy and latency years, Joe was the highlight of his parents' existence. When Joe was eight, his adoptive father began to lose his financial banking empire and became severely depressed about the faltering marriage. In the early years of Joe's life, mother received a great deal of financial security and support from her husband and was in turn able to give Joe a great deal. As her husband fell apart financially and became depressed, the marriage also failed, and they soon separated. From the time Joe was eight until he was thirteen, he became his mother's closest and exclusive love object. She took him to parties as her escort. Joe was an extremely handsome, bright, pseudomature child. Father, likewise, needed the young boy for his own ego and love; he would dress him up in young men's fashion clothes and show Joe off proudly.

Mother's new husband, Bill, entered the picture when Joe was twelve. A successful builder of skyscrapers, he had as a child been severely beaten by a sadistic father who tended to depreciate him. Bill developed a tremendous oedipal rivalry with the very handsome and charming young Joe, the "apple of his new wife's eye." He and Joe constantly fought with each other. When mother and Bill would go away for a weekend, Joe would have sex with girls in his parents' bed, leaving used condoms for mother and Bill to find on their return home.

As his mother began to side with her new husband and reject Joe, the boy became heavily involved in barbiturate and alcohol abuse. Prior to seeking analytic treatment, Joe had befriended a twenty-four-year-old man whom he trusted as a father figure. He felt this man represented the older brother he had always wanted. This man was very supportive and nurturing of Joe, but one day he made a sudden, unexpected homosexual overture. Joe knocked him to the floor, took a handful of barbiturates, and then almost drove his car off a cliff.

Treatment Course

When Joe first came to see me, he had blocked out the homosexual overture. Shortly after Joe's treatment started, mother and her new husband moved 100 miles away, father married a wife who wanted nothing to do with Joe, and Joe was moved to an open residential setting for youngsters with drug problems.

Three months into Joe's three-times-per-week psychoanalytic psychotherapy, he had begun to feel at home in the residential setting in which he was staying. He was particularly fond of the man who directed the setting, but he began to feel that he could not remain there, since other youngsters and the staff made fun of Joe for being in intensive therapy. I called the director of the home, who confirmed that Joe was reporting accurately; the other adolescents were envious of how quickly Joe had stopped using drugs, and there was much pressure on him to give up his analytic treatment.

In his sessions, I underlined the very difficult nature of the dilemma he faced. I told him I was available if he wanted some direct guidance about the conflict. On his own, he decided to leave the center, choosing to continue in analytic therapy. When he announced his choice to his family, his father depreciated him, stating, "You could not make it there; you're no good!" I took a different position, telling him that I felt his father was wrong and that the choice Joe had made showed good judgment on his part, even though I knew he was frightened about not knowing where he would live.

In the next session, Joe presented a memory of a dream sequence from age five. In the dream, there is a giant hiding in his bedroom. He and a six-year-old girl cousin are frightened by the "peevish giant." An Indian youth then puts an ax into his father's back. Joe hooked this dream up with his own inner feelings of depression and, for the first time in treatment, showed outward signs of depression. He related his deep sadness to not having had a close and meaningful relationship with his father. He expressed great disappointment not only in his father's passivity but in the fact that his father always seemed to put him down. I reflected to him that he seemed to be searching for a father with whom he could feel a comfortable identification and with whom he could have a meaningful, nonthreatening, and nondepreciative relationship.

Two sessions later, he expressed a feeling of lacking "masculine stuff." In actuality, Joe had started having intercourse with girls when he was twelve. He had constantly worked at sexually outshining all the other boys, and he had a reputation in his neighborhood and school for being a stud with whom all the girls wanted to go to bed. This macho-acting boy, with a deep seductive voice and pseudomasculine acting out, now brought into his analysis a feeling of lacking in masculinity. He stated he did not know what a man was. I began to talk to him about the complexities of what made a man. He intellectually accepted my remarks that a man could be tender and understanding. I very directly said to him that it did not necessarily have to make him feel more like a woman, or more like his mother, just because he had sensitive feelings.

He then expressed ambivalent pride in his father's successful, self-made business ventures, followed by anger at his father for becoming a passive "slob, who never really took action," but who "manipulated" his way through business and life. In his attempt to find a masculine adult ego ideal, he compared his father with his uncle Karl, an aggressive, at times obnoxious, person. I explained to him that I did not feel either approach was necessarily reflective of a strong man. His depression deepened and for the first time since he started treatment he felt the strong urge to use barbiturates again. He was, however, able to control the urge.

The Adolescent Identifies with Needed Parenting

After he left the residential setting, Joe accepted a job taking care of two children after school while living with them and their mother. Within a few weeks of his working there, the job began to include providing frequent sex to the woman. Joe became overwhelmed. When he first talked about his getting the job, I was unaware of all the complications that were coming. Now that the true nature of the employment became clear, I encouraged Joe to ask his parents to help him find a better place to live. They refused to help him. I told him that I felt he had taken too much responsibility as he felt overburdened by the woman's sexual demands and her children's individual needs. When he decided to leave this setting, his father depreciated him, and his mother told him that he was immature and irresponsible for "leaving a job without seeing it through." When he directly asked me for advice, I declared to Joe that I felt his judgment in the matter was correct and that, even though we did not know where he would go and what would happen to him, I would try to help him and his family find him a new home.

Following my support of his decision to move out of that home, Joe cried openly and told me how frustrated he felt, how lonely he was, and how lost he was. He stated that he was beginning to feel close to me and wanted to lean on me. This feeling triggered within him the urge to either take drugs or miss his next session. The direct guidance I gave to this young man was essential. It represented age-appropriate dependency support. Joe, however, had denied his dependency needs for many years and instead acted them out in self-destructive ways. To be dependent went against the pseudomature image he and his parents had developed for him.

Four months later, Joe began to express feelings of competition toward me. These feelings made him very uncomfortable, to the point where he felt he was not deserving of my care and consideration. He would tell me that he knew I was a successful doctor, a successful father, and a successful husband. He said he wanted to be a better father to a child and a better husband to a wife than I was. This induced such guilt that he considered missing sessions. He said that he was surprised that I did not get angry with him, did not put him down, or "kick him out of therapy." Whenever he made competitive remarks toward mother's new husband, like "you're getting old, Bill," or "I don't see what my mother sees in you, Bill," or, "I bet you're not that good sexually with women, Bill," Bill would depreciate him and throw him out of their home.

Joe again recalled his dream at age five, in which a father is axed in the back by his Indian son. He wondered if his recall had anything to do with his adoptive father's and Bill's rejection of him. I suggested that he felt that he did not deserve his father's affection and that he provoked his father and stepfather to reject him out of guilt. He then reported an incident that had occurred while he was working for the thirty-five-year-old mother of the two boys. One day he became enraged with her. She had a boyfriend sleeping with her one night, and, when her four-year-old walked into the bedroom, catching his mother and her boyfriend having sex, she screamed at him and threw the boy out of the room. The next day, Joe raged at the woman, telling her that she had done a "very terrible thing." She "made her boy feel small and rejected." Joe then instructed her to tell her child that she still loved him, which she proceeded to do. I praised him for his intuition and his preventive psychiatric work. I told him I thought he had done a very fine job in helping that little boy. I said this in a very serious way because I felt it was important to validate some of his growing empathic capacity.

Following this, Joe brought up primal scene impressions from his own childhood. He thought that he may have been "caught" observing his parents having sex, but he was not sure. As he tried to deal with this primal scene material over the next few sessions, he would frequently shift to themes bordering on homosexuality without his having conscious awareness of the homosexual content. He denied any feelings of homosexuality or bisexuality but began to talk about what he considered premature ejaculation. This led to much open discussion and education about sex. It was quite amazing to me to discover what little factual knowledge Joe had about sex, in spite of much overt sexual experience. Whatever sexual education he may have had as a child was completely repressed. Even though he was able to perform the sexual act with great skill, he considered it to be premature ejaculation when he "could not stay in and hard all night." As he talked about feeling inadequate and ashamed, I wondered whether he had some deeper shame regarding certain sexual feelings he might have had as a young child. He jumped up from the couch and reacted with a loud, "Wow! I'm suddenly thinking of my mother!" Incestuous feelings that he did not believe he had were suddenly experienced and reported.

Dependency Crisis of Adolescence

The exquisite confusion around a teenager's acceptance of nurturing and guidance is always highlighted by interruptions in treatment. When Joe first learned that I was going to be away on a vacation, he felt strong urges to return to the use of barbiturates. After I confronted him with his fears and his anger, he talked of a sense of loneliness and despair over not having parents to live with any more. I suggested that he was not only struggling with the loss of his parents but with the impending loss of me as well. He denied this vehemently and proceeded to miss the next two sessions. He subsequently admitted he would miss me, cried openly, after which he again missed a session. The following day, he stated that he knew he was running away from his feeling of needing me. Once again, his thoughts went to his childhood dream of a youth axing his father in the back. I told him that I believed that he must have been angry with his father for making him feel unloved and unwanted, especially as he faced adolescence. He felt confused by his father, who wanted him to be "a sweet little girl" and on the other hand demanded complete grown-up responsibility. Yet, father appeared most nurturing to Joe when father's demands were met.

Five days before the start of my vacation, Joe announced that he was going to stop his analysis. I suggested that he was missing me in advance and was feeling desperate to have to go to such an extreme as to stop his treatment. He admitted "small feelings of desperation" but preferred to take a tranquilizer. I pointed out that he felt critical of himself for longing for an adult parent to take care of him and critical of himself for feeling he would miss me. I further stated that, although it was painful for him to face depressive loneliness, it would help if he stayed in psychotherapy and did not turn to drugs. I offered some educational comments about how severe depression can result from a person's not expressing lonely feelings about losing someone. I told him that, if he could face his sadness, he would not ever again have to hurt himself with drugs. He suddenly expressed much anger at his mother for betraying him and abandoning him. He talked with rage about the woman in whose home he had been working, stating that she, too, abandond her children. Joe said he felt abandoned by both his mother and his father. I clarified that his frustration was even greater since he had had his mother and much parental guidance from her for all of his early years; now he felt she and her guidance had been stolen from him. Toward the end of this particular session, Joe asked, "What will happen to me if I never have treatment any more?"

Joe stated that he was mainly depressed about his father. I related his depression, in part, to his feelings about my coming vacation. He wept loudly, saying he felt "very ashamed of crying, since only babies and girls cry." I told him that it took great strength for a man to be able to show his tears in our culture and that he certainly had a right to feel sad and tearful. My remarks were not just presented to him with educative words. Joe could see that I, too, had tears in my eyes at this point, which I did not try to conceal from him.

Before leaving for vacation, I demanded that both sides of Joe's family come for a series of family therapy sessions. I encouraged them to find Joe a place to live and to help him find a less demanding job. They came through on both of my demands. Although he was very grateful for this, he later shared with me that he felt threatened by my having taken such an active part in his life. It highlighted for him what his parents had not been able to do on their own. I told him they had always meant well but had not had proper guidance in the past.

Dependency Needs versus Dependency Addiction

On return from my three-week vacation, Joe was extremely angry. On the telephone he told me he would not be returning to treatment. He said he felt he would be "weak, falling apart, and in danger" if he were to return to treatment. I suggested that there was no real danger, that I felt he had made great strides. I added that he was not a weak, helpless boy because he needed me and emphasized all the strengths he had exhibited in facing his problems and restructuring his life. While I was gone, he realized that his underlying attachment and dependency had become very strong and he felt frightened by needing me so. His friends made fun of him and depreciated him for needing a "shrink." On the phone, he added that analysis was a "drug addiction" in which the analyst was the "pusher." The analyst-pusher told the patient-addict, "You need me, come on back, I'll give you a little fix of analysis." I told Joe that he was unduly frightened by his feeling of needing me. I stressed how recognizing his need for me, and his fear of that need, would help him not give in to "addiction to me" and would, in fact, help him to continue to develop his strengths and master his problems. When he came in for the next session, he expressed a great deal of anger, stating, "All the bullshit about the importance of three and four times a week analysis, and then you go away for a whole month! . . . I don't ever want to feel that I'm going downhill and that I need you to hold me up!" I told him that his fear of a dependency addiction was blocking him from comfortably and appropriately relying on me when he needed me. He responded with, "I guess I really feel I will always need you." I suggested that he confused his missing me and getting needed help from me with an addiction to me. I further praised his courage in admitting these feelings, which many adolescents his age would not admit. I told him many would say nothing and would instead actually discontinue their treatment or go back to taking drugs.

He raised the issue of fitting analysis into his crowded schedule. I empathized with his full load of activities—school, work, and treatment. I offered to rearrange our appointments to fit his schedule.

I feel it is very important in working with adolescents to see them at times that will least interfere with their activities. These are reality resistances that can never be successfully interpreted as resistance to the developing transference.

Fairly soon, Joe asked for reassurance about the move he had made out of the older woman's house. I again told him that his judgment was correct. He then seemed freer to bring out some of his hidden immature desires. I find that reminding an adolescent of the mature things he has done allows him to bring out his more symbiotic, less mature feelings and needs. Joe talked of wanting to "be a little boy again," of wanting "his mommy and daddy to take care" of him just as they had when he was six and seven years old. He cried as he described fantasies of wanting to be my son—of wishing I could continue to guide him in a way that he felt his parents were failing to guide him. I suggested that his parents really did guide him at one time but were now confused and inconsistent about how much independence or dependence he needed. He soon recognized that denial of his dependency needs was very closely related to his heavy use of drugs. We reviewed many examples of this connection.

Several months later, there was another crisis in his treatment during which he again felt the urge to take drugs. This occurred as I was preparing to be gone for seven days of professional work. Although we dealt with his potential sadness, loneliness, and anger, he was angry and determined to take drugs while I was away. During the time I was gone, I sent him a postcard. In that postcard, I strongly and directly urged him not to take drugs. My card to him read: "You do not need drugs to keep yourself alive in my head while I am gone." When I returned, he greeted me with great joy and pleasure about the postcard. He said that when he read it, he felt the most "healthy connection" that he had ever felt toward anyone before. The card meant a great deal to him, and he no longer felt the desire to take drugs.

Homosexual Themes

On a conscious level, Joe was very hateful and contemptuous of homosexuals. The theme of homosexuality began to play itself out in analysis, as he felt closer to me. First Joe raised the question of whether his competitiveness with his father in his early years may have been what led to his father's financial and emotional decline. In his eyes his father went from being a successful businessman to becoming a weak, depressed, and "castrated" man. He felt his mother had "wiped out" his father and that all women used and abandoned men. He suddenly had the urge to run from therapy, stating that he was beginning to feel "queer." When I asked him what those feelings were, he said that he was feeling sexual feelings toward me and other men. I educated him about the difference between homosexual feelings and being homosexual. He was then able for the first time to directly deal with his confusion around his own sexual identification. His associations raised his concern about whether it was better to be a weak, passive man like his father but nonetheless "a man" or an active, alert, bright, powerful person like his mother. He then recalled the nature of his panicked feelings just prior to starting analysis, after he almost drove his car off a cliff. He reported how he had knocked out the older man who had befriended him after the man made homosexual overtures toward him. In subsequent sessions, he suggested that he thought he had used barbiturates for something other than only ameliorating his depression. He now believed that all those years he had also used barbiturates as a means of "covering up" his homosexual feelings. He recalled how, when he was ten years old, he had become involved in mutual masturbation with a watchman on a construction job near his home. He had kept secret from his parents the fact that he had gone back several times to "hold the man's penis." In fact, what he told his parents was that the man had tried to molest him. Subsequently, the man was arrested by the police. All those years, he carried a sense of guilt for that for which he had felt responsible.

My intervention was primarily educational. I told him that the man— and not Joe—was guilty of taking advantage of a young boy; that a boy's sexual curiosity and his interest in a man's penis was a normal feeling; that the man should have controlled his impulses. Joe associated to several instances in which, as a child, he had been ridiculed by his girl cousin when having an erection. He wondered if he was a "homo." I continued to underline the difference between homosexual feelings and being homosexual. This helped him relate his feeling about his childhood friend Jeff. Jeff was his friend—and later rival—in town. They acted out "who could sleep with more older women in the neighborhood?" Jeff had been his "closest buddy" from age six through twelve. One day, at age twelve, Joe hugged Jeff and kissed him on the cheek the way he had often kissed his father. Jeff screamed and called him a "queer." That ended their friendship. Joe soon anxiously expressed homosexual feelings toward me. I educated him about love between fathers and sons and love between men and their male friends. I explained to him that such love feelings often have sexual components but do not result in sexual actions and do not make the men or boys "queer." I told him that fantasies about sex were not the same as sexual acts. Joe then recalled how his adoptive father let his genitals "rest" on Joe's thigh when the boy occasionally slept in the father's bed prior to age twelve. After these memories came up in the analysis, Joe was able to go on to sort out many of his feelings about men, women, youth, and adulthood.

Conclusions

The analytic treatment of the adolescent frequently requires parenting, education, and guidance in addition to genetic reconstruction and interpretation. In fact, genetic reconstruction with adolescent patients most often follows parenting, education, guidance, and reassurance activities by the therapist.

When the family is not providing the necessary parenting structure, family therapy intervention should aim at helping the parents to carry out their parental supportive roles. If parents are unable to respond appropriately, some authors would argue against the analyst carrying out parenting and educational roles. They might say that such activity was not analysis. Regardless of the treatment approach, an adolescent always needs some teaching, parenting, and guidance. The adolescent is developmentally not fully responsible for his or her own developmental strides, especially in the face of fixation or regression. An adult may have many neurotic problems but, at least, is considered developmentally responsible for himself. For such adults, the analyst's parenting and guidance can become a detour. However, for the adolescent, such guidance becomes—not a detour—but the pathway to insight and growth.

NOTE

Presented as keynote address at the Sixth Pan American Forum on Adolescent Psychiatry, February 24, 1983, Mexico City.

REFERENCES

Blos, P. 1962. *On Adolescence.* New York: Free Press.
Erikson, E. 1968. *Identity: Youth and Crisis.* New York: Norton.
Mahler, M. 1968. *Human Symbiosis and the Vicissitudes of Individuation.* New York: International Universities Press.
Toews, J.; Martin, R.; and Prosen, H. 1981. The life cycle of the family: perspectives on psychotherapy in the adolescents. *Adolescent Psychiatry* 9:189–198.
Williams, F. S. 1973. Family therapy: its role in adolescent psychiatry. *Adolescent Psychiatry* 2:324–329.

10 PSYCHOTHERAPY WITH ADOLESCENTS: THE ART OF INTERPRETATION

JOHN L. SCHIMEL

The notion of interpretation in psychoanalytic theory and practice is close to its dictionary definition: an explanation of that which is obscure (Webster 2). Freud (1900), in *The Interpretation of Dreams*, presented the thesis that explanations (interpretations) of unconscious material result in their being uncovered. This, along with the remembering of early traumatic events and forbidden wishes, leads to recovery. In his study, Freud did not dwell on the style or manner of interpretations—or, for that matter, with the style or manner in which the dreamers' words and affect were reported. In some instances, only a summary of the dream was offered. Such matters also were not emphasized as the study of psychodynamics became more sophisticated and the fate of interpretations was presumed to be related to resistance and transference.

Many of the debates of the time dealt with the meaning of the dream, other symbols, symbolic behaviors, and notions of their correct interpretation, as in the commentaries of Stekel (1943). An early exception, however, was the work of Aichhorn (1925) in *Wayward Youth*. His writings are of particular interest to us since he dealt with adolescence and left glowing testimony to the importance of knowing how to relate to and talk with adolescents. Adler (1956), whose social concerns led him to be one of the first to become involved in child guidance and schools, also noted the importance of the form as well as the content of communications with the young.

What was to be interpreted was also an issue. This is a primary concern for many. For the early Freud (1903), the vicissitudes of instincts and

intrapsychic phenomena were central. Reich (1933) stressed the importance of the psychoanalysis of the character defenses, customary modes
of feeling and relating, as a prerequisite to the analysis of the intrapsychic. Sullivan (1954) focused on the psychoanalysis of interpersonal
factors from both historical and current perspectives. He stressed the
importance of the form as well as the substance of the communications of
both patient and therapist and offered numerous suggestions regarding
the function of various modes of interacting with patients.

Transference-Countertransference in
Adolescent Psychotherapy

A therapist is concerned with acquiring skill in understanding: what the
patient is telling him or her; how the patient is affecting him; how the
patient sees and experiences him; what the patient expects from him both
consciously and unconsciously; what has happened to the patient in the
past and what is happening to him in the present; and how the patient
feels from moment to moment during the interview. The psychotherapist
who works with adolescents also must develop skills in understanding
certain pertinent but less immediately relevant matters—such as the
genetics of the situation; the psychodynamics involved. He also needs to
gauge accurately the effect on the patient of further listening (not necessarily beneficial), of his talking, and of other behavior.

For example: An adolescent patient complains bitterly about the fact
that her parents disapprove of her boyfriend. They are unfair, and,
anyway, she is old enough to choose her own friends. She does not like
their friends either, but she does not try to choose their friends for them.

What do we know from this prototypical encounter between adolescent and therapist? We know that the patient is demanding that the
therapist ally himself with her against her parents, that she sees him as an
adult authority to whom she can appeal, and that she expects or hopes for
sympathy and agreement. This is not the first such encounter with her
parents, nor will it be the last. Sooner or later the therapist will walk a
tightrope on this and other matters. At some point, the patient will be at
least tempted to leave treatment—a prospect more easily contemplated
than leaving her home or her boyfriend.

The therapist observes and feels her near-panic state, recognizing her
massive denial of her own doubts about the boyfriend. He knows that her
mother's remark, "There is more to a relationship than sex," has inten-

sified the rage, self-doubt, and self-loathing in his patient. He inwardly weighs further silence against another form of intervention. He intervenes with a counterprojective maneuver. This is a term that Havens (1976) uses to describe a type of intervention, recommended by Sullivan, when the patient is already in or is likely to be propelled into a highly defended position. The action is moved out, away from the protagonists (therapist and patient) to more or less hypothetical third persons:

T: It is unfortunate that your parents interfered.

P: They mess into everything.

T: Lots of times, when that happens, young women marry out of spite or defiance. [The therapist has attempted to introduce the subject of young women and their parents, rather than this particular young woman—a counterprojective technique.]

P: I know what you're up to. You're just like them, only sneakier. You know I have doubts about John, but that's my problem. I have doubts about everything and everybody. John's different. He's OK. He's nice to me. He's everything a girl could want—lots of the girls want him. But he loves me.

T: You sound like a tigress defending her young.

P: Pretty fancy interpretation. But you're right; I feel fierce.

The following hour, the patient complains bitterly about the way one of her teachers has been treating her and her girlfriend; it is unfair and unjust:

T: This sounds like a rerun of the last hour.

P: What do you mean?

T: It's the same story, just a different cast of characters.

P: You're awful, but it sounds right. It's true that I'm angry a lot of the time and I'm always defending myself or my friends. But I don't get the connection. What are you up to? It's got nothing to do with me and John. What I said is still true. My mother is a bitch and John is OK. All right, you're right. I'm always angry, and here I am mad again with you this time. But what does it mean? I don't get the connection. What does it mean?

T: It means that there are parallel processes at work.

P: (laughs) You're smart today.

[At the end of the hour, as she is leaving, she again turns to the therapist and demands:]

P: All right. It's raining and I lost my umbrella today. What does that mean?

T: I see you're itching to have a go at me, too, but it probably means that you don't carry an umbrella when it's not raining.

P: (laughs) You're very smart today.

What has been happening and what is relevant to the art of interpretation? We must reconsider the notion of interpretation as an explanation of that which is obscure. No interpretation, in that sense, occurred. Something did occur, however, that will make the acceptance of future explanations more likely; a preparation for future interpretations.

Confrontation with the adolescent patient has occurred. Technically, confrontation is the bringing of some aspect of the patient to attention, without explanation. This was done repeatedly. Among the matters confronted, without explanation, were the fact of the patient's own doubts about her boyfriend and other matters, her pattern of rages, her preoccupation with justice and injustice, her clinging and demanding (infantile) behavior, and, perhaps especially, her utilization of denial in dealing with conflictual intrapsychic and/or interpersonal material.

The excerpts illustrate a process of clarification rather than explanation; an exercise in consensual validation between therapist and patient. There is a subtle collusion between patient and therapist. They are playing a game. The patient repeatedly tries to convert the psychotherapist to open support of her position. The therapist refuses. She counters with a defiant challenge to engage him in an argument. The psychotherapist sidesteps this challenge. The patient applauds him. The psychotherapist has introduced a note of playfulness forgotten by the patient, a relationship that her neurosis has precluded previously. The art of the psychotherapeutic encounter lies precisely in such matters.

The therapeutic encounter can be conceptualized as an engagement between two people in which one or the other may operate, from time to time, in a regressed fashion, expressed as resistance or transference manifestations. But this is not quite adequate for our review of the excerpted material. Sullivan's (1954) notion of "the other people in the room" is more helpful. Here is the adolescent (or is it the infant?) warring with authority in the person of the therapist, screaming a challenge:

"What does it mean?" He is the authority, pontificating: "It is unfortunate that your parents interfered." There is also the adolescent who is thoughtful and, one might say, mature, remarking, "It's true; I am angry a lot of the time and I'm always defending myself or my friends." There is the psychotherapist who is less an authority than a thoughtful listener: "You sound like a tigress defending her young." And, there is the adolescent who is an irreverent peer, competitive, and at times, admiring: "Pretty fancy interpretation," and "You're smart today." Here, she is responding to the psychotherapist as competitor who obviously enjoys both her challenges to his authority and his own one-upmanship in those situations.

So we have many people in the room, alternating rapidly, even kaleidoscopically. The pair that bear the main therapeutic burden consists of the thoughtful psychotherapist and the thoughtful patient. The psychotherapist must also utilize his alter ego, expressing authority or competitiveness as indicated. The patient is burdened by her clinging, dependent, demanding infant and rebellious defiant adolescent impulses. While there may be occasional indications for the psychotherapist to exercise his authority or even, on rare occasions, to attempt to discipline his patient, his goal should always be to foster the collaboration of the two thoughtful people in the room.

The interpretation, or, rather, the introduction of an interpretation with adolescent (or other) patients before such a therapeutic alliance is established, often leads to an impasse. The therapist may be completely convinced of the correctness of his interpretation, but the interpretation seems wrong, useless, meaningless to the patient, and, in any event, painful. The resistance interpretation, consoling as it may be to the psychotherapist, simply adds insult to injury for the adolescent patient. Such unresolved confrontations may result in regression to an infantile emotional level manifested by primitive expressions of rage, tearfulness, fearful clinging, or other symptomatic behaviors. Such situations may result from various interventions, including inappropriate silences and premature and other frightening interpretations. Although there may be, as a consequence, the production of suppressed and/or repressed material, the situation approximates that described in Freud's (1910) article on "wild" psychoanalysis. The therapist may be pleased with the deep material uncovered, but it may be experienced as a calamity by the patient.

Greenson (1978) has noted that the procedures of psychoanalysis may

182

seem odd, artificial, and irrational to the patient. This is particularly true for many adolescent patients. I have noted elsewhere (Schimel 1974) the negative therapeutic responses of adolescent patients to strictures against the answering of even innocuous questions, the requests of patients for orientation to the psychotherapeutic process, and the exchange of greetings and pleasantries. I have also noted the importance of the choice of language, the function of the element of surprise, and the timing of interventions. Greenson further notes, "Facility in selecting the right word or language is similar to what one observes in story tellers, humorists, or satirists. I am stressing verbal dexterity rather than literary ability." Alexander (1964) once remarked that, in psychotherapy, "what you plan to do depends upon how good an actor you are." He referred not to pretending but to the degree that thoughts and emotions can be communicated meaningfully and with traction for patients. This is the art of interpretation—an essential element in the art of healing (Grotjahn 1957).

But let us return to our patient, now in a later stage of her treatment. She has become aware of her continuing tendency to integrate situations with others, including a subsequent boyfriend, in a manner in which any frustration of her wishes moves her to attack. She is now aware of her vigilance to any signs of vulnerability in herself to which others may respond with criticism or attack—as well as vigilance to areas of vulnerability in others whom she might attack when frustrated. She knows now that she tends to be blind to defects in others (denial) when things are going well. She knows that at those times her friends can do no wrong; her enemies can do no right. She has some appreciation, in a nontechnical sense, that her world is one of good or bad, black or white (splitting, if you will), and that this is a reflection of an early childlike cognitive and developmental level, a narcissistic orientation. At times, however, she is despairing in contemplating the repetition of infantile patterns.

P: I'm much better than I used to be, sometimes for days on end. I'm getting pretty good marks in school, too. But I still fly off the handle—and sometimes for no reason. OK, OK, I know there's always a reason. You've told me so often enough. But it feels like there's no reason. Like uncontrollable. I know, I know; you always want an example. Well, last night Mother walked into my room and I blew. I blew it. Ranting and raving. She hadn't done anything.

T: Black and white again. She's all right; you're all wrong.

P: Well, she's supposed to knock first. But I don't always blow when she comes in without knocking. She's hopeless, the original Snoopy.

T: So, something was different this time.

P: One plus one equals two. Sure. Yes, something was different. I was supposed to be studying and I was daydreaming—about Bill, I suppose. But she couldn't read my mind. Maybe I reacted as though she had. You once told me that children sometimes believe that their mothers can read their minds. But what if she did read my mind; what's to be ashamed of? It's the matter of intolerance again. I'm getting tired of it. I'm afraid of everybody and what they think of me. And I always imagine the worst. I'm just as bad. Sometimes I feel I don't really have a good word for anybody, at least not for very long. I should be more loving. I'm the most intolerant person in the world.

T: Congratulations.

P: You mean grandiose again! The most intolerant person in the world! OK, but what do I do? This whole thing stinks. I have to do something. What can I do?

T: You already have your own solution.

P: What's that?

T: You know: to become all-wise, all-knowing, all-loving.

P: The same shit again. That's what I expect from others. That's what I expect from myself.

Discussion

The foregoing excerpts were selected to illustrate an ongoing collaboration between patient and psychotherapist in which the interventions are more or less jargon free, even laconic, and in which there are elements of surprise for the patient in the twisting of perspective that permit the appearance of new dimensions of problem areas. Confrontation as a technique is continued. It may be apparent that interpretations—in the sense of explanations of that which is obscure—have been made and have been integrated. Ongoing interpretations are made as the material evolves, once the groundwork has been sufficient to permit collaborative use by patient and therapist. In this context, it may be seen that the psychotherapist's remark, "Black and white again. She's all right; you're all wrong," served to explain what had been obscure. The remark, in addition, served to focus the patient's attention in a particular direction. I believe that the matter of directed associations, Sullivan's (1954) term, is a matter for continual scrutiny by the psychotherapist. I do not believe that there is an escape hatch for the therapist in the notion of free association. Patients find direction in any event. I believe that the issue is one of heightened consciousness on the part of the psychotherapist of the effect of his interventions or presumed noninterventions. Freud once suggested that, when the patient became capable of free association, it was a signal that the therapy was completed.

The laconic or analogic form of the psychotherapist's interpretation does not spell out the psychodynamics for the patient but leaves work to do. The same reasoning applies to his humorous "congratulations" to the patient as a way of bringing to her awareness the grandiose posture she struck with her statement, "I'm the most intolerant person in the world." This matter of leaving work for the patient to do fosters the feeling of the two working together. Similar considerations apply to the use of anecdotes, humor, aphorisms, information giving about childhood modes of perception, and average expectable reactions of people in our culture generally. The patient is offered a conceptual tool, a generalized explanation that she can apply to one or, one hopes, to many situations in which she regularly finds herself.

This is a far different and more dynamic matter than the psychotherapeutic notion of waiting for the material to emerge. I believe that, for the alert psychotherapist, the material is always there. The question is one of timing and appropriate formulation. There is no safety in psychotherapeutic waiting, particularly with adolescent patients. This is not to obviate the exercise of respectful and prolonged listening when appropriate.

No solutions to the patient's problems have been or are currently offered, nor will they be. In fact, the circularity and interdigitations of the neurotic processes are constantly being explored and exposed. Meanwhile, the process of growth achieves a kind of inexorable momentum that is reflected in the content of the excerpts. The foregoing is not meant to preclude the possibility of offering information, coaching, or advice when indicated.

One note: Sullivan (1954) wrote that the supply of interpretations is always greater than the need. I hope this discussion has succeeded in suggesting that there are more important matters than the truth of interpretations. There is the crucial matter of laying the groundwork for interpretations and for the development of a collaborative working relationship with the patient generally. When this is successful, the patient has integrated, in part, the image of the thoughtful psychotherapist. In the final excerpt the patient repeatedly demonstrates that she is listening to herself with the third ear of the psychotherapist. She says, for example, "OK, OK, I know there's always a reason. . . ." Call this an observing ego, if you will.

Conclusions

The analogy of the psychotherapist to the chess player may be a useful one in considering the art of interpretation. Intervention may well be made when the therapist knows the patient reasonably well, with a foreknowledge of future interventions. This follows if our theories of personality and therapy have validity. The psychotherapist need be in no hurry with interpretations. They have to be made in stages as they become applicable and usable. They may have to be made in bits and pieces, endlessly repeated and extended to meet new situations as they arise. They must grow as the patient grows in order to be relevant to progressive developmental stages and the problems that attend them. While being prepared for surprises and detours, the psychotherapist nevertheless may have a clear appreciation of the route that the therapist and the patient must traverse. Human growth and development are relatively predictable and assured when the hindrances are progressively attenuated by the collaborative work of patient and therapist.

REFERENCES

Adler, A. 1956. In H. L. Ansbacher and R. R. Ansbacher, eds. *The Individual Psychology of Alfred Adler*. New York: Basic.

Aichhorn, A. 1925. *Wayward Youth*. New York: Viking, 1974.

Alexander, F. 1964. Quoted by M. Grotjah in *The Newsletter of the American Academy of Psychoanalysis* 8:6.

Freud, S. 1900. *The Interpretation of Dreams*. New York: Modern Library, 1938.

Freud, S. 1910. Observations on "wild" psycho-analysis. *Collected Papers* 2:297–304. London: Hogarth, 1933.

Greenson, R. R. 1978. *Explorations in Psychoanalysis*. New York: International Universities Press.

Grotjahn, M. 1957. *Beyond Laughter*. New York: McGraw-Hill.

Havens, L. 1976. *Participant Observation*. New York: Aronson.

Reich, W. 1933. *Character-Analysis*. New York: Orgone Institute, 1945.

Schimel, J. L. 1974. Two alliances in the treatment of adolescents: towards a working alliance with parents and a therapeutic alliance with the adolescent. *Journal of the American Academy of Psychoanalysis* 2(3): 243–253.

Stekel, W. 1943. *The Interpretation of Dreams*. New York: Liveright.

Sullivan, H. S. 1954. *The Psychiatric Interview*. New York: Norton.

11   THE MEANING OF CULTS IN TREATMENT OF LATE ADOLESCENT ISSUES

KENNETH M. SCHWARTZ

In the past decade a large number of North American youth have turned to charismatic religious groups or cults. Estimates of total U.S. membership range anywhere from three to ten million people, involved in more than 3,000 groups (Clark 1979). Despite the predictions of some, cults do not seem to be a passing phenomenon, and new groups spring up to replace old ones. Although not as numerous, reports of cult happenings, such as the mass marriage of over 4,000 members of the Unification church, still appear in the popular press.

Religion typically provides a special system of belief, worship, and conduct for its members. In the groups under consideration, members display unquestioning loyalty and complete obedience to a dominant charismatic leader or figure who makes absolute claims with respect to his divinity or omniscience.[1]

Although most cults are religious in nature, they need not be. Some proselytize a psychological scheme or philosophy with the same demands for commitment as a religious cult (Galanger 1982). Nor can these movements be easily placed in any one large category. Most of the groups popularly considered to be cults or fringe religions disavow these labels. Yet many of these groups share attributes. Common features include a hierarchical system with a strong figure(s) espousing an ideology that reduces ambiguities for a membership that is actively recruited. The new members subsequently become fervent followers and are preoccupied with the group, which provides unique meeting places, rules, and rituals. There is usually a similar length of stay with personal improvement the ultimate aim. In contrast to North American society, which espouses pluralism, cults are particularist and provide members with only a single reason for their existence. Differences among groups include the use by some of subterfuge in the recruiting, the amount of family ties or outside contacts permitted, and whether the group chooses to call itself a religion. Despite this, the essential matter is, not the orientation of the group or the acknowledgment of itself as a cult, but its practices.[2]

There is much controversy surrounding cults. Levine (1979, 1981) warns that "cults should not be seen as intrinsically evil or dangerous any more than they should be praised indiscriminately." Most of the literature thus far on cults has concentrated on descriptions of cult members and activities. It is generally thought that members are Caucasian, well educated, and from middle- and upper-class intact families. The majority of members are thought not to be more seriously disturbed than their peers. However, it is likely that the popularity of the groups is related to the fact that young people hope to obtain help in their attempt to deal with both normal and pathological conflicts.

Crucial to the understanding of the attraction of youth to cults is an understanding of the normal adolescent process, especially Erikson's (1963) developmental model, with the focus on the stage of identity versus identity diffusion. Erikson (1956) views the adolescent process as complete only "when the individual has subordinated his childhood identification to a new kind of identification which forces the person into choices and decisions which lead to a more final self-definition, role pattern, and commitment." Similarly, Blos (1967) views adolescence as the second individuation process involving the shedding of family dependence and the loosening of infantile object ties to become a member of the adult world.

Levinson (1978) describes in similar terms the two tasks of the early adult transition. The tasks are to terminate the adolescent life structure and to step into the adult world. Vaillant and Milofsky (1980) comment that adult independence derives from "identification and internalization of important childhood figures." Failure at this stage may lead to self-destructive behavior. Cults, in establishing rigid systems of beliefs and controls, take away individual responsibilities, thus preventing future growth and identity formation. Freed (1980) notes that cults create settings where the new member abandons his own identity and instead attaches himself to the group's.

Levine (1978), in his study of group members, comments that "identity resolution, a task they should have been well on their way to achieving or at least grappling with, was a long way off." Gitelson and Reed (1981) report "that the precommitment identity status among adolescent devotees was at either the moratorium or identity diffused level." Maleson (1982) points out that a cult's response to predisposing psychopathological needs involves addressing "severe conflicts over dependency or aggression." Spero (1982) sees members as "having a disposition towards regressive solutions of conflicts." Levine and Salter (1976) view cults as attracting youths who are experiencing distress such as "alienation, demoralization, and low self-esteem; their joining fulfills the needs of believing and belonging." Levin and Zegans (1974) understand the emergence of cults as an attempt of adolescents and young adults "to fashion a meaningful identity and consistent personal code of moral behaviour in a changing culture of uncertain values."

"Countercultists," rather than emphasizing the intraphysic pathology, point to the use of deception, indoctrination techniques, and brainwashing. Lifton (1981) stresses the similarity of the conversion process to techniques of thought control used by the Chinese during the Korean War.

Members leave the groups for a variety of reasons. Much has been written on deprogramming, a controversial method not without its dangers (Parke and Stoner 1977). Little, however, has been written on the clinical managment of cult members who present voluntarily for treatment, particularly with regard to the resolution of conflicts around leaving the group and reintegrating into society. This chapter includes a case report which describes the issues in working with a patient whose central development conflict was manifested in her association with a cult group.

Case Report

A, a twenty-four-year-old female, first presented for treatment with the complaint of anxiety attacks. Past history revealed that her conception was unplanned and her forty-four-year-old father died of leukemia shortly before her birth. From an early age she did not feel a part of her family. With her forty-two-year-old mother out working, she was looked after first by her grandmother and then, after she left following a dispute with the patient's mother, by a succession of baby-sitters. When she misbehaved, her mother would leave the discipline to her two teenage brothers who would, on occasion, pack her in a crate and threaten to send her away. She was a lonely and frightened child, who felt very small in a world of "grown-ups." When upset, she would cry out for her "daddy" to comfort her.

Her family tried to live as if her father had never existed. There were no reminders of him around the house. In order not to upset their mother, her brothers would warn her not to ask any questions about him. She recalls being taken to his grave and feeling guilty at being unable to weep, as she could not conjure up an image of what he was really like.

A obtained good grades in school and was fairly popular. Although unsure of which career she wished to follow, the patient entered university at age nineteen. She found the adjustment difficult and soon became frightened and unhappy. Disillusioned, she quit in her first year to marry a young, unemployed musician whom she had met only a short time before. She felt secure with him even though they shared little or no intimacy. After six months he abandoned her, leaving her panic stricken, and she returned home to live with her mother.

She traveled to Europe in an effort "to find herself." On her return, she unsuccessfully attempted to become reinvolved in the traditional Anglican church. Despite this, and excellent grades at university night courses, she experienced a sense of purposelessness and a sense of being alone.

With a friend, at age twenty-one, A attended a two-day workshop of a group whose programs were based on a mixture of fundamental Christian teachings, Eastern philosophy, and T-group techniques.[3] She felt swept up in the highly charged atmosphere and was easily persuaded to sign up both for the four- and seven-day workshops. During this period of warmth and studied attentiveness, she chased away any "negative" thoughts pertaining to the group and eagerly joined.

Immediately on joining, she began to work in the group office as a secretary and devoted all her free time to doing volunteer work for them. As well, in order to comply with the group's expectations, she became involved with a male member and moved into a community house. Although unhappy with her partner, she stayed because of her immense fear of disobeying the group's charismatic and authoritarian leader. With the leader's permission, she separated from this partner two years later. Still wishing to follow the rules of the organization, A immediately found another male member with whom to live. Since the leader suggested that there should be some marriages, several months later along with other couples she became engaged.

At this point she entered psychotherapy because of anxiety attacks. She feared the group's disapproval and kept secret her psychotherapy. The patient presented as a bright and charming twenty-four-year-old woman and did not show any disturbance of thought process, cognition, or affect. She expressed resentment about her whole life revolving around the group. However, she seemed reluctant to change her involvement lest she incur the wrath of the leader or her fiancé. Several weeks after the therapy began, she married.

She soon began questioning the group's practices, for "it did not seem to be practicing what it was preaching." She wondered if anyone else felt this way and questioned her husband's devotion, for it seemed directed more at the group. She considered therapy to be her primary link with the "outside world."

In the ensuing months, therapy focused on her displeasure with the group and her fears of leaving. This phase culminated in her resigning her position as group secretary and finding work elsewhere. She continued, however, to spend most of her free time on group-related activities and rarely saw her husband. She began establishing new friendships and some semblance of a life apart from the group. This increased the stress on the marriage. She felt less a part of the group and finally, at age twenty-six, left altogether. Her husband remained very devoted to the group and with its encouragement separated from her. Immediately she became involved with a co-worker who, according to her friends, was unsuitable for her. For the first time, she began coming late or missing appointments.

She continued with therapy and began to deal with other intrapsychic issues, such as examining her initial attraction to the group, her difficulties leaving, and her affair. Although she expressed caring feelings for her husband, she wondered whether there was any attraction to him outside of their previous common interest in the group. By establishing new interests and dating other men, she developed a sense of satisfaction with her self-sufficiency. Six months later, because of increasing demands and bizarre behavior by its leader, the group disbanded. Her husband, now out of the group, reapproached her. Unsure of what they had in common, they tentatively began dating. Several months later they decided to move back together, feeling a greater sense of intimacy.

Discussion

Prior to joining the group, A was experiencing feelings of low self-esteem and worthlessness. Attempts throughout her adolescence to make herself feel more attractive and popular were not supported by her mother. Derived from numerous similar interactions with her mother, she developed an image of herself as "bad," "ugly," and "dependent." Unsuccessful attempts at university and marriage reinforced this self-image. Similarly, as a child she believed herself to be a "brat" and responsible for driving away her grandmother and other caretakers, much as she had fantasized she was responsible for her father's death. Not having any opportunity to discuss these issues made it difficult for her to clear up these misconceptions. Her fear of being bad and causing people to leave or be sent away was reinforced unwittingly by her brothers' behavior of packing her in a crate, which symbolically represented a coffin. She became a clinging, compliant child who yearned for attention and love and was fearful of separations.

The home environment did not allow A any opportunity to mourn her absent father and to sort out fact from fantasy, and indeed, any mention of his existence was strongly discouraged. As a child she created an image of her father that would soothe her in times of distress and she continued to search for this father figure in later difficult periods. Her marriages, joining the cult, and finally her turning to psychotherapy perhaps represented such searches. The disturbing effect of object loss in childhood on adult personality structure when mourning has been interrupted and prolonged has been described by Fleming and Altschul (1963). Thus, the patient was encouraged to ask questions and collect as much information as possible about her father in order to reactivate the mourning work and facilitate resumption of arrested development. As well, this helped her finally construct a more realistic image of what her father was really like.

According to Masterson (1976), the achievement of ego autonomy via the normal separation-individuation process lays a foundation that enables the child to take on and master later developmental tasks. Life events that may represent a growth opportunity for the normal individual, however, can precipitate a clinical syndrome in those with a borderline personality disorder. As with many others with borderline symptomatology, A did not encounter difficulties till faced with the tasks of adolescence. After unsuccessful attempts at university, work, and intimacy, she continued to experience depression and general dissatisfaction with her life, common chief complaints in the better-adjusted borderline patients (Masterson 1976). It was at this point A became involved with the group through a friend. Others at this point turn to drugs, alcohol, or other types of more accepted groups, while some turn to psychotherapy. While in the group A was temporarily able to function with minimal impairment by symptoms by adopting a life-style enabling her to avoid the developmental tasks facing her. However, her getting married, an event usually signaling normal progression in the life cycle, even though to a fellow group member, uncovered her special vulnerability and reawoke latent conflicts leading to the onset of anxiety and depression related to her fear of being abandoned and difficulties with intimacy.

In the first phase of therapy, which was approached from the complementary models of Blos (1967), Erikson (1963), and Masterson (1976), the patient attempted to establish a trusting and significant attachment with the therapist. She was fearful of being abandoned by the therapist or causing the therapist to abandon her, in the same manner she fantasied had occurred with her father, her husband, and the group leader. This became apparent early in therapy, when the therapist went on a short vacation and the patient experienced a recurrence of anxiety attacks. The therapist increasingly served as a lifeline to the rest of the world, preventing her from being completely submerged by the cult.

The formal structure of therapy afforded the patient an opportunity to test out her concerns in a safe, nonintrusive setting in the presence of a benign, nonauthoritarian therapist. In contrast, her group's encouragement of externalizing any difficulties and warding off doubts by rituals precluded self-examination. Maleson (1982) has remarked that insight-oriented psychotherapy is "exceedingly difficult when cult commitment remains strong and psychic conflict is perceived as a spiritual deficiency having external sources and solutions."

Although she perceived the group to be helpful initially, she became more aware of the group's shortcomings and of the increasing demands, be they for time, money, or loyalty. Like many other cult members, although disillusioned, she had difficulty leaving. Her regressive dependence on the group for her sense of identity and purpose permitted her to retreat and block engagement in the developmental tasks that faced her. Any move toward separation brought on associated feelings of anxiety, depression, and abandonment.

In treating this type of patient, the therapist actively concentrates on the patient's doubts and resistances to leaving. In this process, the therapist should avoid colluding with the patient's passivity and reluctance to explore painful feelings which are reawakened by the therapeutic focus on the issues of separation and individuation. In accordance with Blos's (1967) view of the normal adolescent process, the patient should be

194

assisted in a regression to an earlier developmental stage in the service of future ego development.

The therapist empathically supported the development of autonomous ideas and behavior. The patient needs to verbalize and examine doubts about the group, feelings of shame regarding joining, and feelings of loss on leaving. Having retraversed this developmental stage of autonomy versus shame and doubt that addressed issues of ambivalence, the patient found the will to leave the group. First she quit her job as group secretary and took the initiative to find work elsewhere. Life now had a purpose apart from the group. Work (industry) provided her with an opportunity to rebuild her sense of competence and take the first step toward establishing an identity separate from the group's. With a firmer sense of identity, the patient no longer needed to engage in "role repudiation" and was able to take tentative steps toward the next stage of development: intimacy (Erikson 1963).

As she became less involved with the group, she established a closer relationship with the therapist, who dealt with her fear of forming yet another attachment involving the loss of her sense of identity and separateness. As well, the therapist remained active, dealing with the patient's guilt about leaving the group and its leader, her fear of their relationship, and her uncertainty as to how she would manage in the outside world—a world she had largely given up. She was able to construct a new view of the world, enabling her to finally leave. This entailed the risk of losing her husband, who continued to be very closely tied to the group.

Therapy supported the patient's separation from the group, her living on her own, and her regaining a sense of personal identity. On the other hand, the therapist served as the object of the patient's wishes to be taken care of. The therapist in the transference came to function as the empathic mother who allowed her child to separate and be her own individual who would not need to rely on a group or ultimately on a therapist. The therapist needs to be empathically aware of the patient's turmoil over separation-individuation and be able to interpret in a way that would allow her to work through this issue at her own speed. The therapist must guard against becoming a substitute for the fantasied solutions to the patient's problems in the same manner as the cult. The therapist should only serve as a stable, sustaining, and continuing contact to whom the patient could voice her anxiety over developmental issues.

Away from the protection of the group and in defense against losses, the patient acted out her disappointment with the therapist by having an affair and missing appointments. Finally, having detached herself totally from the group, she experienced a tremendous surge of anxiety. She both wished for and feared that the therapist would take over, just as the group had done previously.

Her leaving represented an abandonment by the father and thus she turned to the mother and recapitulated the rapprochement phase with the therapist (Mahler 1968). Thus, the acting out in essence represented a rapprochement child testing her world, in this case, the transference, to see whether the therapist-mother would be harsh and judgmental and reject her or would encourage clinging behavior, thereby not letting her separate and leading to the child or patient feeling inadequate and bad.

The handling of this third phase of therapy became crucial as it afforded an opportunity for true intrapsychic exploration of the feelings being awakened by being out of the group and on her own. Spero (1982) has noted that the aim of psychotherapy with the cult devotee "is not simply an exit from the cult, but helping the patient to deal with the perpetual tendencies, ego conflicts, and object relational needs which have partially encouraged his attraction to regressive phenomena like cults." The therapeutic task required the enlistment of the patient's observing ego in order to reinitiate developmental progress. The patient needed to maintain her own separateness and sense of identity without succumbing once more to a more morbid type of attachment, as evidenced by her marriages and cult involvement.

After a number of months of psychotherapy that dealt with her developmental difficulties, and later after she had been on her own for some time, the patient was recontacted by her husband. He had also left the group. In this second trial of testing the marriage, A was better able to attempt to establish an intimate relationship.

Confusion, guilt, and frustrations can and do spring from both personal characteristics and social conditions, particularly in areas of instability that create fertile soil for "revitalistic" cults (Frank 1973). Joining a cult has been viewed as interaction among several factors: a disposition toward regressive solutions to conflicts, the overwhelming difficulties encountered in adapting to modern life, and the indoctrination techniques of cults designed to manipulate such variables (Spero 1982). Schwartz and Kaslow (1979) state that the strength of the father-child relationship appears to be a critical factor in the vulnerability/nonvulnerability of youth to cult recruitment. Those who have had a reasonably satisfying ongoing relationship with a strong father do not need to become part of an organization headed by an omniscient and omnipotent father figure.

Although the cult provides potential benefits of security in a group, the restricted life-style and total obedience to a rigid structure leads to lost opportunity for emotional, social, and intellectual growth in late adolescence or early adulthood. Psychotherapy can aid in the adjustment of youth who have turned to such groups and has been cited by Levin and Zegans (1974) as "suitable if not mandatory for successful deregression from cultic commitment." They state that "only with exploration of unsatisfactory object relations and other deficits in ego functioning, will one minimize the occurrence of subsequent recidivism to cult involvement." Schwartz and Kaslow (1979) advocate using group counseling and community-oriented approaches in conjunction with individual therapy in dealing with ex-cult members.

Despite clear differences between various groups, psychological issues in this patient parallel issues of members in more well-studied cults. Like many others, A turned to a cult at a critical period of her development. She was experiencing difficulty with the late adolescent tasks of individuation and identity formation. The group at first provided her with the support and solutions that more traditional methods (e.g., traveling abroad and involvement with traditional religion) did not.

A differs from others in that she lent only a part of herself to the group and retained another part that always questioned and observed closely the extent of her commitment. This personal strength allowed her to enter and use psychotherapy, despite being in a quasi-therapeutic organization, itself partly an offshoot of the human potential movement. The group she joined, although it frowns on continued contact with family or medical profession, did not insist on a total break with the outside. This perhaps explains her lack of cognitive and affective blunting as described in some long-term cult members (Clark 1979).

It is rare for a person so enmeshed in such a group to seek psychotherapy. It, therefore, provided a unique opportunity, a psychological window, to closely study and treat a member still involved in a cult. Most previous information has come from large studies of members by social scientists, from clinicians treating members referred with specific problems, or from books in the popular press (Conway and Stegelman 1978; Patrick 1976).

It is important to distinguish between group members such as this patient, who was able to retain her observing ego and engage in psychotherapy from members who are not, whether they are in a similar group or in one which imposes more stringent controls with regard to outside contacts. It is perhaps when the individual lacks an observing capacity and adequate self-differentiation that less attractive methods of removing a cult member, such as deprogramming, are attempted. Unfortunately, when attempts to separate are unsuccessful, members cling more strongly to the cult.

Some members stay on in a group and, according to Singer (1979), are gratified to "submerge their troubled selves into a selfless whole." In contrast, Ungerleider and Wellisch (1979) found that some cultists leave voluntarily because their "needs were less intense for safe, structured, predictable environment which would permit relatively conflict-free emotional affiliation with others." Levine (1984) views the "radical departure," that is, the joining of a cult, as a "rehearsal for separation" and feels that most members leave the group within two years better psychologically prepared "to try the painful thrust into adulthood for real." It is likely that issues such as the individual's capacity for self-observation, the needs the cult is meeting, and the methods employed by the group to discourage members from leaving all need to be taken into account.

Conclusions

It is perhaps crucial to distinguish between members such as this particular patient who, though burdened by developmental difficulties, are using cults to help deal with normal adolescent issues and who could more readily benefit from psychotherapy from those more seriously disturbed members who, in a more pathological manner, use the cult as a retreat. This chapter presented a patient who did well. Perhaps this could have been predicted from her life history. For example, her trip abroad, her turning to traditional religion, her joining the cult, and finally her seeking psychotherapy all can be viewed as representing internal thrusts to attempt to deal with the normal adolescent issues of separation, individuation, and identity formation. Unlike cults, therapy can aid these particular types of youth by addressing their developmental issues in a nonauthoritarian and growth-enhancing manner. One such therapeutic approach has been outlined. Further intensive study and treatment of individual cult members will ultimately lead to a better understanding of normal adolescent process.

NOTES

The author thanks Drs. Saul Levine, Elsa Marziali, and Stephen Signer for their kind assistance.

1. Jewish Community Relations Council of Greater Philadelphia: The Challenge of the Cults. January, 1978.
2. Personal communication, Dr. S. V. Levine, 1983.
3. D. G. Hill, June 1980. *Government of Ontario: Study of Mind Development Groups, Sects and Cults in Ontario: Report to the Attorney-General's Office.*

REFERENCES

Blos, P. 1967. The second individuation process of adolescence. *Psychoanalytic Study of the Child* 22:162–186.
Clark, J. G., Jr. 1979. Cults. *Journal of the American Medical Association* 242:279–281.
Conway, E., and Stegelman, J. 1978. *Snapping.* New York: Lippincott.
Erikson, E. H. 1956. The problem of ego identity. *Journal of the American Psychoanalytic Association* 4:56–121.
Erikson, E. H. 1963. *Childhood and Society.* 2d ed. New York: Norton.
Fleming, J., and Altschul, S. 1963. Activation of mourning and growth by psychoanalysis. *International Journal of Psycho-Analysis* 44:419–431.
Frank, J. 1973. *Persuasion and Healing: A Comparative Study of Psychotherapy.* Baltimore: Johns Hopkins University Press.
Freed, J. 1980. *Moonwebs: Journey into the Mind of a Cult.* Toronto: Dorset.
Galanger, M. 1982. Charismatic religious sects and psychiatry: an overview. *American Journal of Psychiatry* 139:1539–1548.
Gitelson, I. B., and Reed, E. J. 1981. Identity status of Jewish youth pre- and post-cult involvement. *Journal of the Jewish Community Service* 57:312–320.
Levin, T. M., and Zegans, L. S. 1974. Adolescent identity crisis and religious conversion: implications for psychotherapy. *British Journal of Medical Psychology* 47:73–82.
Levine, S. V. 1978. Fringe religions: datas and dilemmas. *Adolescent Psychiatry* 6:75–78.
Levine, S. V. 1979. Role of psychiatry in the phenomenon of cults. *Canadian Journal of Psychiatry* 24:593–603.

Levine, S. V. 1981. Cults and mental health: clinical conclusions. *Canadian Journal of Psychiatry* 26:534–539.

Levine, S. V. 1984. *Radical Departures: Desperate Detours to Growing Up.* New York: Harcourt, Brace, Jovanovich.

Levine, S. V., and Salter, N. E. 1976. Youth and contemporary religious movements: psychological findings. *Canadian Psychiatric Association Journal* 21:411–420.

Levinson, D. J. 1978. *The Seasons of a Man's Life.* New York: Knopf.

Lifton, R. J. 1981. *Thought Reform on the Psychology of Totalism.* New York: Norton.

Mahler, M. S. 1968. *On Human Symbiosis and the Vicissitudes of Individuation.* New York: International Universities Press.

Maleson, F. G. 1982. Dilemmas in the evaluation and management of religious cultists. *American Journal of Psychiatry* 138:332–344.

Masterson, J. F. 1976. *Psychotherapy of the Borderline Adult: A Developmental Approach.* New York: Brunner/Mazel.

Parke, J. A., and Stoner, C. 1977. *All God's Children.* Radnor, Pa.: Chilton.

Patrick, T. 1976. *Let Our Children Go.* New York: Dutton.

Schwartz, L. L., and Kaslow, F. W. 1979. Religious cults, the individual and the family. *Journal of Marital and Family Therapy* 5:15–26.

Singer, M. T. 1979. Coming out of the cults. *Psychology Today* 12:72–82.

Spero, M. H. 1982. Psychotherapeutic procedure with religious cult devotees. *Journal of the Nervous and Mental Diseases* 170:332–344.

Ungerleider, J. T., and Wellisch, D. K. 1979. Coercive persuasion (brainwashing), religious cults, and deprogramming. *American Journal of Psychiatry* 136:279–282.

Vaillant, G. E., and Milofsky, E. 1980. Natural history of male psychological health. IX. Empirical evidence for Erikson's model of the life cycle. *American Journal of Psychiatry* 137:1348–1359.

12 TRAUMATIC CONTRIBUTIONS IN THE DEVELOPMENT OF AN OBSESSIONAL NEUROSIS IN AN ADOLESCENT

LORETTA R. LOEB

In 1905, Freud in his *Three Essays on Sexuality* outlined the development of the sexual drive from infancy to adulthood. Freud defined the sexual drive as an instinctual force that seeks gratification and influences both behavior and thoughts. Basic bodily needs of the infant are accompanied by pleasurable sensations, and the gratification of these needs becomes an end in itself and introduces an erotic quality. Freud considered these pleasurable sensations to be sexual gratifications. He used the term libido to refer to the quantitative measure of energy of this sexual drive.

A developmental sequence of phases of libidinal (or sexual) erotogenic zones and behaviors, beginning in infancy and continuing on into adulthood, were found by Freud (1905) to exist in normal psychosexual development. These phases overlap, and the transition from one phase into the next is very gradual. For the first year and a half of life, the mouth, lips, and tongue are the organs of satisfaction. In the next year and a half, the anus and the surrounding areas become the leading zones of erotic pleasure. Gratification is now achieved both through the function of excretion and its eventual mastery. In the third year of life, the genitals assume the leading sexual role as site of gratification and continue in this role thereafter. For both sexes, this phase of development has been called the phallic phase. In the fourth or fifth year of life, during the oedipal phase, the child's three earlier phases of psychosexual development—the oral, the anal, and the phallic—merge into a wish for gratification from the parent of the opposite sex. Following puberty there is a wish for the attainment of mutual sexual gratification with a new partner of the opposite sex; and when this is eventually accomplished, the genital phase of development is attained (Freud 1905; Brenner 1955).

During each of these phases of development, the child's aim is to seek gratification from a person, a sexual object, toward whom its drive is directed (Freud 1905). The first object is the mother, then both parents are objects, and next the parent of the opposite sex is primarily desired. In the normal course of adolescence new objects other than the parents are sought and found.

In each early phase of development, the child's instinctual wish for gratification may come into conflict with a parent's desires. According to Anthony (1967), this external conflict between the parent and the child can be resolved without psychological trauma to the child. He stated that the prognosis is good that the child will work through such conflicts with further development: (1) if earlier developmental phases have proceeded peacefully; (2) if the parents are more helpful than harmful; and (3) if constitutional factors are slight. Most children make the helpful demands of their parents part of themselves by a process of internalization, and these demands are then used by the children to manage their own instinctual (id) wishes so that they can proceed to the next developmental level. This internalization of the parents' desires leads to the gradual formation of the child's superego, which is nearly completed by the end of the phallic-oedipal phase. Once this process of internalization is completed, the child can seek resolution of these former conflicts with the external world within its own mind.

Because of the internalization of these conflicts, an abnormally persistent attachment may occur to the original, phase-specific, object(s) and/or modes of gratification that were associated with the initial external conflict. These abnormally persistent attachments are called fixations and become the individual's primary object(s) and/or mode(s) of gratification. Because of these fixations, the child may not seek new modes of gratification or new objects at the next level of development and, hence, may proceed forward with only partial success in his or her handling of the normal developmental conflicts at the next psychosexual phase. The gratifications attained at each phase of development are never completely abandoned, even if fixations do not occur (Brenner 1955).

The child learns there are dangers associated with the attainment of gratification during each of the psychosexual phases (Freud 1915). These dangers have their origin in fantasies about, and memory traces of, actual childhood experiences. The memories of many of these danger situations, whether or not fixations have occurred, are repressed and thereafter remain in the child's unconscious. The typical danger situation that accompanies the gratifications of the oral phase is a fantasied fear of the loss of the loved one on whom the child is dependent. The real or fantasied anger and disapproval of the parent(s) during the anal phase can result in the fear of parental loss in the child. In both sexes, the fears concomitant with the achievement of genital gratification during the phallic phase are associated with fantasies of parental disapproval together with fantasies of the loss of, or damage to, the genitals. During the oedipal phase, thoughts of oedipal gratification with the parent of the opposite sex lead to fears of disapproval from the parent of the same sex. The child responds to and manages this fear by patterning his behavior after the prohibitions he thinks exist in the parent of the same sex. He incorporates this pattern into his ego as a moral conscience (superego) (Freud 1933). A signal of impending danger, experienced as anxiety, now replaces his fear and then alerts the child to past fantasied and real dangers when he desires the wished for, but prohibited, gratifications he had wished for or experienced during each of his prior phases of psychosexual development (Freud 1926). This anxiety occurs, even when his parents are not present, whenever his unconscious instinctual wishes come into conflict with his now incorporated and unconscious parental prohibitions.

Eventually, as the child works out these normal childhood instinctual conflicts, defensive ego patterns develop that allow either a degree of acceptable direct gratification or a modified expression of the instinctual drive called a sublimation (Freud 1915).

Unfortunately, real losses such as deaths or separations can occur during a child's early development. Furman (1974) found that many children are able to comprehend death and mourning following the loss of a loved object in spite of the immaturity of their thought processes. These children do not necessarily have residual problems for many factors, from within and from without the child's personality, influence the outcome. Among these factors are: (1) the child's instinctual impulses, defensive measures, and attendant anxieties at each developmental phase; (2) the nature of his experiences with death; (3) his adaptation to, or identification with, adult attitudes toward death; and (4) the amount of correct or incorrect information he receives. If the child is not alone in his struggle with the frightening experiences of death and does not arrive at confused conclusions about death, he tends to be able to mourn successfully. If these aids to normal development are not available to these children (Anthony 1967), they use defense mechanisms to aid them in handling their loss. These defense mechanisms, however, according to Furman (1974) impede the process of mourning. Laufer (1966) also stated that object loss itself is not pathogenic but can become the nucleus around which earlier conflicts as well as other unconscious conflicts are organized.

Earlier conflicts take form and later become organized when the balance between the instinctual drive and the normal defensive patterns are traumatically disturbed. Then the repressed drives tend to reenter consciousness; and intense anxiety, beyond the level of a signal, is perceived by the individual. To subdue this anxiety, a compromise between the repressed drives and the superego's defensive patterns results in a disguised, partial (or substitute) gratification of the instinctual wish in the form of a neurotic symptom. Such a psychoneurotic symptom allows the sufferer to avoid some of the anxiety (or superego guilt) that would accompany the undisguised breakthrough of the instinctual wishes (Moore and Fine 1968). The particular neurosis or illness that develops as a consequence of symptom formation is dependent on the nature of the neurotic conflict. This conflict is in turn determined by the interaction of the following factors: (1) the nature and strength of the external stress or traumas; (2) the force of the instinctual drives; (3) the specific defenses used against the instinctual drives; and (4) the strength and weaknesses of the character structure of the individual (Moore and Fine 1968).

Clinically, an obsessive-compulsive neurosis is formed when an individual is unable to resolve and deal with the conflicts he is confronted with during his phallic-oedipal phase of development and so regresses back to using the defenses he had employed to deal with conflicts he had experienced during his anal phase of development. These anal level defenses include isolation, reaction formation, and undoing. The obsessive-compulsive traits of ambivalence, magical thinking, and a rigid, sadistic superego—all major characteristics of a child's thinking during the normal anal phase—reappear with this regression to the fixations of the anal phase and enter into the neurotic syndrome (Moore and Fine 1968).

Characteristic of this neurosis are the unwelcome obsessive and compulsive symptoms. Obsessive thoughts repeatedly intrude into these patients' conscious minds and can be wishes, temptations, impulses, doubts, commands, or prohibitions. When the obsessions and the persistent and meaningless compulsive motor acts are prevented or interfered with in some way, these patients reexperience the anxiety that had been alleviated when the symptoms were first formed. Although these sufferers have some insight into the meaning of their symptoms, they are unable to control them and readily seek help (Moore and Fine 1968).

Clinical Case Study

A case will be presented of Lisa, a thirteen-year-old girl whose parents were unable to provide her with a model of how to deal with the multiple deaths and losses that she suffered during her oedipal and latency periods. In adolescence, her earlier object losses and her defenses against these losses became the nidus around which her earlier infantile conflicts eventually developed into a full-blown obsessive-compulsive neurosis. The analysis of this adolescent patient helped her discover the repressed infantile conflicts behind her obsessive-compulsive neurosis, and this permitted her to mourn, in the manner described by Fleming and Altschul (1963), the lost objects of her childhood.

EARLY DEVELOPMENT

Mother, forty-four, was an attractive, Protestant, only child of a wealthy mining family. Her mother bought her expensive clothing but spent little time with her. Although mother's father gambled, he always had time for Lisa and her mother. Lisa's father, also forty-four, was a handsome Catholic stockbroker. Mother described him as impatient, unhappy, and having a vulgar tongue. His father drank heavily, gambled, and died leaving his family destitute when Lisa's father was seven.

Lisa was born three years after her only sibling, a sister; father blamed his not having had a son on "bad luck." Lisa first walked, gave up her bottle, and refused milk at seven months. According to mother, toilet training was difficult. Lisa wore diapers past age two and one-half and never flushed the toilet. Mother has pictures of Lisa at three sitting on the toilet being toilet trained. Other than entering Lisa in swimming races, father, like mother, spent little time with Lisa; but, unlike mother, he was more aware of her needs and disciplined her. Lisa's earliest memories were: (1) flushing a diaper down the toilet at age three; (2) walking into the kitchen to see what mother was doing at age four; and (3) being permitted by her mother to stay up late against father's objections.

At age five, Lisa felt guilty that her maternal grandfather paid more attention to her than to her sister, that she was able to get away with not napping, and that she competitively won first place in games and swimming races. Lisa wanted to be punished but felt she successively avoided it. At age five, when her grandfather suddenly died, she did naughty things over and over again, but no one paid any attention or spanked her. Mother said that children were perfect and beautiful and would stay that way unless you spanked them. Only Granny occasionally spanked her. Following grandfather's death, Lisa stopped winning swimming races and games, began doubting things, and feared that "everything would go bad." At six, Lisa became self-conscious in her swimsuit and did not want to swim. She recalled sitting in her room, coloring, waiting for her father to come home.

Lisa remembered little about her mother's mother, Granny, who died when she was eight years old. Indeed she remembered little of her latency period except that she did not do as well in school after her grandmother's death, which she did not wish to discuss. According to her mother, Lisa began receiving psychiatric help when she was eight because of difficulty with peers and poor academic performance.

ADOLESCENT DEVELOPMENT

Lisa's father and mother separated when she was eleven years old. She and her sister would spend weekends with their father. Following a fight her sister had with their father, her sister refused to visit, and Lisa began spending weekends alone with her father. Although she did not want to, Lisa became father's confidante. She felt great sympathy when her father complained about how sad he was living alone. Lisa stayed with her father throughout the next summer. She spent her days cleaning his house, for she could not stand to have her father's house "scummy." After work, father would take Lisa out to dinner and a movie. Even though she had always disliked hearing her parents argue, she now began to wish her parents would get back together. During this summer her rituals began. Initially, she would have to open and close the kitchen cupboards in her father's house as a protection against losing her friends. Soon she found herself flushing the toilet five times and tapping five times whenever she went through a doorway. Because of her rituals she "became restless" and felt she should return home to her mother.

When her father returned to live with the family the following fall, he found Lisa preferred to sit alone in a semidark room, had trouble making and keeping friends, and was the last one chosen for school functions. Every night Lisa would now spend fifteen minutes before bed telling her mother repeatedly, "I love you, Mommy." Lisa did not wish to be separated from her mother. She would pry into her mother's whereabouts, activities, and phone calls, and she frequently wanted to sit in her mother's lap. Her mother wondered if this strange new behavior was Lisa's attempt to break away from her. Her mother considered Lisa's symptoms to be a means of keeping her at a distance.

Lisa was embarrassed when her menarche occurred at age thirteen. Her secondary sexual characteristics were slow in developing, but she was not aware of any development until her older sister insisted she begin wearing a shirt and not go bare chested. Other indications of Lisa's isolating her sexual and aggressive feelings were that she told gross, "dirty" jokes and began saying "ugly" hostile things, such as, "eat your shit" and "your chocolate frosting looks like dog pooh" without any expression of embarrassment. After saying such things to her mother, she would always add, "I love you Mommy." Although Lisa had received various types of treatment for these problems from age eleven to thirteen, her symptoms only intensified.

When Lisa entered eighth grade, silence terrified her, and she began having nightmares. Awaking from these dreams, she would go into her mother's bed. At school Lisa worked hard to maintain her grades and would not miss a day of school or do anything that would jeopardize her good grades in an advanced math class. Lisa was now also performing her rituals at school and felt they allowed her to keep her friends and to remain in a three-times-per-week ballet class. In spite of her rituals, Lisa's peer relationships deteriorated. She found herself more comfortable with grown-ups. As she realized she was doing strange things—her rituals and her prying into other people's affairs—her anxiety increased. It was apparent to Lisa and her parents that she was more interested in her mother's activities than in pursuing activities that were fitting to an adolescent. Lisa and her parents now sought help from the author.

COURSE OF THE ANALYSIS

In the first interview Lisa was quick to tell the author that behavior modification and other forms of therapy had failed because no one was going to tell her what to do. Lisa's mother had no awareness that her attractive, slender, well-dressed daughter was unconsciously grieving her many losses, but complained that Lisa sniffed everything, spoke crudely about bodily excretions and sexuality, and intruded into mother's activities. During the evaluation Lisa was embarrassed to discuss personal sexual matters, but her defense of isolation permitted her to swear and to tell "dirty" sexual jokes. She eagerly wanted the therapist to help her learn why she couldn't stop doing "funny things" (her compulsions), which gave her much pain and interfered with her social life and schoolwork. She also complained of difficulty making decisions and overconcern and anxiety about her mother's whereabouts.

Lisa was seen four times a week over a four-year period for the analysis of her obsessive-compulsive neurosis. From the beginning, as Lisa had feared, mother tried to interfere with the analysis by calling the therapist frequently to ask about her daughter. The necessity for confidentiality was explained, but mother continued calling. Lisa was informed of these calls; and this, together with her enjoyment of free association, her natural ability to understand mental phenomena, and her driving need to be rid of her painful symptoms, fostered a strong therapeutic alliance.

During the beginning of the analysis, Lisa transferred onto her therapist the battle over control she had had with her mother. Lisa positioned her chair in exactly the same place each session and objected to changes in her therapist, her therapist's office, or their schedule. She spoke rapidly, changed the subject, made messes in the office, verbally attacked her therapist, and timed the sessions. She eventually recognized these behaviors as attempts to control her therapist. She often insulted her therapist, and then she would compliment her. Analysis of a dream clarified this reaction formation for her. She told her father that her boyfriend had insulted her, and her father wanted to break his arm. That night Lisa dreamed her father and boyfriend were shaking hands. Chuckling insightfully she explained, "It's like my mother talks, and the way I act towards you," and she mocked mother's sweet mode of speech. She then expressed fear of being punished for her angry feelings.

Lisa eventually realized that her compulsions in the office, including her returning after her sessions many times to say good-bye, were both an expression of her anger toward her therapist and a magical defense to prevent her therapist from dying. This awareness of her anger diminished her obsessions and compulsions, but when she began expressing her anger directly to her mother, mother informed Lisa that if she didn't stop she would be sent away. Lisa again became "sweet" to her mother and her tapping increased, but she continued to be able to express anger with her therapist. Lisa saw how she had incorporated her mother's negativism and was expressing it toward both herself and her therapist. Lisa realized she had inhibited her anger because she feared being rejected for it. Lisa now saw that she made her therapist into a policeman and a rejecting person, but that her therapist was neither. This transference reaction was to protect her against her own feared impulses. Lisa then realized she had done this same thing with her mother. Once relieved of these superego restrictions, many long-repressed memories returned, and she began to remember things about her Granny.

Granny had controlled the patient's mother by hanging on to the family money. Lisa described Granny as an asexual lady who was clean, not fashionable, went to church, and was not competitive with her mother. Lisa had great love for Granny and had many times observed her mother being hostile to Granny. Granny set many limits on Lisa; for example, Granny made sure Lisa washed her feet before going to bed. Granny also made Lisa feel sex was bad and dirty, which led Lisa to desire punishment for her sexual impulses.

At Granny's funeral, when Lisa was eight, Lisa noticed that her mother was laughing and not crying. Lisa felt deprived of her limit-setting, caring Granny and felt sad to be without her. Lisa now began to hate being left alone by her mother. Lisa wondered how she might behave at her mother's funeral and immediately felt anxious at the thought that her mother could actually die. Following Granny's funeral, whenever she saw her mother crying, Lisa magically thought that if she, Lisa, cried, her mother would die like Granny did. After the age of eight, whenever Lisa's mother left Lisa alone or did not prepare her dinner, Lisa would feel anxious and would obsessionally have to ask herself three questions: (1) Is the house going to burn down? (2) Am I going to die? (3) Are the headhunters going to get me? Lisa also became horrified of matches and fire sirens. She no longer could light a match for, as we learned later in the analysis, she unconsciously wished that her mother's house would burn down and feared her impulse to set the house on fire.

As Lisa's repression lifted in the analysis, she recalled competing with her sister for her father and her disappointment when her sister was taken to Hawaii by mother's lady friend when Lisa had an appendectomy at age nine. Lisa had wished this lady dead and then, one year later, the lady died of a brain tumor. Recalling her appendectomy, she remembered she had had sexual fantasies about the rectal exam, and she also realized she had had fantasies about parental intercourse since age five. Thoughts of the lady's death led Lisa to realize that her grandmother's death when Lisa was eight precipitated her neurosis. The obsessional fears she had at the time of developing a brain tumor, going blind, and getting fat and dying were both punishments for her hostile wishes and identifications with her loving but strict grandmother, who was obese and going blind before she died.

Throughout the early and middle phases of the analysis, Lisa smeared food and makeup in the office and put her shoes and feet on the desk and in her analyst's face. She connected this behavior both to her ambivalent feelings toward her mother and to her wish for limits and gratification of her dependency wishes when her grandmother washed her feet. Analysis of this behavior made her aware of her wish to force her therapist, in the mother transference, to set limits on her. Lisa realized that her mother, out of guilt, covered her hostility toward Lisa by buying her expensive clothing and by not setting limits and that Granny had done the same thing to mother. Lisa now realized that she had become angry at her mother for not suffering at grandmother's funeral and that she had wished her mother had died instead of her Granny. These thoughts and feelings were first acted out in the transference neurosis. At these times she identified with her mother and acted angrily toward her therapist as her mother had toward her grandmother. After these sessions, she would leave and then anxiously return several times to say "good-bye" and be sure her analyst was still alive. Analysis of this undoing of her magical thinking during this middle phase of the analysis led Lisa to connect her grandmother's death to her parents' separation when she was eleven and to the development of her compulsions. Now, toward the close of the first year of the analysis, Lisa was able to recognize that she was repeating in the transference with her therapist the hostile battle for control that she had seen played out between her mother and her grandmother. Lisa's anxiety now diminished, and she was now able to clean her room for the first time since Granny had died six years before. She had been unable to do this because most of the things in her room had either been given to her by Granny or reminded her of her Granny. It was at Granny's funeral that her unacceptable wish that her mother die instead of her Granny began. Most of Lisa's symptoms had now abated, and she was able to relate to her father with less guilt. Lisa now clearly realized that her conflict was within herself and not between herself and mother or between herself and her therapist. Work on her internalized mother led to further resolution of the transference neurosis.

Lisa now recalled that, at eleven, she felt disgusted when she saw her mother passionately kiss a man who had previously kissed Lisa. Lisa realized she had repressed these memories because she had been sexually aroused and had feared her wish to take this man from her mother. In the transference Lisa relived her competitive feelings toward her mother. She would say her therapist was envious of her body and her clothing, and then complain that her own thighs were too fat. By so putting herself down, she unconsciously punished herself to please her therapist. She both wished to outdo her therapist and was guilty for this wish. She feared that her analyst would be competitive, like her mother, and put her down.

We learned that Lisa's guilt for her wish to outdo her therapist was also determined by her fear that her wish to outdo her sister had magically resulted in her sister's having developed a serious illness when Lisa was eleven. Lisa repeatedly tested her "magical power" in the transference neurosis; when it failed, she felt relieved. Lisa had dreams of being prettier than her therapist and of separating her therapist from her husband. It was now easy for Lisa to see how she was repeating with her therapist patterns of behaviors and thoughts she had had with her parents when she was much younger. She expressed the hope that her analyst would stop her from competing. After having such oedipal wishes toward her therapist, Lisa would regress back to the anal level and mess up her therapist's office. Her rigid sadistic superego would now turn on herself, and she would punitively put herself down.

At fifteen Lisa was able to return to spend the summer with her father without guilt or symptoms. However, Lisa continued to isolate her sexual feelings from her father. She had hostilely wished her parents would separate when she was little for her father was nicer to her than her mother. For this reason Lisa had felt she was responsible for the divorce. By sixteen, she experienced conscious sexual pleasure instead of disgust when she dated. This awareness allowed her to recall the frightening sexual feelings she experienced at age eleven when she lived alone with her father. She was given the only bedroom and continued to sleep naked as she had before her parents separated. Father, wearing only shorts, would sleep on the living room couch. After he thought Lisa was asleep, he would go to her bed and sleep on top of the covers. Lisa, pretending to be asleep, would look at her father and fantasize sexual activity with him. These thoughts made her feel anxious. She tried, without success, to substitute a boyfriend for her father in her fantasies. She then attempted to contain her anxiety by counting the five letters in this boyfriend's name. This is how her obsession to count to five began, and it spread to tapping five times, closing the door five times, and so forth. Gradually she had forgotten this incestuous, sexual origin of her compulsions.

During Lisa's third year of analysis, when she was sixteen, she tried to provoke her therapist into setting limits on her sexuality and her dating. Lisa called her therapist "Dr. Pubic" and told crude sexual jokes. Analysis of this behavior led to further understanding of the transference, which was to see her therapist as a grandmother or mother who set limits. Gradually Lisa came to understand these behaviors to be unconscious reenactments of her early memories of Granny's puritanical, asexual limits. They were also expressions of a wish to have her Granny guide and help her with the sexual feelings she was now dealing with in adolescence. Lisa's isolation of her sexual thoughts and feelings greatly diminished during the analysis once she recognized her need for the control this defense mechanism accomplished. She slowly was able to discuss her sexual feelings without disgust or guilt. Now that she was conscious of her feared sexual wishes, she was no longer overwhelmed by her drives and she now could control them consciously without compulsions. Lisa could now proceed with the major adolescent task of withdrawing her libido (removing her fixations) from her parents and seeking a new object for gratification. Her first boyfriends were either similar to her father or introspective like her analyst. Lisa spent many sessions comparing her behavior with her boyfriends with her mother's behavior and attitudes around and toward her father and stepfather. This enabled her to relinquish her intense attachment to her mother and, in her mind, separate herself from her mother. As Lisa became aware of her oedipal conflict, her attitude toward her parents became more realistic. She saw that her mother's needs were fulfilled by her marrying an older man and that father was afraid of aggressive, competent women like her mother.

Lisa's new individuation frightened her mother, who threatened to take Lisa's car away so that Lisa would be less autonomous. Without her former guilt, Lisa successfully persuaded her stepfather to intervene. Lisa now consciously compromised her own wishes in order to get along with her mother. She no longer accepted money and clothing from her mother. Getting a job was more ego syntonic for Lisa. Resuming ballet lessons, doing better at school, and taking up photography were further evidence of Lisa's ability to separate from her mother and individuate.

Lisa saw her therapist now as a friend from whom she did not fear retaliation. She laughed at having once seen her therapist as a weird "conscience and judge."

Finishing the analysis was an achievement for Lisa, because her past inhibitions had prevented her from completing anything. A date was set to finish in three months, but Lisa worried that she might unconsciously thwart herself. Indeed, Lisa's oedipal guilt resurfaced in the process of termination, and impulses to tap returned intermittently. In the transference neurosis Lisa again made her therapist a superego figure and sought punishment from her therapist whenever she visited her father. This enabled Lisa to work through her having internalized her ambivalent mother and the corrupt superegos of both her parents. She dreamed of driving off with her therapist's husband. This dream was different in that she allowed herself to win over her therapist. She stated she no longer needed to win her therapist's husband or her father but could get her own man. By discerning what she saw as mother's seductive qualities, Lisa could see how mother's behavior with Lisa's father and stepfather had put her into conflict. Mother reacted to Lisa's new strength and success in finishing her analysis by putting Lisa down. Lisa responded by letting her mother know that she never again wanted to be treated like a baby or be put down. Mother acquiesced.

Lisa saw that, in terminating the analysis, she could either separate from her therapist or be cared for by her therapist without guilt. In the last session she thanked her therapist and asked permission to hug her good-bye. She said she no longer feared regressive feelings or the loss of her autonomy, and so could freely express positive feelings to her therapist, a person she had formerly seen as her grandmother, her mother, and her father.

DISCUSSION

Lisa's developmental history, clinical picture, and transference to her analyst all evidenced that she had regressed from the oedipal phase back to earlier points of fixation that developed out of conflict during her anal-sadistic phase. At this phase she had already developed a sense of omnipotence and magical thinking, partially as a result of not having significant external limits set on her. By age five, she demonstrated a rigid, sadistic, and self-depreciating conscience. When her grandfather died during this oedipal phase, she became anxious, for she felt punished and retaliated against for having won her grandfather. Her oedipal guilt increased toward all her internalized, ambivalent, parental objects— especially her mother. The loss of her grandfather therefore enhanced her oedipal conflict, and she defensively regressed back to her earlier unresolved anal-sadistic conflicts and could no longer be successful and win races.

In his "Notes upon a Case of Obsessional Neurosis," Freud (1909) said that the defense of doubting occurs when, "The thought-process itself becomes sexualized, for the sexual pleasure which is normally attached to the content of thought becomes shifted onto the act of thinking itself, and the satisfaction derived from reaching the conclusion of a line of thought is experienced as a *sexual* satisfaction. . . . But procrastination in *action* is soon replaced by lingering over thoughts. . ." (p. 245). Freud went on to say that when a patient, out of oedipal anxiety, regresses to the anal-sadistic phase, the affects of the oedipal phase are isolated and repressed. The trauma, Freud said, instead of being forgotten, is deprived of its feelings.

Thus Lisa could consciously and without anxiety discuss the multiple losses in her life because the thoughts of these losses were isolated from and, therefore, devoid of feelings. She knew of her traumatic losses, but they had no affective significance for her. In the transference to her therapist, Lisa repeated the trauma of her losses and was then able to reexperience the formerly isolated feelings associated with these losses. It was as a result of her transference to her therapist that Lisa became aware of both her defenses and her unresolved conflicts. She became aware of the isolation, reaction formation, and undoing that she used to defend against her ambivalence, magical omnipotent thinking, and sexual and aggressive wishes.

Lisa had been able to maintain her unconscious, infantile, conflicted wishes in a state of relatively asymptomatic equilibrium until her grand-mother's death. Then Lisa could no longer keep her hostile, anal-sadistic impulses toward her mother from disturbing her conscious mind. When this hate emerged into consciousness, she had opposing feelings of love and hate for her mother and experienced intense anxiety. Lisa then developed exaggerated obsessional symptoms that were a conscious, unrecognizable form of her ambivalent love-hate feelings toward her internalized objects, particularly her mother.

Fleming and Altschul (1963), in their article "Activation of Mourning and Growth by Psychoanalysis," stated that psychoanalytic treatment could activate a delayed mourning process by facilitating the resumption of arrested development. Once Lisa was able to look at the anger she had experienced toward her mother at the time of her grandmother's funeral, she could see that this anger was only a feeling and not a deed. She also realized that just because she had had a hostile wish that her mother would die did not mean that it would happen. Lisa knew she really was not so omnipotent as to be able to have her mother die by wishing it. Yet the anxiety she felt when her unwelcome hostile wishes entered her conscious thoughts continued and perpetuated her defenses against these wishes. This was reenacted in the transference when she had angry thoughts toward her therapist and then compulsively returned five times to be sure that her therapist had not died. Once Lisa was able to see in the transference how her compulsions were connected to her hostile and sexual wishes and work this through, she was able to mourn her grandmother. She did this in the process of cleaning her room, which she had not cleaned since her grandmother's death. She went over and de-cathected each of grandmother's gifts to her and each item in her room that connected her with her grandmother and thereby put both her room and her mind in order.

Furman (1974) said, "The degree of ambivalence and the relationship with a dead loved one was particularly important." Lisa had more love than hate for Granny and identified with the limit-setting aspect of Granny that her own mother despised. As a result, this identification with Granny allowed Lisa to have an incorporated object that set a limit on herself. However, because of Lisa's early pathology, she became inhibited after her grandmother's death as a result of the conflict within herself between Granny's restrictiveness and mother's permissiveness. Lisa's love for Granny led her to identify with Granny, and manifestations of Granny's illness formed an important aspect of Lisa's self-representation. Furman also observed cases where this type of identification with the lost object was self-punitive. Furman mentions that the identification with the healthy aspects of the deceased loved one's personality were present alongside the pathological ones. As Furman stated, adults as well as children who suffer from unresolved conflicts have difficulty mourning, depending on the stage of development at which the loss occurred and the relationship they have with their surviving objects. Understanding the source of Lisa's concerns about dying, going blind,

215

and getting fat completed her mourning process for her Granny. Grandmother died when Lisa was in the third grade. Lisa's grades had been good until her Granny's death; then they precipitously fell because her obsessive thinking prevented her from concentrating. After she had mourned the loss of her grandmother and detached herself from her identification with her grandmother (and mother), Lisa's psychic energy was free to be reinvested in other things such as her schoolwork, ballet, and photography. In the analysis she was now able to work through the loss of her father when her parents separated. In the process of doing this she attained further insight into her compulsions and they stopped.

Lisa's unresolved anal-sadistic conflicts had prevented her from mourning her grandparents following their deaths. By working through these internalized conflicts in analysis, Lisa was able to mourn and proceed on to the task of resolving her oedipal conflict.

Conclusions

The four-year analysis of an adolescent girl with an obsessive-compulsive neurosis demonstrated that her symptoms were in part determined by her being unable to deal with multiple deaths and losses during her oedipal and latency periods. Lisa's earlier object losses and her defenses against these losses had become a nidus around which her infantile conflicts eventually developed into a full-blown obsessive-compulsive neurosis during adolescence. Once Lisa recognized her defenses of isolation, reaction formation, and undoing as they manifested themselves in the transference, she was able to work through her unresolved anal conflicts and reactivate her delayed mourning process. Thus, once Lisa was aware that both her healthy and her pathological identifications with her lost objects existed alongside each other, she was able to understand her ambivalence toward these objects and could complete her task of mourning (Furman 1974). Lisa's fixated psychic energy was now freed through the process of analysis and could be sublimated and reinvested in new objects more appropriate to adolescence. With the resolution of her oedipal conflicts Lisa understood her feelings about the loss of her father when her parents separated. This new insight led Lisa to discover the unconscious origins of, and mechanisms behind, her compulsions; and they stopped.

NOTE

I wish to express my thanks to Rudolf Ekstein and Peter Manjos for their consultations, which facilitated the therapeutic outcome in this case. Presented in an earlier version to the American Society for Adolescent Psychiatry, Seattle, Washington, September 25, 1982.

REFERENCES

Anthony, J. E. 1967. Psychiatric disorders of childhood. II. Psychoneurotic disorders. In M. Freedman and H. Kaplan, eds. *Comprehensive Textbook of Psychiatry*. Baltimore: Williams & Wilkins.
Brenner, C. 1955. *An Elementary Textbook of Psychoanalysis*. New York: International Universities Press.
Fleming, J., and Altschul, S. 1963. Activation of mourning and growth by psychoanalysis. *International Journal of Psycho-Analysis* 44:419–31.
Freud, S. 1905. Three essays on the theory of sexuality. *Standard Edition* 7:125–244. London: Hogarth, 1961.
Freud, S. 1909. Notes upon a case of obsessional neurosis. *Standard Edition* 10:153–251. London: Hogarth, 1961.
Freud, S. 1915. Instincts and their vicissitudes. *Standard Edition* 14:105–140. London: Hogarth, 1961.
Freud, S. 1920. An autobiographical study. *Standard Edition* 20:3–74. London: Hogarth, 1961.
Freud, S. 1926. Inhibitions, symptoms and anxiety. *Standard Edition* 20:72–175. London: Hogarth, 1961.
Freud, S. 1933. New introductory lectures. *Standard Edition* 22:3–158. London: Hogarth, 1961.
Furman, E. 1974. *A Child's Parent Dies*. New Haven, Conn.: Yale University Press.
Laufer, M. 1966. Object loss and mourning during adolescence. *Psychoanalytic Study of the Child* 21:269–293.
Moore, B., and Fine, B. 1968. *A Glossary of Psychoanalytic Terms and Concepts*. New York: American Psychoanalytic Association.

PART III

AN OVERVIEW
OF
EATING DISORDERS

INTRODUCTION:
AN OVERVIEW OF EATING DISORDERS

ARTHUR D. SOROSKY

A central theme of the history of man has been the eternal search for sufficient food. Yet, the psychological aspects of the particular eating disorders are the manifestations of luxury and plenty rather than of deprivation. Rather than being concerned with getting enough calories to survive, people are preoccupied with the taste and atmospheric aspects of eating and dining. Paradoxically, while food ads or stories in magazines, newspapers, and television are tempting us to try newer and better recipes, models, actresses, and centerfold pinups are demonstrating that "thinness is beautiful." Such double messages are extremely confusing to vulnerable young women who are struggling with identity issues relating to sexuality and body image. The failure to control excessive eating and to maintain thinness often leads to a sense of embarrassment, shame, and guilt. At the same time, studies have shown that up to 70 percent of adolescent and young adult women in the United States and Europe believe that they are overweight, even though their weight is normal according to their height and body build.

The three primary eating disorders (obesity, bulimia, and anorexia nervosa) exist in a continuum in which there is considerable overlapping. Of the three, obesity is the easiest to differentiate, but it is highly multidetermined, with psychological factors being only one aspect of an etiology including genetic predisposition as well as hormonal and other metabolic or physiological factors. Bulimia is the most perplexing of the eating disorders as it may coexist with either obesity or anorexia nervosa or occur as a distinct entity. In the recent literature, anorexia nervosa has been divided into restrictor and bulimic subtypes. The restrictor anorectics are involved in typical self-starvation practices, whereas a certain percentage of anorectics suffer from concomitant symptoms of bulimia, and others develop bulimia in the later stages of their illness. Causing further confusion in the literature is the contention by some investigators that eating disorders are secondary to mood disturbances, especially depression, while still others view the mood distubances as a secondary manifestation of the primary eating disorder.

During the 1960s and 1970s there appeared a plethora of books and articles on the eating disorders, especially anorexia nervosa. During the 1980s, especially after the special demarcation given to bulimia in DSM-III, there have been an equally large number of publications on bulimia. As is typical with all of the psychological literature, the earlier articles focused on historical reviews, descriptions of symptoms, and various explanations of the psychodynamics involved. More recently, the emphasis has shifted to treatment techniques, although there remains a diversity of opinion about which methods work and why. It will take the still remaining step of well-controlled prospective longitudinal studies to determine the true delineation of the three primary eating disorders, enabling us to be more effective in predicting the natural course of the illness and the effects of intervening with the various forms of treatment available.

The diagnosis of anorexia nervosa requires a weight loss of greater than 25 percent of the original body weight in patients with no known medical or psychiatric illness. Typically, patients manifest a denial of the illness, an apparent enjoyment of the weight loss, body image disturbances, and bizarre hoarding or handling of food. Secondary symptoms include amenorrhea, lanugo body hair, bradycardia, periods of overactivity, depression, and episodes of bulimia. The restrictor subtypes are typically obsessive and overcontrolled, whereas the bulimic subtypes are more impulsive, chronic, and difficult to treat. Finally, anorectic symptoms can be seen in association with hysterical, obsessive, or phobic symptomatology, or with patients suffering from more serious psychopathology, that is, narcissistic or borderline personality disorder or schizophrenic disorder.

Reports of cases of anorexia nervosa date back to the fourth century;

however, the first clinical descriptions were written in the 1600s. The three classic papers on the subject are Morton's "Of a Nervous Consumption" in 1694, and Gull's "Anorexia Nervosa (Apepsia Hysterica, Anorexia Hysterica)" and Lasegue's "On Hysterical Anorexia," both of which were written in 1873. The landmark investigations made during this century were by Hilde Bruch, who has published her views in previous issues of this publication. Currently, meticulous research on anorexia is being undertaken in a multitude of university and hospital centers throughout the United States and Western world.

The outcome of the widespread dissemination of knowledge on anorexia nervosa has resulted in earlier diagnosis and treatment, with a consequent decrease in mortality. Investigators have also isolated certain vulnerable subpopulations predisposed to developing anorexia nervosa: models, ballet dancers, jockeys, flight attendants, and others whose jobs or careers require constant attention to weight control. Furthermore, the treatment of the medical complications of anorexia has become more sophisticated, especially the concern with electrolyte imbalance and consequent cardiac arrhythmia. Likewise, the use of antidepressants for those anorectics also suffering from major depressive disorder has resulted in a lowering of the suicide rate among these patients.

Although bulimia was commonly observed among the more affluent citizens of the Roman world, during subsequent centuries with the emphasis on asceticism, binge-eating became viewed as a form of gluttony that was to be condemned. The bulimic syndrome resurfaced in the late 1900s, with the first detailed account of the illness appearing in the 1940s. However, until the past decade the term bulimia referred primarily to neurologic disorders causing episodes of overeating, that is, hypothalamic hyperphagia. Today, bulimia, like anorexia, has become almost a household term. Confusing matters, however, are the variety of other terms used in the lay and professional literature to describe the bulimic syndrome: "bulimarexia," "binge-purge syndrome," "bulimia nervosa," "the compulsive eater syndrome," and "thin-fat people." The term "normal-weight bulimia" is now being widely employed as a means of differentiating the primary syndrome from the bulimic subtype of anorexia nervosa.

Bulimia is characterized by repeated episodes of rapid ingestion of large amounts of food during a discrete period of time, typically less than two hours. Patients are typically aware that their eating binges are abnormal, and they fear the inability to terminate their eating voluntarily. Following these episodes they often experience a depressed mood and self-deprecating thoughts. Similar to individuals with addiction to drugs, alcohol, tobacco, or gambling, bulimic individuals keep trying to convince themselves that the most recent episode is going to be the last. The eventual inability to rationalize or deny the severity of the problem often leads to a confession to a parent or friend, resulting in the subsequent referral to a mental health specialist, eating disorder treatment program, or one of the proliferating self-help groups.

In both anorectic and bulimic patients the outset of the illness is typically triggered by a pursuit of thinness, which eventually leads to a morbid fear of becoming obese. The determinants of which of the two illnesses develops may be more related to underlying premorbid personality features rather than to distinct psychodynamic phenomenology. There are many features that are common to both syndromes. Both are more prominent among middle- and upper-middle-class young women, a group that is particularly preoccupied with weight and caloric intake. These women have either learned or are predisposed to use food as a means of dealing with stress or emotional conflicts. In the case of the restrictor anorectic, the symptom provides a sense of control in at least one aspect of the patient's life. In the normal-weight bulimic, the symptoms provide a sense of immediate gratification while beating the physiologic system of weight gain secondary to excessive caloric intake. In both the bulimics and anorectics, the eating disorder enables the patient to block out or repress the typical age-specific conflicts, which now become buried underneath the massive energy and focus of attention given to food or the avoidance of food.

Both anorexia nervosa and bulimia are associated with serious medical complications. Although the mortality rate in anorexia nervosa has declined significantly, clinicians must never become lax as this illness is potentially fatal at any time. Careful attention must be given to electrolyte balance, cardiac rhythm, endocrine function, and the patient's overall health. Even though patients rarely die from bulimia they frequently suffer from salivary gland enlargement, erosion of dental enamel, and a variety of gastrointestinal disturbances. The rare causes of death in these patients result from rupture of the stomach or tearing of the esophageal wall.

In this special section of chapters on eating disorders, special emphasis has been given to diagnosis and the various forms of treatment available. The goal has not been to provide a minitextbook but to provide an

224

overview of a most contemporary problem in adolescent psychiatry. The emphasis has been more weighted on normal-weight bulimia because of the preponderance of previous papers on anorexia and obesity in this, as well as other publications. Barton J. Blinder and Kristin Cadenhead review the literature on bulimia from an historical perspective. They trace the evolution of this entity from its more generalized usage in ancient times, to its inclusion as part of the anorexia syndrome, and finally to its place as a diagnostic classification in DSM-III.

Richard L. Pyle and James E. Mitchell have presented an epidemiological review of the prevalence of bulimia as defined in DSM-III. They conclude that the true prevalence is around 1–2 percent of females in the age range of eighteen to thirty. A rather small percentage of these patients seek out treatment, and unlike anorectics they are often able to conceal their symptoms and avoid referral for professional assistance. The apparent increase in prevalence is not entirely evident in recent studies and may be more a reflection of wider publicity of the illness, with a greater willingness of patients to "come out of hiding" and discuss the intimate details of their binge-purge habit disturbance. Statistical surveys of the syndrome are dependent on self-report questionnaires with all of their inherent limitations. Furthermore, bulimic patients, as a group, may have a tendency to distort their responses either by underreporting to conceal the severity of symptoms or by overreporting in an attempt to please the examiner.

Craig Johnson and Karen L. Maddi conceptualize bulimia as a paradigmatic psychosomatic disorder that is multidetermined in its etiology. Their chapter synthesizes current knowledge of how the interrelationship of biological, familial, and sociocultural factors predispose predominantly adolescent and young adult women to develop bulimia. The authors believe that young women who are at risk for developing bulimia have a biological vulnerability for affective instability. This affective instability is exacerbated by both a conflicted and disorganized family environment as well as a sociocultural environment that is in a confused state of transition. Such youngsters suffer from a lowered self-esteem and self-regulatory difficulties, which they attempt to remedy through the achievement of thinness. However, the physiological and psychological side effects of semistarvation result in a "psychobiological impasse" that, paradoxically, results in an exacerbation of the original difficulties of affective instability and low self-esteem. The ultimate goal of this research project is to develop a risk-factor model for bulimic behavior that can facilitate earlier detection and a more sophisticated means of assessment.

C. Philip Wilson differentiates anorexia nervosa into restrictor and bulimic subtypes. Both groups have similar underlying psychodynamics in which there is not a lack of appetite, or anorexia, but rather a struggle to avoid being overwhelmed by impulses, including voraciousness. Another common denominator is a retreat from the development of adult sexuality via a regression to the prepubertal relationship with the parents. The restrictor anorectics are more perfectionistic and controlling, whereas the bulimic anorectics have ineffective impulse controls where the slightest gain in weight produces panic, exercising, starving, and vomiting. The author presents five clinical case studies in which intensive psychoanalytic or psychoanalytically oriented therapy is used to treat these youngsters, often associated with conjoint therapy of the parents. The methods described are similar to those used by many clinicians treating borderline and narcissistic patients.

Laura L. Humphrey presents a study of bulimia as viewed from a family systems perspective. The illness is conceptualized as a homeostatic mechanism that enables family members, especially the parents, to avoid dealing with severe psychopathology. Dyadic dynamics are delineated in an attempt to explain the effects each of the family members has on the others. In many of the families, the child's eating disorder may be equated with explosive outbursts of anger evidenced in the parents or siblings. The author also proposes that different family dynamics are responsible for the development of the various subtypes of bulimia. Such findings point out the need for parental involvement in the treatment program, either through family therapy or collaborative therapy methods.

Harold Leitenberg and James C. Rosen have devised a behavioral treatment approach for patients suffering from bulimia. Their group of patients have been involved in uncontrollable binge-eating and self-induced vomiting while suffering from an intense dread of weight gain or change in body appearance. These patients are contrasted with anorectic patients by: (1) eating excessively while out of control, whereas the latter group is overcontrolled and engaged in self-starvation; (2) attempting to achieve a stereotyped or idealized conception of a perfect feminine and sexually attractive appearance, whereas the anorectic patients are denying their sexuality; (3) being a generally older age group—early twenties, instead of anorectics, who are typically in their low teens; and (4) being more secretive about their illness, yet being less likely to minimize or deny the problem, whereas anorectics "advertise" their disorder through their appearance.

The authors describe how binge-eating is triggered by an antecedent event, dysphoric feelings, or lapses from a rigid diet. They believe most of these individuals would never continue to binge-eat unless they developed the technique of vomiting afterward. Once self-induced vomiting is learned, this becomes the driving force that sustains the binge-eating rather than the opposite phenomenon. It is as if the addition of the vomiting frees the bulimic patients from the normal inhibitions against binge-eating. They propose a form of treatment that relies heavily on anxiety reduction. The patient's anxiety-provoking feelings are explored, whereas the behavior modification methods concentrate or focus on minimizing the vomiting aspect of the bulimic syndrome. This approach contrasts with other behavioristic approaches that have concentrated more specifically on diminishing the loss of control or desire to binge-eat.

David M. Garner has evolved a form of cognitive therapy for patients with bulimia without a history of emaciation—a group clearly distinguishable from those with the bulimic subtype of anorexia nervosa. His approach involves the following steps: (1) teaching the patient to monitor her own thinking or heighten awareness of her own thinking; (2) helping the patient to recognize the connection between certain dysfunctional thoughts and maladaptive behaviors and emotions; (3) examining with the patient evidence for the validity of particular beliefs, especially cultural and societal emphasis on dieting and maintaining a perfect shape; (4) assisting the patient in gradually substituting more realisitic and appropriate interpretations based upon the evidence; and (5) establishing, as the ultimate goal, a modification of underlying assumptions that are fundamental determinants of specific dysfunctional beliefs. For some, such a treatment program may be highly successful within a short period of time. For others, especially those with a history of anorexia nervosa, multiple treatment failures, or extremely chaotic eating patterns, treatment may have to be of a much longer duration.

Katherine N. Dixon reviews the utilization of homogeneous group therapy methods for the treatment of bulimia. Such an approach is widely used for other specific disorders including alcoholism, drug abuse, homosexuality, and anorexia nervosa. The author stresses that group therapy should be prescribed only if it is part of an overall systematic and comprehensive treatment program. Treatment goals include both alleviation of symptoms and gaining insight into internal and familial conflicts. The chapter addresses the selection of members, treatment techniques, problems encountered, and treatment outcome. Objective studies of bulimic groups have demonstrated a significant reduction or cessation of symptoms as well as increased self-esteem and improved impulse control, along with a decrease in anger, somatization, anxiety, and depression.

James C. Sheinin has presented a thorough overview of the medical complications resulting from anorexia nervosa and bulimia. Although anorexia nervosa is a potentially life-threatening disorder, bulimia is also capable of inducing severe physical damage. The author emphasizes the crucial importance of careful clinical and laboratory monitoring of patients suffering from either of these eating disorders. In anorectic patients attention must be given to the hypothalamic-pituitary-thyroid axis, as well as gonadal dysfunction, fluid balance alterations, electrolyte imbalance, cardiac arrhythmias, orthostatic hypotension, renal and hepatic problems, and various gastrointestinal difficulties. The bulimic patient characteristically has evidence of enlarged salivary glands with erosion of dental enamel induced by repeated forced vomiting of acidic fluids. These bulimic patients are also vulnerable to developing irreparable damage to the GI tract, cardiac arrthymias and conduction abnormalities, skeletal and smooth muscle weakness and paralysis induced by severe protein and potassium depletion, and fluid depletion. Ignoring these potential medical complications in a well-conceived treatment program would be a grave error.

Enrique J. Friedman describes the neuroendocrine aspects of bulimia. Neuroendocrinological studies of anorexia nervosa are readily found in the literature. Only recently has attention been given to similar physiological changes in normal-weight bulimic patients. The author proposes that problems in the hypothalmic-pituitary-thyroid-adrenal axis are common to both anorexia nervosa and bulimia. Furthermore, he has focused on the specific role of neurotransmitters and gastrointestinal tract hormones. Although preliminary in its scope and speculative in its content, the chapter provocatively outlines directions for future research in the highly enigmatic field of eating disorder pathophysiology.

David B. Herzog reviews the published studies of normal-weight bulimics and the relationship of the syndrome to affective illness, particularly depression. The findings are rather inconsistent, and it is unclear as to whether the depression is a mood, a symptom, or a syndrome. There

228

are basically four hypotheses: (1) depression causes bulimia; (2) bulimia leads to a depressive state; (3) bulimia and depression are essentially distinct and separate entities; and (4) both bulimia and depression are an outgrowth of similar genetic, biochemical, and psychodynamic predispositions. The available data do not allow for any definitive conclusions. It will be necessary to clearly delineate the various subtypes of bulimia and follow afflicted individuals through longitudinal studies. Such investigations will help clarify the association between bulimia and depression and allow for a more specific and successful treatment of the syndrome.

B. Timothy Walsh explores the use of medication in the treatment of bulimia. Initially, anticonvulsant drugs were used because it was believed the problem might be the manifestation of a seizure disorder. The results were equivocal, and these drugs are rarely used anymore. More recently, antidepressant drugs have been utilized because of the apparent link between bulimia and affective illness. Although the outcome has been quite positive, the use of these drugs is not without problems in this particular patient population. Their impulsivity and tendency to act out increases the risk of overdose and suicide. Monitoring plasma levels can be very helpful in assuring compliance, attaining therapeutic levels, and detecting overdoses. Although the MAO-inhibitor antidepressants may be quite effective, they are potentially more dangerous because of the required dietary restrictions. It is preferable to commence treatment with one of the tricyclic antidepressants and switch over to an MAOI antidepressant if the former drugs are not effective or if side effects are unacceptable.

13 BULIMIA: A HISTORICAL OVERVIEW

BARTON J. BLINDER AND KRISTIN CADENHEAD

In ancient times Romans prepared large banquets in which the participants, after lounging and gorging, would tickle their throats with feathers or take emetics after each course, vomit, and return to their gluttony (Fischer 1976). This practice led to the use of vomitoria and possibly the beginning of the use of the term "bulimia" to describe such behavior. The term "bulimia" derives from *bulimy* in Greek, meaning ravenous hunger (Kaplan and Garfinkel 1984; Siegel 1973). Literally, it derives from the Greek meaning "ox" and "hunger" and the Latin words meaning "canine hunger." Galen (Siegel 1973) described *boulimia* as also being called *kynos orexia* or dog's hunger. He considered boulimia to be caused by an abnormal humor that provoked an exaggerated desire for nutrition and frequent feedings that may also be associated with severe vomiting and copious bowel movements. In the *Talmud* (400–500 A.D.) the term *boolmut* is used to describe a syndrome in which a person is overcome with hunger to the point that both his judgment concerning food and his level of awareness of outside events is impaired. Boolmut was considered to be life threatening. It is possible that certain medical conditions (for example, insulinoma) were included under this descriptive term (van der Eycken 1985).

In medical dictionaries of the eighteenth and nineteenth centuries bulimia was often described as a medical curiosity or symptom of other diseases (Forsyth 1826; Hooper 1825; James 1743; Morris and Kendrick 1807; Porter 1829). James (1743) described *"boulimus"* in association with *"caninus appetitus"* and *"fames canina"* to describe how the person would vomit like a dog to ease the stomach after eating too much food. Hooper (1825) described "bulimia emitica," "bulimia canina," and "cynorexia" to designate a voracious appetite followed by vomiting (Loudon 1984).

Much of the early literature describing bulimia is in association with anorexia nervosa (Casper, Eckert, Halmi, Goldberg, and Davis 1980; Gull 1873; MacKenzie 1888; Marshall 1895; Osler 1892; Playfair 1888; Sollier 1891; Soltman 1894). Gull (1873), who was the first to use the term "anorexia nervosa," described overeating in a patient who would think of "putrid cat pudding" while eating, causing her to vomit. Others (MacKenzie 1888; Marshall 1895; Playfair 1888; Sollier 1891) describe cases of vomiting attributed to gastric pain in anorexia nervosa patients. Janet (1903) presented a subgroup of anorectic patients whom he described as "obsessionals" (in contrast to "hysterics"), who were distinguished by the persistence of hunger sensations, a more intense loathing of the body, and ruminative thinking centered on food and the control of appetitive drives. Berkman (1939) found that vomiting occurred in 66 percent of patients with anorexia nervosa, in association with the sensation of fullness. Waller and Kaufman (1940) described two case histories of women who would first overeat on candy and then, in reaction, starve themselves because of magical ideation connecting pregnancy to eating. Binswanger's (1944) study of Ellen West describes a patient with partially remitted anorexia nervosa who began to struggle with bulimia, occasionally followed by violent vomiting and laxative abuse. Bond (1949), Nemiah (1950), and Bruch (1962) were also aware of overeating and laxative and enema abuse as well as self-induced vomiting in anorexia nervosa patients but considered the bulimia to be a variant in the eating and dieting pattern of anorexia nervosa patients rather than a distinct syndrome.

The clinical symptoms of bulimia have been described in nonanorectic patients for many years (Abraham 1916; Bruch 1962; Kirshbaum 1951; Lindner 1955; Stunkard 1959; Wulf 1932), but they have generally been regarded as rare neurotic conditions rather than a distinct syndrome. Abraham (1916) described a condition of excessive eating that was more common in women. He considered it to be a neurotic hunger derived from anxiety and internalized conflict rather than determined by a full or empty stomach. Abraham suggested that the condition was associated with repression of libido and resembled an addictive process. Lindner (1955) described the case of "Laura" who binged but did not vomit. Lindner proposed that Laura's bulimia was the result of an active oedipal wish to be impregnated by her father, who had left the family when she

232

was a preadolescent. The protruding abdomen produced by the binge symbolized her father's infant growing inside of her. Wulf (1932) described five cases of periodic "eating and sleeping mania" in which enormous quantities of sweet things, cakes, unappetizing remnants, scraps of paper, etc., were devoured, while persistent unrefreshed sleep, disturbed by erotic dreams or masturbation, accompanied the process of digestion. These manias and cravings were said to differ from the compulsions in obsessional neurosis by affording direct rather than substitute gratification and by exhibiting less manifest anxiety. He considered them to be closely allied to drug addiction and to be intermediate between addiction and melancholia. Stunkard, Grace, and Wolff (1955) were the first to describe a bulimia pattern in obese patients that they called "the night eating syndrome." The syndrome involved consumption of large amounts of food during the evening and night, sleeplessness, and morning anorexia in obese patients. It was also during this period that Kirshbaum (1951) described "hyperorexia" as a symptom of organic brain disease in the hypothalamus and frontal lobes.

The recognition of bulimia as a distinct syndrome did not occur until it became evident that binge-eating and vomiting behavior occurred in individuals who did not have histories of weight disorders such as anorexia nervosa or obesity (Boskind-Lodahl and White 1978; Strangler and Prinz 1980; White and Boskind-White 1981). In 1976, Boskind-White coined the term "bulimarexia" to describe an eating disorder, prevalent in young women, that was characterized by alternating episodes of eating and rigid dieting, accompanied by low self-esteem, body image devaluation, and a fear of rejection in heterosexual relationships. Their results indicated the "importance of sociocultural factors in female role definition and the view of bulimarexia as related to the struggle to achieve a 'perfect' female image in which women surrendered their self-defining power to others" (Boskind-Lodahl and White 1978). It has been suggested that a trend developed in the 1940s both in clinical descriptions of eating disorders and in societal concerns emphasizing attention to body shape (Casper 1983). It culminated in the 1960s into what Bruch (1973) labeled "the pursuit of thinness" and Selvinni-Palazzoli (1978) called "the desperate need to grow thinner." These ideas were further validated by the Garner, Garfinkel, Schwartz, and Thompson (1980) study that showed the decreasing weights and body-contour measurements of Miss America contestants and *Playboy* magazine centerfolds over a period of several decades. Increasing clinical experience

233

led to the classification of bulimia as a disorder distinct from anorexia nervosa in the third edition of the DSM-III (1980) of the American Psychiatric Association.

Bulimia, as defined in DSM-III, is characterized by repeated episodes of rapid ingestion of large amounts of food in a discrete amount of time, typically less than two hours. The individual is aware that the eating binges are abnormal, fears the inability to terminate eating voluntarily, and experiences depressed mood and self-deprecating thoughts following the episodes. Also characteristic of bulimia is inconspicuous eating; weight fluctuations of greater than ten pounds; consumption of high-caloric, easily ingested food during the binge-purging behaviors; and the termination of binges by pain, sleep, social interruption, or self-induced vomiting. The DSM-III stipulation that the bulimic episodes not be due to anorexia nervosa or any physical disorder limits the syndrome to those individuals who are at or above normal weight.

The inclusion of the symptom picture in DSM-III has resulted in a newly developing area of research. There is growing evidence that the incidence and prevalence of bulimia exists to a significant degree among women with no history of weight disorder (Halmi, Falk, and Schwartz 1981; Hawkins and Clement 1980; Johnson, Lewis, Love, Lewis, and Stuckey 1984; Nagelberg, Hale, and Ware 1984; Pyle, Mitchell, and Eckert 1981; Russell 1979). Halmi et al. (1981) found the prevalence of bulimia to be 13 percent among 355 college students (87 percent female, 13 percent male). Pyle et al. (1981) also surveyed a college population and found that 4.1 percent of 355 students (7.8 percent female, 1.4 percent male) met the criteria for bulimia. Johnson et al. (1984) found that 4.9 percent of 1,268 female high school students met the criteria for bulimia.

The typical bulimia patient has been found to be a single, white female in her early twenties who is well educated and of average weight for her height (Johnson et al. 1984). Results show that these individuals are more vulnerable to anxiety, depression, impulsive behavior, mood fluctuation, obsessive-compulsive traits, confused sex-role identity, poor self-esteem, and severe food and weight preoccupations in response to a cultural norm of thinness than women with no evidence of eating pathology (Boskind-Lodahl 1976; Johnson and Larson 1982; Pyle et al. 1981; Weiss and Ebert 1983).

Because there have been so many individuals who fit into the current DSM-III criteria for bulimia, there has been some confusion as to whether the criteria can distinguish clinically pathological levels of bulimic behavior. It remains to be demonstrated which criteria are sufficient or necessary to identify individuals whose bulimic behavior is in some way so significantly interfering with their functional adequacy and physiologic integrity as to be designated as a disorder (Johnson et al. 1984).

Another clinical issue concerning the DSM-III criteria for bulimia is that the symptoms of bulimia occur along a continuum of weight disorders including anorexia nervosa (Casper et al. 1980; Garfinkel, Moldofsky, and Garner 1980; Russell 1979) and obesity (Stunkard 1959). According to the DSM-III criteria, any history of anorexia nervosa precludes a primary diagnosis of bulimia. However, recent research (Beaumont, George, and Smart 1976; Casper et al. 1980; Garfinkel et al. 1980; Strober 1981; Strober, Salkin, Burroughs, and Morrell 1982) has suggested that anorexia nervosa patients who manifest bulimic symptoms represent a subgroup distinct from those who are typically referred to as "restrictors" or "starvers." Russell (1979) designated the term "bulimia nervosa" to describe a subgroup of patients who, in contrast to restrictors, have been found to have an older age of onset, a more chronic outcome, and a higher incidence of premorbid and family obesity (Beaumont et al. 1976; Casper et al. 1980; Garfinkel et al. 1980; Strober 1981; Strober et al. 1982). These patients manifest greater anxiety and depression, report a higher incidence of impulsive behavior (substance abuse and kleptomania), more evidence of premorbid instability, a greater body image distortion, and more extensive family conflict (Casper et al. 1980; Garfinkel et al. 1980; Katzman and Wolchik 1984; Strober 1980). Also, first- and second-degree relatives of bulimic anorectics show a higher prevalence of affective disorders as well as of drug and alcohol abuse than do restrictors (Strober et al. 1982). Thus, symptoms of bulimia in anorexia nervosa patients may have important etiologic, prognostic, and clinical implications. Furthermore, bulimic anorectics have been found to be more like normal-weight bulimics than they are like restricting anorectics (Garner, Garfinkel, and O'Shaughnessey 1985; Johnson and Larson 1982; Johnson et al. 1984). Garner et al. (1985) note that because of the similarities between bulimic women with anorexia nervosa and bulimic normal-weight women, the distinction between the two groups according to DSM-III may be imprecise.

Studies of bulimia in association with affective disorders suggest that 20 percent may meet the criteria for major depression (Blinder, Chaitin, and Hagman 1984; Herzog and Copeland 1985). Abnormalities of the hypothalamic-pituitary-adrenal axis (specifically, failure to suppress cortisol in response to dexamethasone) have been found in bulimia as well as in depression (Blinder et al. 1984; Gwirtsman, Roy-Byrne, Yaeger, and Gerner 1983). Studies of bulimia also suggest possible central neurochemical abnormalities of the serotonergic and noradrenergic systems (Herzog and Copeland 1985). The restrictive and bulimic forms of anorexia have been differentiated on the basis of the accumulation of the serotonin metabolite 5-hydroxyindolacetic acid in the cerebrospinal fluid after probenecid administration in patients after weight recovery (Kaye, Ebert, Gwirtzman, and Weiss 1984). The level of 5-hydroxyindolacetic acid is lower in bulimic anorectics, suggesting decreased serotonin turnover, which may indicate a disrupted satiety mechanism that predisposes the patient to binge.

Further work must still be done to fully understand and classify the syndrome of bulimia. It appears that multiple factors are involved in both the etiology and persistance of the disorder. Further studies are needed to evaluate treatment protocols (pharmacologic, individual and group psychotherapy, behavioral intervention, nutritional approaches) on the basis of long-term clinical course. Investigations of the developmental line of eating and the neurobiology of appetite and eating may provide the data to further define bulimia as a disorder in a broader psychobiologic context (Blinder 1980; Blinder, Chaitin, and Goldstein 1986).

REFERENCES

Abraham, K. 1916. The first pregenital stage of the libido. In *Selected Papers of Karl Abraham*. New York: Basic, 1954.

Beaumont, P. J.; George, G. C.; and Smart, D. E. 1976. Dieters and vomiters and purgers in anorexia nervosa. *Psychological Medicine* 6:617–622.

Berkman, J. M. 1939. Functional anorexia and functional vomiting: their relation to anorexia nervosa. *Medical Clinics of North America* 23:901–912.

Binswanger, L. 1944. The case of Ellen West: an anthropological-clinical study. In R. May, E. Angel, and H. Ellenberg, eds. *Existence*. New York: Basic, 1958.

Blinder, B. J. 1980. Developmental antecedents of the eating disorders: a reconsideration. *Psychiatric Clinics of North America* 3(3): 579–592.

Blinder, B. J.; Chaitin, B.; and Goldstein, R. 1986. *The Eating Disorders*. New York: Spectrum.

Blinder, B. J.; Chaitin, B.; and Hagman, J. 1984. Two diagnostic correlates of dexamethasone nonsuppression in normal weight bulimia. Presented at the Second International Conference on Eating Disorders, September, Wales.

Bond, D. D. 1949. Anorexia nervosa. *The Rocky Mountain Medical Journal* 46:1012–1019.

Boskind-Lodahl, M. 1976. Cinderella's stepsisters: a feminist perspective on anorexia and bulimia. *Signs: Journal of Women in Culture and Society* 2:342–356.

Boskind-Lodahl, M., and White, W. C. 1978. The definition and treatment of bulimarexia in college women—a pilot study. *Journal of the American College Health Association* 27:84–86.

Bruch, H. 1962. Perceptual and conceptual disturbances in anorexia nervosa. *Psychosomatic Medicine* 24:187–194.

Bruch. H. 1973. *Eating Disorders: Obesity, Anorexia and the Person Within*. New York: Basic.

Casper, R. C. 1983. On the emergence of bulimia as a syndrome: a historical view. *International Journal of Eating Disorders* 2:3–16.

Casper, R. C.; Eckert, E. D.; Halmi, K. A.; Goldberg, S. C.; and Davis, J. M. 1980. Bulimia: its incidence and clinical significance in patients with anorexia nervosa. *Archives of General Psychiatry* 37:1030–1035.

Diagnostic and Statistical Manual of Mental Disorders, 3d ed. (*DSM-III*). Washington, D.C.: American Psychiatric Association.

Fischer, M. F. K. 1976. *The Art of Eating*. New York: Vintage.

Forsyth, J. S. 1826. *The New London Medical and Surgical Dictionary*. London: Sherwood, Gilbert & Piper.

Garfinkel, P. E.; Moldofsky, H.; and Garner, D. M. 1980. The heterogeneity of anorexia nervosa: bulimia as a distinct subgroup. *Archives of General Psychiatry* 37:1036–1040.

Garner, D. M.; Garfinkel, P. E.; and O'Shaughnessey, B. S. 1985. The validity of the distinction between bulimia with and without anorexia nervosa. *American Journal of Psychiatry* 142(5): 581–587.

Garner, D. M.; Garfinkel, P. E.; Schwartz, D. M.; and Thompson, M. G. 1980. Cultural expectations of thinness in women. *Psychological Reports* 47:483–491.

Gull, W. W. 1873. Anorexia hysterica (apepsia hysterica). *British Medical Journal* 2:527.

Gwirtsman, H. E.; Roy-Byrne, P.; Yaeger, J.; and Gerner, R. H. 1983. Neuroendocrine abnormalities in bulimia. *American Journal of Psychiatry* 140:559–563.

Halmi, K. A.; Falk, J. R.; and Schwartz, E. 1981. Binge-eating and vomiting: a survey of a college population. *Psychological Medicine* 11:697–706.

Hawkins, R. C., and Clement, P. F. 1980. Development and construct validation of a self-report measure of binge-eating tendencies. *Addictive Behaviors* 5:219–226.

Herzog, D. B., and Copeland, P. M. 1985. Eating disorders. *New England Journal of Medicine* 313(5):295–303.

Hooper, R. 1825. *Lexicon Medicum.* London: Bliss & White.

James, R. 1743. *Medical Dictionary.* London: Osborne.

Janet, P. 1903. *Obsessions et la psychasthenie.* Paris: Alcan.

Johnson, C., and Larson, R. 1982. Bulimia: an analysis of moods and behavior. *Psychosomatic Medicine* 44:333–345.

Johnson, C.; Lewis, C.; Love, S.; Lewis, L.; and Stuckey, M. 1984. Incidence and correlates of bulimic behavior in a female high school population. *Journal of Youth and Adolescence* 13:15–26.

Kaplan, A. S., and Garfinkel, P. E. 1984. Bulimia in the *Talmud. American Journal of Psychiatry* 141(5): 721.

Katzman, M. A., and Wolchik, S. A. 1984. Bulimia and binge eating in college women: a comparison of personality and behavioral characteristics. *Journal of Consulting and Clinical Psychology* 52(3): 423–428.

Kaye, W. H.; Ebert, M. H.; Gwirtzman, H. E.; and Weiss, S. R. 1984. Differences in brain serotonergic metabolism between nonbulimic and bulimic patients with anorexia nervosa. *American Journal of Psychiatry* 141:1598–1601.

Kirshbaum, W. R. 1951. Excessive hunger as a symptom of cerebral origin. *Journal of Nervous and Mental Disease* 113:95–115.

Lindner, R. 1955. *The Fifty Minute Hour.* New York: Rinehart.

Loudon, I. 1984. The diseases called chlorosis. *Psychological Medicine* 14:27–36.

MacKenzie, S. 1888. Anorexia nervosa vel hysterica. *Lancet* 1:613–614.

Marshall, C. F. 1895. A fatal case of anorexia nervosa. *Lancet* 1:149–150.

Morris, R., and Kendrick, J. 1807. *The Edinburgh Medical and Physical Dictionary.* Edinburgh: Bell & Bradfut.

Nagelberg, D. B.; Hale, S. L.; and Ware, S. L. 1984. The assessment of bulimic symptoms and personality correlates in female college students. *Journal of Clinical Psychiatry* 40(2): 440–445.

Nemiah, J. C. 1950. Anorexia nervosa: a clinical psychiatric study. *Medicine* 29:225–268.

Osler, W. 1892. *Principles and Practice of Medicine.* New York: Appleton.

Playfair, C. 1888. Note on the so-called anorexia nervosa. *Lancet* 1:817–828.

Porter, D. R. 1829. A case of bulimia. *London Medical and Surgical Journal* 3:83.

Pyle, R. L.; Mitchell, J. E.; and Eckert, E. D. 1981. Bulimia: a report of 34 cases. *Journal of Clinical Psychiatry* 42:60–64.

Russell, G. F. M. 1979. Bulimia nervosa: an ominous variant of anorexia nervosa. *Psychological Medicine* 9:429–448.

Selvinni-Palazzoli, M. P. 1978. *Self Starvation.* New York: Aronson.

Siegel, R. E. 1973. *Galen on Psychopathology and Function and Diseases of the Nervous System.* New York: Karger.

Sollier, P. 1891. Anorexie hysterique (sitiergie hysterique). *Revue medicale* 11:625:650.

Soltman, O. 1894. Anorexia cerebralis und centrale nutritione Neurose. *Jahrbuch der Kinderheilklinik* 38:1–13.

Strangler, R. S., and Prinz, A. M. 1980. DSM-III: psychiatric diagnosis in a university population. *American Journal of Psychiatry* 137:937–940.

Strober, M. 1980. Personality and symptomatological features in young, nonchronic anorexia nervosa patients. *Journal of Psychosomatic Research* 24:353–359.

Strober, M. 1981. The significance of bulimia in juvenile anorexia nervosa: an exploration of possible etiological factors. *International Journal of Eating Disorders* 1:28–43.

Strober, M.; Salkin, B.; Burroughs, G.; and Morrell, W. 1982. Validity of the bulimia-restrictor distinction in anorexia nervosa and parental personality characteristics and family psychiatric morbidity. *Journal of Nervous and Mental Diseases* 170:345–351.

Stunkard, A. J. 1959. Eating patterns and obesity. *Psychiatric Quarterly* 33:289–294.

Stunkard, A. J.; Grace, W. J.; and Wolff, H. G. 1955. The night eating syndrome: a pattern of food intake among certain obese patients. *American Journal of Medicine* 19:78–86.

239

van der Eycken, W. 1985. Bulimia has different meanings. *American Journal of Psychiatry* 142:141–142.

Waller, J. V., and Kaufman, M. R. 1940. Anorexia nervosa: a psychosomatic entity. *Psychosomatic Medicine* 2:3–16.

Weiss, S. R., and Ebert, M. H. 1983. Psychological and behavioral characteristics of normal weight bulimics and normal weight controls. *Psychosomatic Medicine* 45:293–303.

White, W. C., and Boskind-White, M. 1981. An experimental behavioral approach to the treatment of bulimarexia. *Journal of Psychotherapy, Theory, Research, and Practice* 2:342–356.

Wulf, M. 1932. Über einen interessanten oral symptomen Komplex und seine Beziehung zur Sucht. *International Zeitschrift P.S.A..* 18:281–301.

14 THE PREVALENCE OF BULIMIA IN SELECTED SAMPLES

RICHARD L. PYLE AND JAMES E. MITCHELL

Bulimia, as described in *DSM-III* (1980), is characterized by an abnormal eating pattern of surreptitious uncontrolled episodic binge-eating usually accompanied by self-induced vomiting, laxative abuse, or restrictive dieting to eliminate unwanted food. The bulimic episodes are followed by low mood and self-deprecatory thoughts. Individuals with this disease who present for treatment are most often women in their mid twenties who developed the illness in their later teens. The illness occurs primarily in white females of all socioeconomic classes (Mitchell and Pyle 1982; Pyle, Mitchell, and Eckert 1981; Russell 1979). With the increasing demand for more treatment resources for bulimia, determination of the prevalence of bulimia in the general population is essential if we are to know what the needs for treatment may be. A related question of major importance is whether the incidence of bulimia is increasing.

There are two areas of controversy regarding bulimia research in general that have a major impact on the design of prevalence studies. One is the problem of defining binge-eating, and the other is choosing the proper inclusion criteria to define the bulimia syndrome. While there is agreement that binge-eating consists of eating an unusually large quantity of food over a brief period of time, researchers differ on whether the subjective definition of binge-eating should be quantified in terms of amount of food consumed. Although many researchers include loss of control over eating in operationalized criteria for binge-eating, this factor is not always included.

Selection of appropriate inclusion criteria has become more difficult for those investigators who wish to include criteria to address the concerns of researchers who believe that the current diagnostic criteria for the bulimia syndrome may be too broad. Future revisions of diagnostic criteria may well include the addition of a minimum frequency criterion for binge-eating episodes and the criterion of self-induced vomiting and/or laxative abuse.

Since reports attempting to adequately describe and classify the bulimia syndrome are relatively recent (*DSM-III* 1980; Mitchell and Pyle 1982; Pyle et al. 1981; Russell 1979), optimally designed epidemiologic studies have not yet been published. The purpose of this chapter is to examine our existing knowledge about the frequency of bulimic behaviors and the prevalence of the bulimia syndrome.

The Definition and Frequency of Bulimic Behaviors

The studies of Halmi, Falk, and Schwartz (1981) and of Hawkins and Clement (1980) called attention to the high frequency of bulimic behaviors in the student population. In this section, we will review the frequency of the behaviors that are associated with the operationalized DSM-III criteria for bulimia and discuss the specific questions from self-report questionnaires that were used to define those inclusion criteria. This will assist the reader to better understand and evaluate data on the prevalence of bulimia.

Inclusion criteria for prevalence studies in the United States are most often designed to elicit the prevalence of bulimia. The DSM-III criteria for bulimia are listed in table 1. Those studies that state that the prevalence of bulimia is based on all the essential features of bulimia indicate that criteria A, C, and D have been included (Halmi et al. 1981; Johnson, Lewis, Love, Stuckey, and Lewis 1983). Criterion B is not considered to be an essential feature, since only three of five behaviors need to be endorsed. More recent prevalence studies have included criterion B (Katzman, Wolchick, and Braver 1984; Pope, Hudson, and Yurgelien-Todd 1984a, 1984b; Pyle, Mitchell, Eckert, Halvorson, Neuman, and Goff 1983).

Some investigators have further limited the number of subjects who meet the inclusion criteria by quantifying binge-eating behavior and adding other quantifying and qualifying criteria such as the presence of weekly self-induced vomiting and/or laxative abuse (Johnson et al. 1983; Katzman et al. 1984; Pyle et al. 1983). The addition of weekly self-induced vomiting and/or laxative abuse as inclusion criteria identifies a

242

RICHARD L. PYLE AND JAMES E. MITCHELL

TABLE 1
Diagnostic Criteria for Bulimia (DSM-III)

A.* Recurrent episodes of binge-eating (rapid consumption of a large amount of food in a discrete period of time, usually less than two hours).
B. At least three of the following:
1. Consumption of high-caloric, easily ingested food during a binge.
2. Inconspicuous eating during a binge.
3. Termination of such eating episodes by abdominal pain, sleep, social interruption, self-induced vomiting.
4. Repeated attempts to lose weight by severely restrictive diets, self-induced vomiting, or use of cathartics or diuretics.
5. Frequent weight fluctuations greater than ten pounds because of alternating binges and fasts.
C.* Awareness that eating pattern is abnormal and fear of not being able to stop eating voluntarily.
D.* Depressed mood and self-deprecating thoughts following eating binges.
E. The bulimic episodes are not due to anorexia nervosa or any known physical disorder.

*Essential features of bulimia for the purposes of prevalence studies.

group of subjects more like those individuals who have been described in series of patients with bulimia (Pyle et al. 1983). This quantification may be important if we are to better identify the number of individuals who are potential treatment candidates. However, there is no assurance that the group of subjects identified by these more restrictive criteria desire treatment or view their behavior as problematic (Fairburn 1983; Fairburn and Cooper 1982).

Many researchers developing inclusion criteria for self-report questionnaires on bulimic behaviors have introduced the element of loss of control into questions relevant to inclusion criteria for binge-eating (DSM-III criterion A). Hawkins and Clement (1980) in their original study used three qualifying phrases: "uncontrolled excessive eating," "rapid eating," and "eating until painfully full." Two studies used "eating an enormous amount of food over a short period of time" and "uncontrollable urges to eat and then eating until physically ill" (Halmi et al. 1981; Johnson et al. 1983). Our research group (Pyle et al. 1983) approached loss of control by using the phrase, "eating a *large* amount of food at one time in a way which you would be embarrassed about if others saw you." While the problem of quantifying the amount of food consumed during a binge remains unresolved, it has been addressed by few researchers reporting prevalence studies (Katzman et al. 1984). These varying definitions of binge-eating for questionnaire studies make com-

243

parison of frequencies for this behavior difficult; however, it is apparent that binge-eating is a frequent behavior in both males and females. The frequency of binge-eating in American female students ranges between 56 percent and 79 percent, with the lower percentage reported by high school students (Halmi et al. 1981; Hawkins and Clement 1980; Johnson et al. 1983; Pyle et al. 1983). On the other hand, a higher percentage of female high school students (21 percent) report weekly binge-eating than do female college students (17 percent) (Johnson et al. 1983; Pyle et al. 1983). A recent study (Katzman et al. 1984) found that 7.2 percent of 485 female subjects engaged in binge-eating (at least 1,200 calories in less than two hours) at least eight times monthly. Two studies cite a somewhat lower frequency of binge-eating for males (42–45 percent) (Hawkins and Clement 1980; Pyle et al. 1983), while one noted very little difference between males and females (Halmi et al. 1981). Weekly binge-eating has been reported by 11 percent of males (Pyle et al. 1983).

The DSM-III criterion C really has two components. Questions that have been used to address this criterion include "Do you consider yourself a binge-eater?" and "Are there times when you are afraid you cannot stop eating voluntarily?" (Halmi et al. 1981; Johnson et al. 1983) or "Do you think your eating habits are unusual?" and "Do you fear not being able to stop eating voluntarily?" (Katzman et al. 1984). Review of data-reporting responses to questions relevant to DSM-III criterion C reveals that women are much more apt than males (35 vs. 8 percent) to consider themselves binge-eaters (Halmi et al. 1981). Fifteen percent of female high school students endorsed this statement (Johnson et al. 1983). Fear of loss of control over eating was reported by 11 to 29 percent of females and 0 to 15 percent of males (Halmi et al. 1981; Hawkins and Clement 1980). One-fourth of high school females reported a fear that they would lose control over their eating behavior (Johnson et al. 1983).

Criterion D regarding depression and self-deprecatory thoughts has also been addressed in different ways, such as being "miserable and annoyed after binge-eating" (Halmi et al. 1981; Johnson et al. 1983), being "depressed and down on yourself after binge-eating" (Pyle et al. 1983), or "Do you feel depressed or think negative thoughts about yourself following an eating binge?" (Katzman et al. 1984). Hawkins and Clement (1980) use two statements to address this criterion: "I hate myself after binge-eating"; and "I feel very depressed after binge-eating." The feeling of being depressed and self-deprecatory after binge-eating is much more common in women than men, with 45–62 percent of women and 11–30 percent of men endorsing this item. Hawkins and Clement (1980) found that, while 29 percent of females endorsed being depressed after binge-eating and 21 percent endorsed hating themselves after binge-eating, neither statement was endorsed by any of the males ($n = 54$) in the study.

DSM-III criterion E is rarely discussed in prevalence studies because of difficulties with establishing coincidence between low weight or diagnosed anorexia nervosa and the behaviors used to satisfy the inclusion criteria for bulimia. However, the presence of low weight or anorexia nervosa is considered by authors of prevalence studies by asking subjects whether they have been treated for anorexia nervosa (Pyle et al. 1983), have been diagnosed as having anorexia nervosa in the last year (Katzman et al. 1984), have met weight criteria (Halmi et al. 1981; Johnson et al. 1983; Pyle et al. 1983), or answer affirmatively questions assessing diagnostic criteria for anorexia nervosa (Pope et al. 1984a, 1984b). While subjects satisfying criteria for both diagnoses may be identified (Pope et al. 1984a, 1984b), only one study has excluded subjects from the bulimia group on the basis of reports of a recent diagnosis of anorexia nervosa (Katzman et al. 1984).

Four studies (Katzman et al. 1984; Pope et al. 1984a, 1984b; Pyle et al. 1983) have included DSM-III criterion B questions. Our group (Pyle et al. 1983) also reported the frequency of the nonessential features of bulimia included in this category. It was found that 20 percent of female students reported binge-eating on high-carbohydrate food; 8 percent preferred to eat in secret; 5 percent ate until interrupted by pain, self-induced vomiting, or other people; 51 percent used some form of weight control to lower their weight; and 20 percent had frequent weight fluctuations of ten pounds or more. These behaviors occurred at similar rates in males except for weight control measures and frequent weight fluctuations, which were reported approximately twice as often by women.

Concerns about the current lack of specificity in the DSM-III diagnostic criteria for the bulimia syndrome have encouraged some researchers to include self-induced vomiting or laxative abuse as a way of restricting inclusion criteria. Studies to date have demonstrated that 6–16 percent of the female population have reported self-induced vomiting (Halmi et al. 1981; Hawkins and Clement 1980; Johnson et al. 1983; Pyle et al. 1983). The 16 percent figure was somewhat alarming in that it occurred in high school females who also reported a higher frequency of weekly binge-eating (Johnson et al. 1983). The prevalence of self-induced vomiting in males has been reported at 6 percent (Halmi et al. 1981; Pyle et al. 1983). Weekly self-induced vomiting has been reported in the range of 2–4 percent for females and 1 percent for males (Johnson et al. 1983; Pyle et al. 1983). English studies indicate that women report a smaller percentage of weekly self-induced vomiting (from 0 to 1 percent) (Clarke and Palmer 1983; Cooper and Fairburn 1983).

To summarize, binge-eating is a common problem. Self-induced vomiting to control weight is less common. However, an even smaller number of individuals engage in bulimic behaviors on a weekly or daily basis. Bulimic behaviors and attitudes, more often reported by females than males, are the pattern of being depressed and self-deprecatory after binge-eating, fear of loss of control over eating, seeing oneself as a binge-eater, and fear of being fat. The feelings and cognitions of the individuals who engage in bulimic behavior merit further study—particularly the role of anxiety, which has been thus far neglected. Having reviewed the process for development of operationalized criteria for the diagnosis of bulimia, we may proceed to our discussion of the prevalence of the bulimia syndrome.

The Prevalence of Bulimia

The secretive nature of the bulimia syndrome and the ease with which cases may be overlooked are illustrated by the early work of Wermuth, Davis, Hollister, and Stunkard (1977). They found that there was only one case of "compulsive eating" in a retrospective chart review of 650 medical cases. Our clinical impression is that patients with the bulimia syndrome may visit physicians often but are more likely to complain of physical problems or depression than bulimia. For this reason, the diagnosis is easily overlooked. The study by Stangler and Printz (1980) first brought to our attention the high frequency of bulimia. This retrospective chart review to check DSM-III diagnoses determined that 5.3 percent of 318 women and 1.4 percent of 282 men coming to a university student psychiatric clinic for treatment met the DSM-III diagnostic criteria for bulimia. The authors suggested that this figure was underreported since a number of cases were revealed during treatment which were not diagnosed at evaluation. The same pattern was true of the development of interest in bulimia nervosa in England. Russell's (1979) original group of thirty cases was collected over a period of six years from 1972 to 1978. It was not until Fairburn and Cooper (1982) brought attention to the frequency of this problem and the small number of individuals who entered treatment that the high prevalence of this illness was suspected.

Table 2 summarizes the current work on the prevalence of bulimia, using self-report questionnaires. The prevalence of bulimia as defined in the questionnaires ranges between 8 and 19 percent for female students, with the higher percentage reported in studies involving Eastern populations (Halmi et al. 1981; Pope et al. 1984b) and the lower percentage in two Midwestern studies (Johnson et al. 1983; Pyle et al. 1983). The wide variation in prevalences (6–19 percent) noted in female students by Pope et al. (1984b) indicates that the type of school surveyed (i.e., private vs. public) may be an important variable in prevalence of the bulimia syndrome. A recent survey of a nonstudent sample demonstrated that 10 percent reported behaviors which met operationalized DSM-III criteria for bulimia (Pope et al. 1984a). The authors of this study also suggested that the increased prevalence of bulimia in lower age groups may represent an increasing incidence of the disorder. Lower prevalence results with even minimum quantification of binge-eating (Katzman et al. 1984; Pyle et al. 1983). In fact, when self-induced vomiting is added as a qualifying criterion, the resulting prevalence of bulimia is very close to that reported for bulimia nervosa in England. The 2 percent prevalence for bulimia nervosa in adult women, according to the criteria of uncontrollable binge-eating, self-induced vomiting, and often terrified of being fat (Cooper and Fairburn 1983) closely resembles the 1 percent prevalence figure in women who meet the diagnostic criteria for bulimia and also meet the more restrictive criteria of weekly binge-eating and weekly self-induced vomiting or laxative use (Johnson et al. 1983; Pyle et al. 1983). The percentage of males with "bulimia" ranges from 0 to 6 percent with less than one of 300 meeting the more restrictive criteria of weekly binge-eating and self-induced vomiting (Halmi et al. 1981; Pope et al. 1984b; Pyle et al. 1983).

The use of more restrictive inclusion criteria, such as weekly binge-eating or self-induced vomiting, has been advocated as a method of identifying individuals who more closely resemble bulimic patients (Pyle et al. 1983). This quantification was initiated when we found that the student sample defined as "bulimic" students without weekly binge-eating or self-induced vomiting as inclusion criteria differed from bulimic patients in that they tended to be overweight binge-eaters, using fasting

TABLE 2

The Prevalence of Bulimia Based on Subject Self-Report

Source	Population	Response Rate (%)	Inclusion Criteria*	Responding Sample	Prevalence for Bulimia (%)	Bulimia with Weekly Binge-Eating (%)	Bulimia and Weekly Binge-Eating; Vomiting/ Laxative Abuse (%)
Halmi et al. (1981)	Eastern college summer school	66	DSM-III A,C,D	212 female 119 male	19 6	2	... ...
Pyle et al. (1983)	Midwestern college freshman	98	DSM-III A,B,C,D	575 female 780 male	8 1	4 .4	1 .3
Johnson et al.† (1983)	Midwestern public high school	98	DSM-III A,C2,D	1,268 female	8	5	1

Study	Population		Diagnostic criteria	Sample			
Katzman et al. (1984)	Freshman students	100[‡]	DSM-III A,B,C,D,E	485 female	. . .	3.9[‖]	. . .
Pope et al.[§] (1984a)	Shopping center patrons	99	DSM-III A,B,C1,D	300 female	10	. . .	. . .
	Urban public college	50	DSM-III A,B,C1,D	102 female	19	. . .	. . .
				47 male	None	. . .	. . .
Pope et al.[§] (1984b)	Private women's college seniors	64	DSM-III A,B,C1,D	287 female	13	. . .	. . .
	Suburban high school	84	DSM-III A,B,C1,D	155 female	6	. . .	. . .
				107 male	None	. . .	. . .

*See table 1.
[†]Omits "awareness that the eating problem is abnormal" (criterion C).
[‡]Of 147 female binge-eaters, 105 were contacted (100% completed the study).
[§]Omits "fear of not being able to stop voluntarily" (criterion C).
[‖]Binge-eating eight times monthly.

249

as a weight-control measure. However, clinic patients with bulimia were more likely to be of normal weight and to use self-induced vomiting as their primary method of weight control (Pyle et al. 1983).

Discussion

Ideally, prevalence studies involve the administration of a standardized, validated questionnaire to a sample, representative of the general population, through a structured interview. Unfortunately, such rigorous methodology has not been used thus far for bulimia research. Studies to date have been limited by the use of self-report questionnaires. Another limitation has been that most of the published questionnaire studies involve samples of high school or college students. Only recently have other samples been surveyed (Cooper and Fairburn 1983; Pope et al. 1984a). A multitude of problems may confound results reported in questionnaire studies. Researchers must select wording that the surveyed population will understand and, at the same time, correctly represent the diagnostic criteria on which the inclusion questions are based. Questionnaires designed to operationalize DSM-III diagnostic criteria are often kept brief to maximize response rate (Fairburn 1983; Pope et al. 1984a). However, this may preclude the detail necessary to measure lifetime prevalence for the disorder and hinder the search for details about the psychopathological features of bulimia. The method of administration of a questionnaire can also greatly affect the response rate, with the lowest response rate usually obtained by direct mailings (Pope et al. 1984b) and the highest by administration of the questionnaire by individuals who are in some way directly involved with the participants (Cooper and Fairburn 1983; Johnson et al. 1983; Pyle et al. 1983). Many researchers prefer anonymous questionnaires since the response rate is higher and the degree of honesty in response may also be greater (Fairburn 1983). With few exceptions (Pope et al. 1984a, 1984b; Pyle et al. 1983), questionnaires used in reported studies were not validated by administration to eating-disordered populations to determine their sensitivity and specificity for identifying clinically significant eating disorders. Also, questions persist as to whether bulimics overreport on questionnaires to please researchers (Cooper and Fairburn 1983) or underreport because they wish to keep their illness a secret (Clarke and Palmer 1983; Halmi et al. 1981; Stangler and Printz 1980).

Conclusions

While there have been several useful studies reported on the prevalence of bulimia in the general population, their research design has not been sufficiently rigorous to encourage definitive statements regarding the prevalence of bulimia in the general population. Taking these limitations into consideration, we are led by information available to us to conclude that the bulimia syndrome as it is seen in patients probably occurs in 1–2 percent of females in the target age of eighteen to thirty. The higher-prevalence figures reported may represent an earlier stage of the illness, may be identifying individuals who have a predisposition to develop the illness, or may be identifying eating abnormalities that are clinically insignificant. Prevalence studies may also be identifying a significant number of overeaters. While some data suggest that prevalence of the bulimia syndrome may be increasing, documentation by repeated studies over time in samples representative of a specific target population would be helpful. Even though evidence exists that very few women with bulimia or bulimia nervosa seek treatment, the high prevalence reported for bulimia suggests that the potential number of people who may seek treatment is high.

REFERENCES

Clarke, M. G., and Palmer, R. L. 1983. Eating attitudes and neurotic symptoms in university students. *British Journal of Psychiatry* 142:299–304.

Cooper, P. J., and Fairburn, C. G. 1983. Binge-eating and self-induced vomiting in the community: a preliminary study. *British Journal of Psychiatry* 142:139–144.

Diagnostic and Statistical Manual of Mental Disorders. 3d ed. (*DSM-III*). 1980. Washington, D.C.: American Psychiatric Association.

Fairburn, C. G. 1983. Bulimia: its epidemiology and management. In A. J. Stunkard and E. Steller, eds. *Eating and Its Disorders*. New York: Raven.

Fairburn, C. G., and Cooper, P. J. 1982. Self-induced vomiting and bulimia nervosa: an undetected problem. *British Medical Journal* 284:1153–1155.

Halmi, K. A.; Falk, J. R.; and Schwartz, E. 1981. Binge-eating and vomiting: a survey of a college population. *Psychological Medicine* 11:697–706.

Hawkins, I. I., and Clement, P. F. 1980. Development and construct validation of a self-report measure of binge-eating tendencies. *Addictive Behaviors* 7:435–439.

Johnson, C. L.; Lewis, C.; Love, S.; Stuckey, M.; and Lewis, L. 1983. A descriptive survey of dieting and bulimic behavior in a female high school population. *Understanding Anorexia Nervosa and Bulimia.* Columbus, Ohio: Ross Laboratories.

Katzman, M. A.; Wolchick, S. A.; and Braver, S. L. 1984. The prevalence of frequent binge-eating and bulimia in a non-clinical college sample. *International Journal of Eating Disorders* 3(3): 53–61.

Mitchell, J. E., and Pyle, R. L. 1982. The bulimia syndrome in normal weight individuals: a review. *International Journal of Eating Disorders* 1:61–73.

Pope, H. G.; Hudson, J. I.; Yurgelun-Todd, D. 1984a. Anorexia nervosa and bulimia among 300 suburban women shoppers. *American Journal of Psychiatry* 141:292–294.

Pope, H. G.; Hudson, J. I.; Yurgelun-Todd, D.; and Hudson, M. 1984b. Prevalence of anorexia nervosa and bulimia in three student populations. *International Journal of Eating Disorders* 3(3): 45–51.

Pyle, R. L.; Mitchell, J. E.; and Eckert, E. D. 1981. Bulimia: a report of 34 cases. *Journal of Clinical Psychiatry* 42:60–64.

Pyle, R. L.; Mitchell, J. E.; Eckert, E. D.; Halvorson, P. A.; Neuman, P. A.; and Goff, G. M. 1983. The incidence of bulimia in freshman college students. *International Journal of Eating Disorders* 2:75–85.

Russell, G. F. M. 1979. Bulimia nervosa: an ominous variant of anorexia nervosa. *Psychological Medicine* 9:429–448.

Stangler, R. S., and Printz, A. M. 1980. DSM-III: psychiatric diagnosis in a university population. *American Journal of Psychiatry* 137:937–940.

Wermuth, B. M.; Davis, R. L.; Hollister, L. E.; and Stunkard, A. J. 1977. Phenytoin treatment of the binge-eating syndrome. *American Journal of Psychiatry* 134:1249–1253.

15 THE ETIOLOGY OF BULIMIA:
BIOPSYCHOSOCIAL PERSPECTIVES

CRAIG JOHNSON AND KAREN L. MADDI

The recent increase in the incidence of bulimia has generated significant curiosity regarding the factors that contribute to the onset and perpetuation of the disorder. Although large data-based research is still in preliminary stages, there is an emerging consensus among investigators that bulimia is a paradigmatic psychosomatic disorder that is multidetermined.

The task of this chapter is to synthesize our current knowledge of how the interrelationship of biological, familial, and sociocultural factors predispose predominantly adolescent and young adult women to develop bulimia. Essentially, the study presents an etiological model of how these factors may have contributed to a characteristic personality profile and how the pursuit of thinness and subsequent bulimic behavior emerges as an adaptation to difficulties characteristic of these patients. (See fig. 1.)

The value of this paper lies in the attempt to synthesize the factors that would place an individual at risk for developing psychopathology. Risk-factor models also have significant clinical utility as they facilitate early detection and highlight how important assessment of etiological factors is for prescribing various treatment strategies.

Biological Factors

The contribution of organic factors to the onset of bulimia is unclear. Although there are often medical side effects associated with bulimia, including electrolyte abnormalities, dehydration, edema, parotid gland enlargement, dental decay, anemia, gastrointestinal problems, and men-

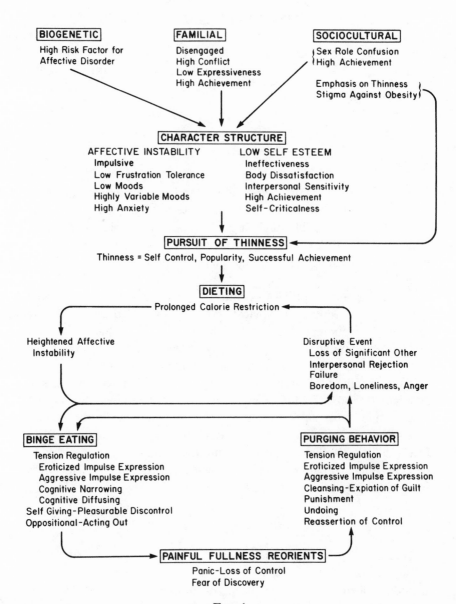

FIG. 1

strual difficulties (Ahola 1982; Gallo and Randel 1981; Hasler 1982; Mitchell and Bandle 1983), to date there has not emerged any consistent endocrine finding of etiological significance. Over the last several years, there has been, however, an increasing body of literature that suggests bulimia may be a symptom expression of a biologically mediated affective disorder. Several converging pieces of evidence have been offered in support of this hypothesis.

The first line of evidence is related to preliminary findings that a large number of bulimic patients report symptoms characteristic of unipolar and bipolar illness. These symptoms include a persistence of low and highly variable mood states, low frustration tolerance, anxiety, and suicidal ideation (Glassman and Walsh 1983; Hudson, Pope, Jonas, and Yurgelun-Todd 1983; Johnson and Larson 1982; Pyle, Mitchell, and Eckert 1981; Russell 1979). Although these early reports suggest that bulimic patients present with vegetative symptoms similar to those of patients with major depression, the etiology of the depressive experience remains unclear. It is possible that the depressive symptoms may be either physiological side effects from weight loss or fluctuations in nutritional status or psychological side effects from repeated exposure to a pattern of thoughts and behavior that results in feelings of helplessness, shame, guilt, and ineffectiveness.

The most compelling evidence for the depression hypothesis comes from family studies that indicate a high incidence of major affective disorder among first- and second-degree relatives of bulimic patients. Using the family history method among a sample of seventy-five patients with bulimia, Hudson and his colleagues (Hudson, Laffer, and Pope 1982; Hudson et al. 1983) found that 53 percent had first-degree relatives with major affective disorder. Likewise, substance abuse disorder was found to be highly prevalent (forty-five of 350 relatives). Results further indicated that the morbid risk factor for affective disorder in relatives was 28 percent, which was similar to that found in families of patients with bipolar disorder. Strober and his colleagues (Strober 1981; Strober, Salkin, Burroughs, and Marrell 1982) found strikingly similar results among anorexic patients who manifested bulimic symptoms. Their findings indicated a 20 percent morbid risk factor for affective disorder in the bulimic families. They also noted that 18 percent of the first- and second-degree relatives reported histories of alcoholism.

There has also been a preliminary attempt to identify biological markers that are associated with depression and bulimia. Although consistent markers have not been isolated that are predictive of affective disorder, two under consideration are suggestive of major depression among bulimic patients.

The dexamethasone suppression test and the thyroid releasing hormone stimulating test have been found positive in bulimic patients with the same frequency as in patients with major depression and much more frequently than would be expected in normal control populations (Gwirtsman, Roy-Byrne, and Yager 1983; Hudson et al. 1982). Sleep-laboratory research has also recently indicated that a subgroup of bulimics at normal weight (with previous histories of anorexia nervosa) displayed sleep disturbance (shortened REM latency) characteristic of patients with affective disorders (Katz, Kuperberg, Pollack, Walsh, Zumoff, and Weiner 1984).

Finally, support is marshaled for this hypothesis by early findings regarding the effectiveness of antidepressant pharmacotherapy. Both open trials and double-blind placebo controlled studies of tricyclic and MAO-inhibitor treatment has resulted in significant improvement in frequency of bulimic symptoms (Brotman, Herzog, and Woods 1984; Jonas, Pope, and Hudson 1983; Mendels 1983; Pope and Hudson 1982; Pope, Hudson, Jonas, and Yurgelun-Todd 1983; Sabine, Yonace, Farrington, Barratt, and Wakeling 1983; Walsh, Stewart, Wright, Harrison, Roose, and Glassman 1982).

Although further research is necessary to substantiate the prevalence of affective disorders among bulimic patients, it is clear that, overall, the group experiences significant affective instability that may have predated the onset of the bulimic symptoms. Furthermore, given the high incidence of affective disorder and substance abuse among the parents of these patients, we can speculate that the family environment is likely to reflect some of the instability the parents experience.

Family Characteristics

Few studies have investigated the nature of the family environment among bulimic patients. Results from preliminary studies are promising, however, in that there appears to be some agreement about what characterizes these families. Most investigators have used self-report measures of family interaction style. Johnson and Flach (1985) and Ordman and Kirschenbaum (1984) have reported that, compared with normal

CRAIG JOHNSON AND KAREN L. MADDI

control families: the families of normal weight bulimics expressed greater anger, aggression, and conflict; they used a more indirect pattern of communication; they gave less support and commitment to each other; they placed less emphasis on assertiveness and autonomy; and they were less interested in political, social, cultural, and recreational events despite expressing higher achievement expectations. Strober (1981) found similar results when he compared the families of anorexic bulimics with those of anorexic restrictors. In addition, he reported higher levels of discord between the parents, higher overall level of life stresses within the family, and more alienation between the anorexic-bulimic patient and the family, especially the father. Mothers of anorexic bulimics were described as more hostile and depressed, while the fathers were more impulsive and irritable, showed poorer frustration tolerance, and were more often alcoholic (Strober et al. 1982). Humphrey (1985) compared anorexic-bulimic families with normal control families and also found virtually the same results.

Garner, Garfinkel, and Olmsted (1983a) compared normal-weight bulimic families with families of anorexics who binged and to families of restricting anorexics. These investigators found that normal-weight bulimics' families were strikingly similar to the anorexic-bulimics' families on six of eight measures of family interaction style including communication, affective expression, affective involvement, control, values and norms, and social desirability. In addition, they reported that the degree of problems in these areas suggested significant overall pathology, well above that of the families of the restricting anorexics.

Two recent investigations have utilized direct observational measures of bulimics' family interaction style. Humphrey (1984) and Humphrey, Apple, and Kirschenbaum (1984) reported that, compared with normal control families, the families of bulimic-anorexics were more belittling and appeasing, and less helping, trusting, nurturing, and approaching. In addition, these parents gave more negative, less positive, more contradictory (double-bind) messages to their daughters, especially around issues of taking control versus autonomy. These direct observations are consistent with and provide validation of the self-report data.

Taken together, these early studies suggest that the bulimics' families can be generally characterized as disengaged, chaotic, highly conflicted, and with a high degree of life stress. Further, they use indirect and contradictory patterns of communication, they are deficient in problem-solving skills, they are less supportive, and they are less intellectually and less recreationally oriented—despite their higher achievement expectation.

At this point in the etiological model we have a child who is at risk for affective instability, who has a high probability of being in a family that is volatile and disorganized with parents who themselves may have difficulty with affective disorder. Unfortunately, as we move to the broader sociocultural context, we find that, particularly for young women, it is a milieu that simultaneously exacerbates feelings of instability and suggests an adaptation to the instability they are experiencing.

Sociocultural Factors

Biological and familial factors alone could not explain why we would be observing an increase in a specific symptom picture among a rather homogeneous cohort (fifteen- to twenty-five-year-old, middle- to upper-class, Caucasian, college-educated women in Westernized countries). Consequently, one has to turn to the broader sociocultural context to see whether any events occurred during the period of increased incidence that would selectively bias the group at risk as well as the specific symptom expression. Retrospectively, it appears that two cultural events occurred simultaneously that could account for this.

The mean age of the patient population indicates that they are the first generation of young women who were raised at the onset of the feminist movement. Several authors have observed that during these years the sociocultural milieu for young women was in substantial transition, which appears to have contributed to role and identity confusion among at least a subpopulation of this age group (Bardwick 1971; Lewis and Johnson 1984; Palazzoli 1974; Schwartz, Thompson, and Johnson 1982). Garner et al. (1983a) review evidence that these shifting cultural norms forced contemporary women to face multiple, ambiguous, and often contradictory role expectations. These role expectations included accommodating more traditional feminine expectations, such as physical attractiveness and domesticity, incorporating more modern standards for vocational and personal achievement, and taking advantage of increased opportunity for self-definition and autonomy. Garner and his colleagues suggest that "while the wider range of choices made available to contemporary women may have provided personal freedom for those who were psychologically robust, it may have been overwhelming for the field-dependent adolescent who lacked internal structure." Consequently, this cohort appears to represent a transitional group within which at least a subgroup may be at increased risk for experiencing anxiety (affective instability) in reaction to the shifting role expectations and increased demand for achievement.

A second cultural shift emerged concomitantly with the feminist movement that appears to have biased the specific symptom expression of food- and body-related behavior. More specifically, during the mid-1960s, an emphasis on thinness for women emerged. In a milieu of increasing focus on achievement and confusion about how to express the drive to achieve, it appears that the pursuit of thinness emerged as one vehicle through which young women could compete among themselves and demonstrate self-control. In fact, the accomplishment of thinness has increasingly become a very highly valued achievement that secures envy and respect among women in the current culture.

Conversely, the absence of weight control, leading to even moderate obesity, leads culturally to social discrimination, isolation, and low self-esteem. Wooley and Wooley (1979) reviewed numerous studies that document the stigma of obesity in childhood and adolescence. They assert that the overweight child is regarded by others as "responsible" for his or her condition and that failure to remediate the situation is viewed as "personal weakness." Both normal-weight and overweight children themselves describe obese silhouettes with pejorative labels such as stupid, lazy, dirty, sloppy, mean, and ugly. Female children add worried, sad, and lonely to the list of adjectives, which suggests that for them obesity carries connotations of social isolation (Allon 1975; Staffieri 1967, 1972).

This negative attitude toward endomorphic children prevails for both sexes. In adolescence and adulthood, however, there is increasing evidence that females are more affected than males by this antifat prejudice. Empirical research has shown that obese girls have greatly reduced chances of being admitted to college compared with nonobese applicants (Canning and Mayer 1966); obese job applicants are less likely to be hired than their slimmer counterparts (Roe and Eickwort 1976); once hired their job performance is more likely to be negatively evaluated (Larkin and Pines 1979); they are less likely to make as much money or to get top spots when promotions come around. Finally, compared with nonobese women, overweight women are much more likely to achieve a lower socioeconomic status than their parents (Goldblatt, Moore, and Stunkard 1965; Mayer 1968).

Against the backdrop of confusing cultural expectations and high achievement expectations, it appears that the pursuit of thinness (which can be scaled and measured) and avoidance of obesity emerged as constituting one very concrete activity through which young women could compete and obtain consistently favorable social responses that held the possibility of enhancing self-esteem. It is extremely important to note, however, that not all young women who were exposed to this cultural milieu developed eating disorders. Therefore, one must attempt to look more closely at the personality characteristics thought to be associated with patients who develop bulimia.

Personality Factors

Although personality trait findings among this group are quite variable, two consistent factors seem to emerge. First, as mentioned, there is substantial evidence that bulimics experience significant affective instability that is manifested in depressed and highly variable mood states, impulsive behavior frequently including drug and alcohol abuse, low frustration tolerance, and high anxiety. Although data-based research has not clearly indicated that the reported affective instability predated the onset of the bulimic symptoms, clinical observations suggest that affect regulation difficulties are long-standing side effects resulting from both biogenetic vulnerabilities and maladaptive parenting styles. Consequently, these patients have long histories of feeling somewhat out of control and perhaps helpless in relation to their bodily experience. This undoubtedly contributes significantly to the second prominent personality trait among bulimics; low self-esteem (Boskind-Lodahl 1976; Conners, Johnson, and Stuckey 1984; Garfinkel and Garner 1982).

Although low self-esteem is commonly associated with any genre of psychopathology, there appear to be certain features that are characteristic of bulimic patients. Several investigators have observed that many bulimic patients have difficulty identifying and articulating different internal states (Bruch 1973). This incapacity appears to contribute to a feeling of being undifferentiated (Lewis and Johnson 1984) that leads to feelings of ineffectiveness and helplessness in controlling these internal states. It is interesting to note that, in addition to the sociocultural factors that might contribute to women feeling dissatisfied with their bodies (imperfect appearance), women who experience difficulty modulating internal states may feel more dissatisfaction, perhaps even rage, at bodies they experience as being defective containers of their affects. Further exacerbating self-esteem problems is that bulimic patients are quite sensitive to rejection, which results in feelings of social discomfort and nonassertive behavior (Boskind-Lodahl 1976; Connors et al. 1984; Johnson, Stuckey, Lewis, and Schwartz 1982; Norman and Herzog 1983; Pyle et al. 1981; Schneider and Agras 1985). Finally, amid these various vulnerabilities, these patients have high expectations of themselves resulting in persistent shame, guilt, and self-criticalness over the repeated discrepancy they feel between their actual self and ideal self (Goodsitt 1984; Kohut 1971).

At this point in the etiological model, we have a situation where the biological, familial, and sociocultural milieus have combined to shape an individual that is at high risk for feeling fundamentally out of control of her internal life. Given these circumstances, it is likely that the person will begin to seek some external adaptation in an attempt to gain control of her internal discomfort. Given the issues related to bodily experience, it seems that the adaptation would need to be focused in that arena. This raises the question as to why food-related or dieting behavior would be selected rather than other potential behaviors such as drug abuse, promiscuity, delinquent behavior, or a more primitive form of self-mutilatory behavior. The following section presents comments on how the pursuit of thinness could emerge for these patients as a viable adaptation to the self-regulatory deficits that have been reviewed.

The Pursuit of Thinness as an Adaptation of Self-Regulatory Deficits, Interpersonal Sensitivity, and Achievement Expectations

Clinical observations and data-based research have documented that an early and primary source of feelings of mastery for children comes from successful control of bodily functions and movements. As suggested, biogenetic and parental factors appear to have predisposed these patients to have long-standing difficulty in identifying and modulating internal affective states. Further, these repeated difficulties might result in feelings of helplessness, ineffectiveness, and being out of control. Over the last several decades an emphasis has emerged on women taking control of their bodies. A demonstration of being in control of one's body appears to have become, more generally, a demonstration that one is in control of one's life. More specifically, for this group of patients the accomplishment of thinness, or control of amount and distribution of fat, has become a demonstration to themselves that they can control the container that houses their affective states. Furthermore, in the absence of knowing how to determine whether they are in control or not, they simply have to weigh themselves to obtain some external, concrete indicator of their level of control.

It was also suggested earlier that many bulimic patients lack confidence interpersonally and feel self-conscious and unattractive. The accomplishment of thinness among these women not only enhances self-confidence but also often results in significant social transformations. Many women report dramatic increases in their social desirability (popularity) as a result of weight loss.

Finally, the pursuit of thinness has also become a vehicle to express achievement. As mentioned, one dimension of change that has occurred during the time frame of increased incidence has been an increased emphasis on achievement for young women. Unfortunately, at the time of increased emphasis on achievement there were relatively few avenues for young women to directly compete that were socially valued. It appears that the pursuit of thinness emerged as one way in which young women could compete and demonstrate intrapsychic and interpersonal achievement. This avenue for achievement and competition not only appeared benign but was also socially sanctioned.

Therefore, there are several reasons why the pursuit of thinness would become a functional adaptation to the personality vulnerabilities mentioned. While it seems clear how the pursuit of thinness and accompanying dieting behavior would increase in incidence, it remains unclear how the symptoms of bulimia also increase in incidence. The following section presents a synthesis of how the symptoms of bulimia might emerge.

The Adaptive Context of Binge-Eating

Over the last two decades a cultural milieu has progressively emerged, particularly for women: if one can control weight (body) and achieve thinness, this will be a demonstration of self-control that will be intrapsychically and interpersonally reinforcing. Thinness, of course, results from extended calorie restriction. Consequently, the increase in the incidence of bulimic behavior occurred during the period when large numbers of adolescent and young adult women were pursuing thinness through highly restrictive dieting.

Predictably, research has indicated that the onset of bulimic symptomology is often caused by periods of prolonged calorie deprivation (Johnson et al. 1982; Pyle et al. 1981). Over the last several years a growing body of research has been documented showing that both physiological and psychological side effects result from semistarvation and that counterregulatory behaviors such as binge-eating also occur in reaction to prolonged states of calorie deprivation. (Garfinkel and Garner 1982; Garner, Rockert, Olmsted, Johnson, and Coscina 1984; Glucksman and Hirsch 1969; Herman and Mack 1975; Herman and Polivy 1980; Keys, Brozek, Henschel, Mickelson, and Taylor 1950; Rowland 1970). The physiological side effects that have been reported include gastrointestinal discomfort, decreased need for sleep, dizziness, headaches, hypersensitivity to noise and light, reduced strength, poor motor control, edema, hair loss, decreased tolerance for cold temperatures, visual disturbances, auditory disturbances, and paresthesias. Additional side effects include persistent tiredness, weakness, listlessness, fatigue, and lack of energy. Psychological symptoms include increased depression, irritability, rage outbursts, increased anxiety, social withdrawal, and loss of sexual interest. Specific increases in food-related behavior, which occur from semistarvation states, include an increased obsession with food, food hoarding, prolonged eating behavior during mealtimes, peculiar taste preferences, and hyperconsumption of substances such as coffee and gum.

The explanation offered for the appearance of these side effects is that as the body drops below a minimal biogenetically mediated (set point) range of weight for an individual, the body initiates a variety of compensatory behaviors designed to conserve energy and to begin to increase the individual's body weight to the internally prescribed weight range (Garner et al. 1984; Keesey 1980, 1983; Mrosovsky and Powley 1977; Nisbett 1972). This is particularly true for women, who must maintain approximately 13 percent adipose tissue in order to menstruate (Frisch 1983). Any time the body fat threatens to drop below this range, a specific biological imperative ensues which involves a persistent and intense drive toward caloric intake. Foremost among the compensatory behaviors that emerge in reaction to caloric deprivation is an increased vulnerability to binge-eating (rapid consumption of a large quantity of food in a short space of time).

Consequently, as figure 1 depicts, at this point in the etiological model, we have an individual who has attempted to compensate for a variety of self-regulatory and self-esteem deficits by attaining thinness. If success in attaining thinness drops the individual's weight near the set point range (menstrual threshold), a variety of physiological and psychological side effects occur that not only exacerbate the original affective instability but threaten the self-esteem developed through the achievement of low weight. Unfortunately, at this point the individual is at what could be referred to as a psychobiological impasse. Essentially, the psychological adaptation developed is at odds with biology. In fact, it is likely that the individual experiences the body's relentless drive to consume calories as the body once again being out of control. As figure 2 demonstrates, a belief system that is logically consistent could emerge that would result in the individual interpreting the internal experience of hunger as a signal that she was out of control and failing at her appointed task. This guarantees that multiple times a day she would have an internal experience (hunger) that she would interpret as evidence that she was ineffective and a failure. Paradoxically, then, the effort at compensation results in an exacerbation of the original difficulties.

Against this backdrop of heightened affective instability, lowered self-esteem, and semistarvation, any stressful life event would be taxing to the failing defensive adaptation (thinness = control and achievement). If disinhibition occurred, given the semistarved state, binge-eating would be the most likely expression of the breakdown in defenses, and, despite the fact that most bulimic patients feel that their episodic binge-eating is a shameful and humiliating experience of being out of control, the act of binge-eating can offer a number of compensatory adaptations that become quite reinforcing.

AFFECT REGULATION

Given the evidence for affective instability, it is easy to see how binge-eating could emerge as a relatively safe mechanism for regulating different tension states. As noted, research studies have indicated that bulimics often experience a wide range of highly variable mood states that they have difficulty identifying, articulating, and controlling. These moods include anxiety, panic, depression, boredom, irritability, anger,

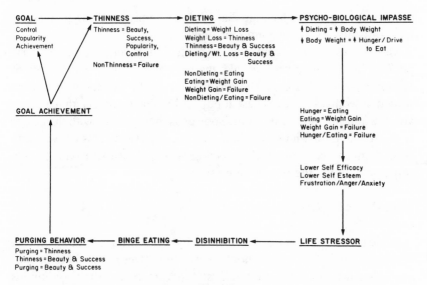

FIG. 2

and euphoria. Throughout the day the variability, range, and seeming unpredictability of the different mood states may become overwhelming and disorganizing for the patient. The concrete and repetitive acts of binging and purging can serve an integrating function for these patients, allowing them to reliably create a predictable affective and cognitive state through the behavioral sequence. Essentially, when overwhelmed by confusing and variable mood states, the binging and purging become both an explanation of the dysphoria ("I am feeling bad because I have binged") and a mechanism for actually helping to regulate the dysphoria ("I feel relieved after I have binged").

IMPULSE EXPRESSION

Bulimic patients are vulnerable to impulsive behavior. Episodic binge-eating can be a relatively safe mechanism for being impulsive, since binge-eating does not carry significant moral, legal, or medical consequences—as does promiscuity, delinquent behavior, or drug abuse. More specifically, bulimic patients can eroticize the binge-eating episodes, thus offering an alternative response to sexual feelings if they are conflicted about masturbation or heterosexual activity. Similarly, binge-eating and subsequent purging behavior can become an effective mechanism for expressing aggressive feelings that research indicates these individuals have difficulty expressing interpersonally.

More obsessive, overcontrolled patients also use binge-eating to temporarily be out of control or have the phenomenological experience of letting go or spacing out. These patients create an experience of controlled discontrol. They invest food, an inanimate object that has no volition and can have only as much power as they grant it, with the power to overcome them and make them become impulsive. This allows some relief from an overcontrolled psychological world without having to take responsibility for the impulsive episodes.

SELF-NURTURANCE

Some bulimic patients are tormented by a profound sense of guilt that results in a belief that they should deny themselves pleasurable or self-enhancing activities. They are quite self-sacrificing, and their continuous efforts to care for others often leave them feeling depleted and exhausted. The act of binge-eating (with the attendant attribution that the event was externally determined) among these patients can serve as a mechanism for briefly feeding themselves or greedily and selfishly consuming for themselves.

Along similar lines, some bulimic patients experience a basic mistrust of others that prevents them from receiving emotional supplies from the outside. Consequently, they will invest food and the act of binge-eating with the ability to soothe, comfort, and gratify themselves. In this regard, they will often project onto the food human-like qualities that allow them the illusion of receiving emotional supplies from a source other than themselves. The fact that food (an inanimate object) can behave only as they desire allows them to simultaneously refuel and yet be protected from potential disappointment in human relationships.

OPPOSITIONALITY

Binge-eating can also serve as a mechanism for expressing oppositionality. For patients who feel that external authority figures have imposed significant restraint on them, binge-eating can become an expression of acting out or of defiance. This is particularly true of bulimics who were raised in families where weight control and dieting were highly emphasized by the parents. The act of binge-eating for these patients becomes a statement of protest and an expression of autonomy.

Whatever specific adaptation binge-eating serves, once an episode has ended, the patients generally feel some combination of guilt, shame, disgust, and fear of being discovered. These feelings become concretely manifested in a sense of panic that they will gain weight, which would be an observable indication that they are out of control, disorganized, undisciplined, greedy, etc. Consequently, the use of evacuation techniques such as self-induced vomiting, laxative abuse, and enemas emerges as a viable mechanism for undoing the binge-eating.

PURGING BEHAVIOR

Like binge-eating, purging behavior can serve a variety of different adaptive functions, some of which may become more important than the actual act of binge-eating in the psychic economy of the bulimic. As with binge-eating, the act of purging can serve as a mechanism for tension regulation. This is particularly true of aggressive feelings. Self-induced vomiting can be a rather violent act, and the physical process of vomiting can be quite cathartic around aggressive feelings. For patients who feel especially guilty and self-critical around the binge-eating episodes, the purging can serve as a self-punishment and an act of undoing or penitence that pays for the crime of impulse expression. For the oppositional patient, it allows them to get away with something without "getting caught" or having to pay the price of overeating.

For more borderline patients, the act of purging (primarily laxative abuse) appears to serve an integrating function similar to other forms of self-mutilatory behavior. The intense pain created by the persistent diarrhea appears to make them feel alive and in touch with reality.

Most important, as figure 2 depicts, the purging behavior becomes highly reinforcing because it allows the individual to avoid the psychobiological impasse of restrained eating. Essentially, purging allows the individual to eat in any compensatory way she desires without the negative consequence of weight gain. Several investigators have noted that the purging behavior can become so highly reinforcing that for some patients a transformation occurs from purging so that they can binge-eat to binge-eating so that they can purge (Johnson and Larson 1982; Rosen and Leitenberg 1984).

Unfortunately, similar to the adaptive effort of the pursuit of thinness, the purging adaptation simultaneously creates and solves a problem. In the absence of immediately apparent negative consequences, the binging and purging progressively increase until the individual is using the cycle to regulate a variety of affective and cognitive states. Eventually the individual feels addicted to, and controlled by, the process that again results in lower self-esteem and heightened affective instability.

Conclusions

The purpose of this chapter is to synthesize our current knowledge of how biological, familial, and sociocultural factors predispose predominantly adolescent and young adult women to develop bulimia. An etiologic model is proposed indicating that young women who are at risk for developing bulimia appear to have a biological vulnerability to affective instability. This affective instability was exacerbated both by a family environment that was conflicted and disorganized and by a sociocultural environment that was confusing as a result of being in transition. It was suggested that these factors contributed to a personality profile that included self-esteem and self-regulatory difficulties. It was further proposed that the sociocultural milieu suggested to young women that the achievement of thinness would help remedy their self-esteem and self-regulatory problems. Evidence was reviewed regarding the physiological and psychological side effects of semistarvation and how the belief system associated with the pursuit of thinness results in a psychobiological impasse that, paradoxically, eventually exacerbates the original difficulties of affective instability and low self-esteem. The binge-eating was presented as a counterregulatory reaction to the psychobiological impasse, and the variety of psychological adaptations that the binge/purge sequence could eventually serve were reveiwed. The value of this study lies in the attempt to develop a risk-factor model for bulimic behavior that would facilitate early detection and more sophisticated assessment.

NOTE

Accepted for publication March 1985.

REFERENCES

Ahola, S. J. 1982. Unexplained parotid enlargement: a clue to occult bulimia. *Connecticut Medicine* 46(4): 185–186.

Allon, N. 1975. Latent social services in group dieting. *Social Problems* 32:59–69.

Bardwick, J. 1971. *Psychology of Women: A Study of Bio-Cultural Conflicts.* New York: Harper & Row.

Boskind-Lodahl, M. 1976. Cinderella's stepsisters: a feminist perspective on anorexia nervosa and bulimia. *Signs: Journal of Women in Culture and Society* 2:342–356.

Brotman, A.; Herzog, P.; and Woods, S. 1984. Antidepressant treatment of bulimia: the relationship between bingeing and depressive symptomatology. *Journal of Clinical Psychiatry* 45(1): 7–9.

Bruch, H. 1973. *Eating Disorders: Obesity, Anorexia Nervosa, and the Person Within.* New York: Basic.

Canning, H., and Mayer, J. 1966. Obesity: its possible effect on college acceptance. *New England Journal of Medicine* 275:1172–1174.

Connors, M.; Johnson, C.; and Stuckey, M. 1984. Treatment of bulimia with brief psychoeducational group therapy. *American Journal of Psychiatry* 141(12): 1512–1516.

Frisch, R. E. 1983. Fatness and reproduction: delayed menarche and amenorrhea of ballet dancers and college athletes. In P. L. Darby, P. E. Garfinkel, D. M. Garner, and D. V. Coscina, eds. *Anorexia Nervosa: Recent Developments.* New York: Liss.

Gallo, L., and Randel, A. 1981. Chronic vomiting and its effect on the primary dentition: report of a case. *Journal of Dentition Child.* 48: 383–384.

Garfinkel, P. E., and Garner, D. M. 1982. *Anorexia Nervosa: A Multi-dimensional Perspective.* New York: Brunner/Mazel.

Garner, D. M.; Garfinkel, P. E.; and Olmsted, M. 1983a. An overview of sociocultural factors in the development of anorexia nervosa. In *Anorexia Nervosa: Recent Developments in Research.* New York: Liss.

Garner, D. M.; Garfinkel, P. E.; and O'Shaughnessy, M. 1983b. Clinical and psychometric comparison between bulimia and anorexia and bulimia in normal-weight women. In *Understanding Anorexia Nervosa and Bulimia.* Columbus, Ohio: Ross Laboratories.

Garner, D. M.; Rockert, W.; Olmsted, M. P.; Johnson, C.; and Coscina,

D. V. 1984. Psychoeducational principles in the treatment of bulimia and anorexia nervosa. In D. M. Garner and P. E. Garfinkel, eds. *A Handbook of Psychotherapy for Anorexia and Bulimia*. New York: Guilford.

Glassman, A. H., and Walsh, B. T. 1983. Link between bulimia and depression unclear. *Journal of Clinical Psychopharmacology* 3:203.

Glucksman, M. L., and Hirsch, J. 1969. The response of obese patients to weight reduction. *Psychosomatic Medicine* 31:1–7.

Goldblatt, P. B.; Moore, M. E.; and Stunkard, A. J. 1965. Social factors in obesity. *Journal of the American Medical Association* 192:1039–1044.

Goodsitt, A. 1984. Self-psychology and the treatment of anorexia nervosa. In D. M. Garner and P. E. Garfinkel, eds. *A Handbook of Psychotherapy for Anorexia Nervosa and Bulimia*. New York: Guilford.

Gwirtsman, H. E.; Roy-Byrne, H. E.; and Yager, J. 1983. Neuroendocrine abnormalities in bulimia. *American Journal of Psychiatry* 140:559–563.

Hasler, J. 1982. Parotid enlargement and presenting symptom in anorexia nervosa. *Oral Surgery, Oral Medicine, Oral Pathology* 53(6):567–573.

Herman, C. P., and Mack, D. 1975. Restrained and unrestrained eating. *Journal of Personality* 43:647–660.

Herman, C. P., and Polivy, J. 1980. Restrained eating. In A. J. Stunkard, ed. *Obesity*. Philadelphia: Saunders.

Hudson, J. I.; Laffer, P. S.; and Pope, H. G., Jr. 1982. Bulimia related to affective disorder by family and response to the dexamethasone suppression test. *American Journal of Psychiatry*. 139(5): 685–687.

Hudson, J. I.; Pope, H. G., Jr.; Jonas, J. M.; and Yurgelun-Todd, D. 1983. Family history study of anorexia nervosa and bulimia. *British Journal of Psychiatry* 142:133–138.

Humphrey, L. L. 1984. A comparison of bulimic-anorexic and nondistressed family processes using structural analysis of social behavior. Northwestern University Medical School, unpublished.

Humphrey, L. L. 1985. Family relations in bulimic-anorexic and nondistressed families. *International Journal of Eating Disorders*, in press.

Humphrey, L. L.; Apple, R.; and Kirschenbaum, D. S. 1985. Differentiating bulimic-anorexic from normal families using an interpersonal and a behavioral observation system. *Journal of Consulting and Clinical Psychology*, in press.

Johnson, C., and Flach, R. A. 1985. Family characteristics of bulimic and normal women: a comparative study. *American Journal of Psychiatry*, in press.

Johnson, C., and Larson, R. 1982. Bulimia: an analysis of moods and behavior. *Psychosomatic Medicine* 44(4): 333–345.

Johnson, C.; Stuckey, M. K.; Lewis, L. D.; and Schwartz, D. 1982. Bulimia: a descriptive survey of 316 cases. *International Journal of Eating Disorders* 2(1): 3–16.

Jonas, J. M.; Pope, H. G., Jr.; and Hudson, J. I. 1983. Treatment of bulimia with MAO inhibitors. *Journal of Clinical Psychopharmacology* 3:59–60.

Katz, J. L.; Kuperberg, A.; Pollack, C. P.; Walsh, B. T.; Zumoff, B.; and Weiner, H. 1984. Is there a relationship between eating disorder and affective disorder? New evidence from sleep recordings. *American Journal of Psychiatry* 141(6): 753–759.

Keesey, R. E. 1980. A set point analysis of the regulation of body weight. In A. J. Stunkard, ed. *Obesity*. Philadelphia: Saunders.

Keesey, R. E. 1983. A hypothalamic syndrome of body weight regulation at reduced levels. In *Understanding Anorexia Nervosa and Bulimia*. Report of the Fourth Ross Conference on Medical Research. Columbus, Ohio: Ross Laboratories.

Keys, A.; Brozek, J.; Henschel, A.; Mickelson, O.; and Taylor, H. L. 1950. *The Biology of Human Starvation*, vol. 1. Minneapolis: University of Minnesota Press.

Kohut, H. 1971. *The Analysis of the Self*. New York: International Universities Press.

Larkin, J. E., and Pines, H. A. 1979. No fat persons need apply. *Sociology of Work Occupations* 6:312–327.

Lewis, L., and Johnson, C. 1985. A comparison of sex-role orientation between women with bulimia and normal controls. *International Journal of Eating Disorders*, in press.

Mayer, J. 1968. *Overweight: Causes, Cost and Control*. Englewood Cliffs, N. J.: Prentice-Hall.

Mendels, J. 1983. Eating disorders and antidepressants. *Journal of Clinical Psychopharmacology* 3:59–60.

Mitchell, J., and Bandle, J. 1983. Metabolic and endocrine investigations

271

in women of normal weight with the bulimia syndrome. *Biological Psychiatry* 18(3): 355–365.

Mrosovsky, N., and Powley, T. L. 1977. Set points of body weight and fat. *Behavioral Biology* 20:205–223.

Nisbett, R. E. 1972. Eating behavior and obesity in men and animals. *Advances in Psychosomatic Medicine* 7:173–193.

Norman, D. K., and Herzog, D. B. 1983. Bulimia, anorexia nervosa and anorexia nervosa with bulimia: a comparative analysis of MMPI profiles. *International Journal of Eating Disorders* 2(2): 43–52.

Ordman, A. M., and Kirschenbaum, D. S. 1985. Bulimia: assessment of eating, psychological, and familial characteristics. *International Journal of Eating Disorders*, in press.

Palazzoli, M. S. 1974. *Self-Starvation*. London: Chaucer.

Pope, H. G., and Hudson, J. I. 1982. Treatment of bulimia with antidepressants. *Psychopharmacology* 78:176–179.

Pope, H. G.; Hudson, J. I.; Jonas, J. M.; and Yurgelun-Todd, D. 1983. Bulimia treated with imipramine: a placebo-controlled, double-blind study. *American Journal of Psychiatry* 140(5): 554–558.

Pyle, R. L.; Mitchell, J. E.; and Eckert, E. D. 1981. Bulimia: a report of 34 cases. *Journal of Clinical Psychiatry* 42(2): 60–64.

Roe, D. A., and Eickwort, K. R. 1976. Relationships between obesity and associated health factors with unemployment among low income women. *Journal of the American Medical Women's Association* 31:193–204.

Rosen, J., and Leitenberg, H. 1984. Exposure plus response prevention treatment of bulimia. In D. M. Garner and P. E. Garfinkel, eds. *A Handbook of Psychotherapy for Anorexia and Bulimia*. New York: Guilford.

Rowland, C. V. 1970. Anorexia nervosa: a survey of the literature and review of 30 cases. *International Psychiatry Clinics* 1:37–137.

Russell, G. F. M. 1979. Bulimia nervosa: an ominous variant of anorexia nervosa. *Psychological Medicine* 9:429–448.

Sabine, E. J.; Yonace, A.; Farrington, A. J.; Barratt, A.; and Wakeling, W. 1983. Bulimia nervosa: a placebo-controlled therapeutic trial of mianersin. *British Journal of Clinical Pharmacology* 15:195S–202S.

Schneider, J. A., and Agras, W. S. 1985. A cognitive behavioral group treatment of bulimia. *British Journal of Psychiatry*. 146:66–69.

Schwartz, D. M.; Thompson, M. G.; and Johnson, C. 1982. Anorexia nervosa and bulimia: the sociocultural context. *International Journal of Eating Disorders* 1(3): 23–25.

Staffieri, J. R. 1967. A study of social stereotype of body image in children. *Journal of Personality and Social Psychology* 7:101–104.

Staffieri, J. R. 1972. Body build and behavior expectancies in young females. *Developmental Psychology* 6:125–127.

Strober, M. 1981. The significance of bulimia in juvenile anorexia nervosa: an exploration of possible etiological factors. *International Journal of Eating Disorders* 1(1): 28–43.

Strober, M.; Salkin, B.; Burroughs, J.; and Marrell, W. 1982. Validity of the bulimia-restricter distinction in anorexia nervosa: parental personality characteristics and family psychiatric morbidity. *Journal of Nervous and Mental Disease* 170(6): 345–351.

Walsh, T.; Stewart, J.; Wright, L.; Harrison, W.; Roose, S.; and Glassman, A. 1982. A treatment of bulimia with monoamine oxidase inhibitors. *American Journal of Psychiatry* 139:1629–1630.

Wooley, S., and Wooley, O. 1979. Obesity and women—I: a closer look at the facts. *Women's Studies International Quarterly* 2:69–79.

16   THE PSYCHOANALYTIC PSYCHOTHERAPY
OF BULIMIC ANOREXIA NERVOSA

C. PHILIP WILSON

During the past thirty years there has been increasing evidence that anorexia nervosa, a generic term that I use to include both the bulimic and restrictor syndromes, is a psychosomatic disorder (Bruch 1978; Sours 1980; Sperling 1978; Thoma 1967; Wilson, Hogan, and Mintz 1983). Specifically, the bulimic patient has strict but ineffective ego controls that are unable to regulate the impulse to eat (Wilson 1982, 1983a). This defect in self-control is so threatening to the patient that the slightest gain in weight may produce panic, excessive exercising, starving, and vomiting. The bulimic patient, unable to control eating, is also unable to control other impulses, so that one sees sexual promiscuity, delinquency, stealing, lying, and running away more frequently than in the starving anorexic patient. This defect in ego controls arises in part from identifying with parents who frequently argue, fight, and act out destructively more often than parents of starving anorexics.

Restrictor and bulimic anorexia nervosa are symptom complexes that occur in a variety of character disorders: hysterical, obsessive-compulsive, borderline, and, in some cases, conditions close to psychosis. However, even in the most disturbed cases, there are areas of relatively intact ego functioning and a capacity for a transference relationship.

For the diagnosis of bulimic anorexia nervosa, gorging and vomiting as well as amenorrhea are necessary. Some cases begin with a restrictor anorexic syndrome and then develop bulimia. Other patients are predominantly restrictive in their eating behavior, with infrequent episodes of bulimia. Many bulimics can keep their weight at near normal range by balancing their starving, gorging, vomiting, and laxative use.

I concur with Thoma's delineation of the syndrome: (1) the age of onset is usually puberty; (2) the patients are predominantly female (although male cases have been reported by Falstein, Feinstein, and Judas [1956], Mintz [1983], and Sours [1980]; (3) the reduction in nutritional intake is psychically determined; (4) when spontaneous or self-induced vomiting occurs, the diagnosis of bulimia is made; (5) amenorrhea (which is psychically caused) generally appears either before or, more rarely, after the beginning of the weight loss; (6) constipation, sometimes an excuse for excessive consumption of laxatives, speeds up weight loss; (7) the physical effects of undernourishment are present, and, in severe cases, death may ensue (7–15 percent die [Sours 1969]). Hogan (1983) added three further observations: (8) there is commonly a tendency toward hyperactivity, which may be extreme; (9) in females there is often a disproportionate loss of breast tissue early in the disease; and (10) the symptom complex is often accompanied by or alternates with other psychosomatic symptoms (or psychogenic equivalents such as depressions, phobias, or periods of self-destructive acting out that may include impulsive sexual behavior, stealing, or accident-prone behavior). With successful psychodynamic treatment, Wilson et al. (1983) have found that all the physical signs and symptoms of bulimic anorexia nervosa return to normal except for irreversible tooth and gum damage caused by gorging and vomiting. However, menstruation may not resume, even though the patient's weight returns to normal limits, if significant conflicts about pregnancy have not been resolved.

I recently (Wilson 1980a, 1982, 1983a) presented hypotheses about the diagnosis, etiology, psychodynamics, and technique of treatment of anorexia nervosa. My research indicates that fat phobia should replace anorexia as a diagnostic term. These patients do not suffer from lack of hunger but from the opposite, a fear of insatiable hunger as well as of impulses of many other kinds (Sours 1980; Sperling 1978; Thoma 1967; Wilson et al. 1983). Psychodynamic work with these restrictor and bulimic anorexics focused on their intense fear-of-being-fat body image disturbance and their fear-of-being-fat complex. Neurotic analysands also evidenced less intensely cathected but clear-cut fear-of-being-fat obsessions and body image disturbances. These findings, coupled with nonanalytic research, lead to the conclusion that in our culture most women and certain men, those with unresolved feminine identifications, have a fear of being fat. Normal women readily admit to the fear. No matter how "perfect" a woman's figure may be, if she is told she is fat she will have an emotional reaction out of all proportion to reality. On the other hand, if she is told she looks thin or has lost weight, she will be inordinately pleased.

It is a central hypothesis of my research that restrictor and bulimic anorexia symptoms are caused by an overwhelming terror of being fat that has been primarily caused by an identification with a parent or parents who have a similar fear of being fat, and that anorexia (fat phobia) is secondarily reinforced by the general irrational fear of being fat of most other women and many men in our culture (fig. 1). Ceaser (1977) noted the role of maternal identification in three bulimics and one restrictor anorexic.

The Family Psychological Profile
and Its Therapeutic Implications

Psychodynamic research with the families of 100 anorexia nervosa patients[1] revealed a parental psychological profile that appears to be etiologic in establishing a personality disorder in their children that later manifests itself as anorexia nervosa. Sperling's (1978) analysis of anorexic children and their mothers laid the groundwork for this research with her findings that the predisposition for anorexia nervosa is established in early childhood by a disturbance in the mother-child symbiosis. Four of the six features of the psychological profile correlate with parental attitudes and behavior described by Bruch (1978) in fifty cases and by Minuchin, Rosman, and Baker (1978) in fifty-three cases. Sours (1980, personal communication) confirms these features in his family research. The two features of the profile not described by these authors are usually uncovered only by psychoanalysis, a modality they do not utilize (Wilson et al. 1983). In our original studies (Wilson 1980c) and in those of Bruch and Minuchin et al., there was no differentiation of the families of restrictor and bulimic anorexics. Our recent findings on the differences in parental attitudes are detailed in the next section.

The Psychological Profile of the Restrictor
and Bulimic Anorexic Family

Although the psychiatric diagnosis in anorexia nervosa cases ranges from neurosis to psychosis and the symptoms offer dramatic evidence of

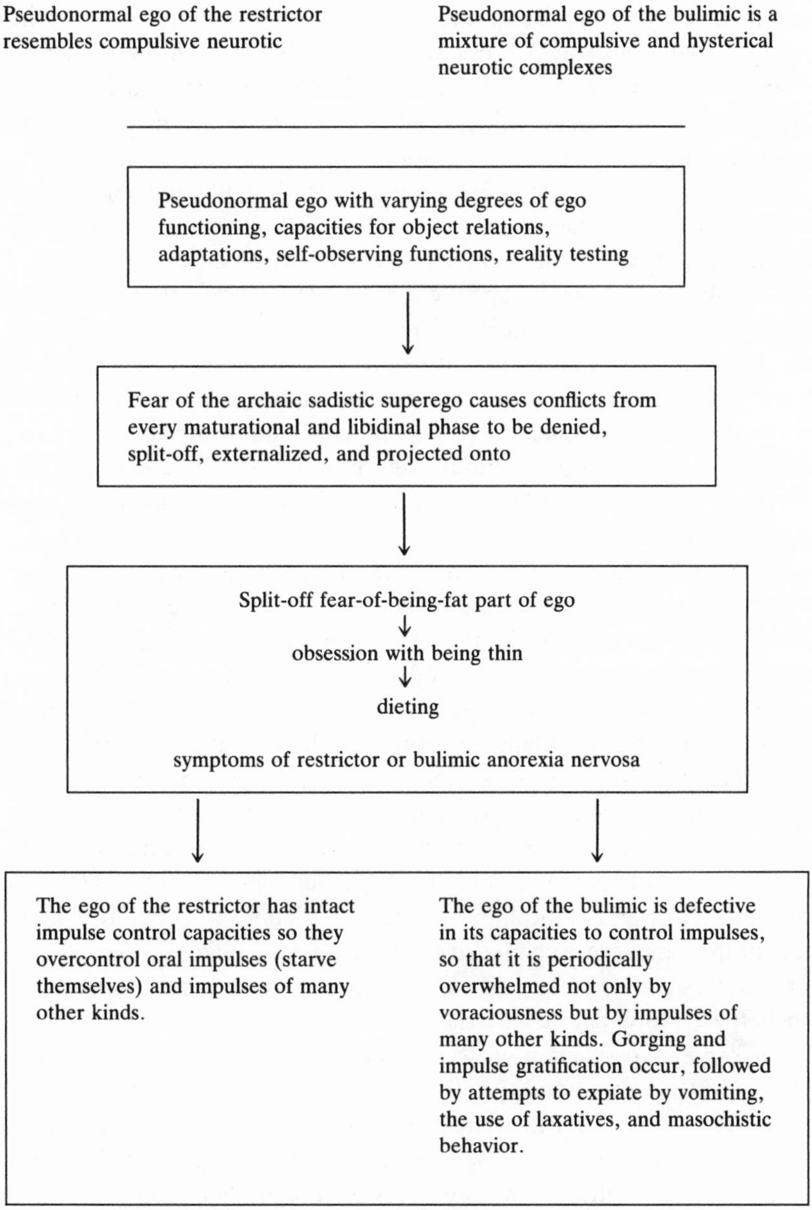

Pseudonormal ego of the restrictor
resembles compulsive neurotic

Pseudonormal ego of the bulimic is a
mixture of compulsive and hysterical
neurotic complexes

Pseudonormal ego with varying degrees of ego
functioning, capacities for object relations,
adaptations, self-observing functions, reality testing

Fear of the archaic sadistic superego causes conflicts from
every maturational and libidinal phase to be denied,
split-off, externalized, and projected onto

Split-off fear-of-being-fat part of ego
↓
obsession with being thin
↓
dieting

symptoms of restrictor or bulimic anorexia nervosa

The ego of the restrictor has intact
impulse control capacities so they
overcontrol oral impulses (starve
themselves) and impulses of many
other kinds.

The ego of the bulimic is defective
in its capacities to control impulses,
so that it is periodically
overwhelmed not only by
voraciousness but by impulses of
many other kinds. Gorging and
impulse gratification occur, followed
by attempts to expiate by vomiting,
the use of laxatives, and masochistic
behavior.

Fig. 1.—Differences in ego structure of the restrictor and bulimic anorexic

conflict, usually anorexic girls vehemently deny their conflicts. Most often unhappy parents bring them in for consultation. These parents are usually highly motivated, well-meaning people who will do everything they can for their sick child. It is healthy for a child to grow up in a home where there are rules, limits, a parental example of impulse control, responsibility, and ethical behavior. However, in their overconscientiousness, the parents of anorexics overcontrol their child. The adolescent anorexic girl is in a situation of realistic and neurotic dependence on her family, so that changes in the parents' behavior and attitudes toward her can be crucial for therapeutic success. Parents may try to withdraw their daughter from treatment prematurely because they cannot tolerate the rebelliousness and antisocial behavior that surfaces when the anorexic symptoms are resolved. They may need therapy themselves in order to accept the emotional changes in their daughter and to understand certain pathological interactions they have with her. Research on the anorexic families yielded the following six-part anorexic family psychological profile.[2]

1. All the families showed perfectionism. The parents of restrictor anorexics were overconscientious and emphasized good behavior and social conformity in their children. Most were successful people who gave time to civic, religious, and charitable activities. Many were physicians, educators, business executives, or religious leaders, that is, pillars of society. The parents of bulimic anorexics, although they are perfectionistic, seem to have a greater incidence of neurosis, marital conflict, divorce, and addiction than the parents of restrictors. In other respects this psychological profile with variations that are noted applies to both groups. For example: The mothers of two bulimics were addicts (one to alcohol, the other to morphine), but their addictions were family secrets, and both women were compulsive, perfectionistic college professors who tried to be perfect mothers. Their addictions expressed a rebellion against their hypermoral character structure.

2. *Repression* of emotion was found in every family group; it was caused by the hypermorality of the parents. In several cases, parents kept such strict control over their emotions that they never quarreled in front of the children. The loss of temper, quarreling, and conflict that were characteristic of the bulimics' parents were ego alien. Aggressive behavior in the children was not permitted, and aggression in general was denied (e.g., one father's volunteer military service was disdained by his family). Most families laughed at the father's assertive male behavior and

saw him as the "spoiler" in the sexual relation; the mother was the superior moral figure. The father's authority was diminished further by his busy schedule, which left him little time for his children.

3. The overconscientious perfectionism of the parents in these families resulted in infantilizing decision making and overcontrol of the children. In some of the families, fun for fun's sake was not allowed. Everything had to have a noble purpose; the major parental home activity was intellectual discussion and scholarly reading. It was no surprise that the anorexic daughter hated the long hours of study she felt compelled to do. In therapy, it was difficult for anorexics to become independent and mature and to get rid of the humiliating feeling that they were puppets whose strings were pulled by mother and father.

4. Parental overconcern with fears of being fat and dieting was apparent in every case. The mother and/or the father and other relatives were afraid of being fat and dieted. In some families there was a predominance of the father's fear-of-being-fat complex.

My research (Wilson 1980a, 1982, 1983a) has confirmed Sperling's (1978) observations that specific conflicts and attitudes of the mother and/or father predispose a child for the development of psychosomatic symptoms (e.g., a mother's overconcern with bowel functions may predispose a child for ulcerative colitis). The specific etiological factor in anorexia is the parental preoccupation with dieting and the fear of being fat, which is transmitted to the daughter by identification. The other features of this profile are also found in the parents of patients suffering from psychosomatic symptoms such as asthma, migraine headaches, and colitis. The last two features of the profile are usually uncovered only by psychoanalysis.

5. *Exhibitionistic parental sexual and toilet behavior*, whose significance was completely denied, was found in every family. Doors in these homes were not locked, and bedroom and toilet doors often were left open, which facilitated the curious child's viewing of sexual relations and toilet functions. The children frequently witnessed parental sexual intercourse. Such experiences, coupled with parental hypermorality and prudishness, caused an inhibition in normal psychosexual development in the anorexic daughters. Many were virginal, sexually repressed girls who feared boys.

Sours (1980, personal communication) confirmed the anorexic family psychological profile but did not observe as much exhibitionistic behavior in families of self-starving young anorexics. However, he notes exhibitionistic parental behavior in families of gorging, vomiting anorexics, including frequent seductive sexual behavior by the fathers.

6. In these families, there was an emotional selection of one child by the parents for the development of anorexia. This child was treated differently than the other children. Such a choice may result from: (*a*) the carryover of an unresolved emotional conflict from the parents' childhood (e.g., the infant may represent an unconsciously hated parent or brother or sister); (*b*) an intense need to control the child, so that the child is treated almost as a part of the body of one parent; (*c*) a particular psychological situation and emotional state of the parent(s) at the time of the child's birth that seriously damaged the parent-child relationship (e.g., the child may be infantilized because he or she is the last baby or may be overcathected by a parent who has suffered a recent loss).

Exceptions to the Family Psychological Profile

Hogan (1983a), although confirming the difference in character structure of the restrictor and the bulimic, questions any validity to a family psychological profile. He notes a restrictor anorexic who grew up with alcoholic parents. Sperling detailed the analysis of a restrictor anorexic whose mother was psychotic (Wilson 1983a). I have also seen exceptions to this profile. One restrictor anorexic came from a family where the father, mother, and siblings were all obese. Another restrictor's family included a father who was an alcoholic gambler. I realize that the number of cases we have seen is limited, and the complexities of early development are multiple. Moreover, in some families one child may be a restrictor, another bulimic. Nevertheless, in the great majority of cases the family psychological profile is applicable. In many adolescent cases, conjoint or individual therapy of the bulimic parents that focuses on aspects of the family psychological profile is absolutely necessary for therapeutic success.

Psychodynamics

Much has been written about the psychodynamics of anorexia nervosa. It generally has been observed by analytic authors that there is a flight from adult sexuality accompanied by a regression to more primitive defenses (e.g., Fenichel 1954; Gero 1953, 1984; Lorand 1943; Masserman

1941; Moulton 1942; Selvini Palazzoli 1961, 1978; Sperling 1953, 1968, 1978; Thoma 1967; Waller, Kaufman, and Deutsch 1940). This regression involves conflict around primitive sadistic and cannibalistic oral fantasies (Selvini Palazzoli 1961, 1978; Sperling 1953, 1968, 1978). Typical pregenital defense mechanisms are at work (Fenichel 1954; Masterson 1977; Sperling 1953, 1968, 1978; Risen 1982; Volkan 1976; Wilson 1983a).

I and my colleagues (Wilson et al. 1983) have confirmed Sperling's (1978) findings that unresolved preoedipal fixations to the mother contribute to difficulties in psychosexual development and that anorexic girls displace sexual and masturbatory conflicts from the genitals to the mouth, thus equating food and eating with forbidden sexual objects and activities.

Most analytic authors agree that the regression of anorexic patients is a flight from their own insatiable instinctual needs, which are defended against with primitive defenses of equal force. Sperling (1978) has correctly labeled anorexia nervosa "an impulse disorder."

The role of unconscious pregnancy fantasies in the genesis of this illness is almost universally recognized by psychoanalytic authors. The anorexic patient fears and denies these fantasies.

VOMITING AND PURGING

Vomiting and laxatives are greatly overdetermined symptoms. They are attempts to undo the preceding phase of gorging and to placate the archaic superego. Vomiting is resorted to for purposes of control. Many bulimics report feeling at peace with themselves after vomiting or using laxatives. Various unconscious fantasies and the ejection of internalized objects are carried out through these symptoms. Vomiting has more oral meanings, whereas laxative use has anal connotations (Wilson et al. 1983).

I and my colleagues (Wilson et al. 1983), along with Sperling (1978), do not agree with Bruch (1962, 1965, 1970, 1978), Crisp (1965, 1968), Dally (1969), and Selvini Palazzoli (1961, 1978) that a psychoanalytic approach to these patients should be avoided. The experience of our group agrees with Mushatt (1982), Blitzer, Rollins, and Blackwell (1961), Jessner and Abse (1960), Lorand (1943), Masserman (1941), Mogul (1980), Risen (1982), Rizzuto, Petersen, and Reed (1981), Sours (1980), Sperling

(1958, 1968, 1978), Thoma (1967), and Waller et al. (1940) that psychoanalytic investigation is of the utmost importance in understanding this illness as well as the treatment of choice in most cases.

Psychodynamics of Bulimic Anorexia Nervosa

In psychodynamic terms,[3] this complex is rooted in unresolved sadomasochistic oral-phase conflicts that result in an ambivalent relationship with the mother. Fixation to this phase of development, with its accompanying fears of object loss, is caused by maternal and/or paternal overcontrol and overemphasis on food and eating functions as symbols of love. This unresolved conflict influences each subsequent maturational phase so that anal, oedipal, and later developmental conflicts are unresolved.

The unresolved preoedipal fixation on the mother contributes to the difficulty in psychosexual development and the intensity of the oedipal development. Bulimic anorexia nervosa, fat phobia, can be considered a specific pathological outcome of unresolved oedipal conflicts in a child whose preoedipal relationship to the mother has predisposed her to this particular reaction under precipitating circumstances.

The genetic influences on this complex are parental conflicts about weight and food specifically and about aggressive and libidinal expression generally. In addition, the neurotic and/or addictive parents are perfectionistic, significantly denying the effect on the developing child of their exhibitionistic toilet, bedroom, and other behavior. Other genetic factors are cultural, societal, and general medical influences, as well as secondary identification with women and/or men who share the fear-of-being-fat complex.

From an economic point of view, the unremitting pressure of repressed, unsublimated aggressive and libidinal drives, conflicts, and fantasies is a central issue for these inhibited patients. The terror of loss of control (i.e., of becoming fat) comprises the conscious fear of overeating and the unconscious fear of incorporating body parts, smearing or eating feces, bleeding to death, mutilating or being mutilated, or masturbating and/or becoming nymphomaniacal, which could result in orgastic pleasure.

All these feared drive eruptions are held in check by the terror of retaliatory punishment from the archaic sadistic superego. These conflicts are displaced onto and condensed into the fear of being fat. The defective bulimic ego is unable to contain impulses to gorge; there is a giving in to voraciousness and then an attempt at self-punishment and undoing by vomiting and/or the use of laxatives. In the bulimic there are also parallel attempts by the ego to suppress and repress libidinal and aggressive fantasies, drives, and impulses—a surrender to these impulses and masochistic behavior that also expresses self-punishment and undoing.

From a structural point of view, ego considerations are central. In the preoedipal years, the ego of the bulimic anorexia–prone (fat-phobic) child becomes split. One part develops in a pseudonormal fashion: cognitive functions, the self-observing part of the ego, adaptive capacities, and other ego functions appear to operate normally. While the restrictor anorexics in childhood are most often described as "perfect" and have excellent records in school, the bulimic anorexics have more evidence of disobedience and rebellion at home and school. In adolescence there is more antisocial behavior, sexual promiscuity, and addiction. The ego represses, denies, displaces, externalizes, and projects conflicts onto the fear-of-being-fat complex. In many cases, conflicts are displaced onto habits such as thumb-sucking, enuresis, encopresis, nail-biting, head banging, and hair pulling. In other cases, there is a concomitant displacement and projection of conflict onto actual phobic objects. In some patients, bulimia anorexia alternates with other psychosomatic disease syndromes, such as ulcerative colitis (Sperling 1978), migraine, and asthma (Mintz 1983). This split in the ego manifests itself in the intense, psychotic-like denial of the displaced wishes, conflicts, and fantasies. In other words, the split-off neurotic part of the personality is denied in the fear-of-being-fat complex.

From an adaptive point of view, conflicts at each maturational and libidinal phase are denied, displaced, and projected onto the fear-of-being fat complex. Conflicts in separation-individuation (Mushatt 1975 1982) are paramount and are denied by the parents and developing child. Normal adaptive conflict is avoided and denied. Many parents of bulimics raise them in an unreal, overprotected world. Perfectionistic parents impair the ego's decision-making functions with their infantilizing intrusions into every aspect of their child's life. In each case a focus of therapy is on the pregenital object relations that have been caused by the unresolved parental relationships and conflicts in separation-individuation.

Unlike Sperling (1978), I, along with Hogan (1983) and Mintz (Wilson et al. 1983), include males under the diagnostic category of anorexia nervosa. Mintz (1983) has shown that male bulimic anorexics have oedipal and preoedipal fixations and unresolved problems in separation-individuation, severe latent homosexual conflicts and a feminine identification, and the same fear-of-being-fat complex seen in the females, caused by an identification with the mother and/or the father's fear-of-being-fat complex.

The Relationship of Bulimia to Addiction and Childhood Habits

To understand and treat bulimic anorexics, it is necessary to understand the impulse disorder, the addictive personality structure (Wilson 1981; Wurmser 1980), and the habits of childhood that are frequently the developmental forerunners of bulimia. I have emphasized that bulimia is a food phobia, an addiction. In bulimics I have noted the frequent occurrence of thumb-sucking, nail-biting, cuticle chewing and eating, head banging, hair pulling and eating, and other childhood impulse disorders such as encopresis and enuresis. In certain cases, there is a childhood history of excessive good behavior. However, therapy uncovers isolated episodes or phases of rebelliousness. The ego utilizes the same defenses in its struggle with a childhood habit or a childhood impulse disorder as it uses later in trying to cope with bulimic anorexia nervosa or the other eating disorders. Thus the defenses of denial, splitting, displacement, externalization, withholding, and lying are deeply ingrained in the ego structure of the bulimic anorexic. In some cases, we see a chaotic ego structure, as when a childhood habit coexists with bulimia and an addiction.

In my research on the fear-of-being-fat complex (Wilson et al. 1983), I found that usually this fear becomes intense in adolescence, the period when bulimia most often occurs. The fear of giving in to a habit, of not being able to control it, is the forerunner of the fear-of-being-fat complex. When a habit or an addiction is interrupted, patients are afraid of becoming fat, of overeating, but also are afraid of losing control in other ways, for example, losing their temper and/or acting out.

BODY IMAGE

In the terror of being fat (anorexia), the basic conflict is rooted in a massive preoedipal repression of sadomasochistic oral-phase conflicts

284

that have been elaborated by the ego with new defensive structures at each subsequent libidinal and maturational phase of development. It is the surface of the mother's breast, and by extension her figure, that has been projected in the anorexic's body image. The fear of being fat reflects the terror of oral sadistic incorporation of the breast of mother and later of other objects (Wilson et al. 1983).

A few restrictors and a number of bulimics do not evidence a clear-cut body image disturbance, although they are all fat phobic. In these cases, the ego is healthier and the psychopathology primarily oedipal.

Split in the Ego

To further understand the bulimic anorexic ego structure, one has to keep in mind the split in the ego. Wilson et al. (1983) noted that, from a structural point of view, ego considerations are central. In the preoedipal years, the ego of the anorexia-prone child becomes split. One part develops in a pseudonormal fashion; cognitive functions, the self-observing functions of the ego, adaptive capacities, and other ego functions appear to operate normally. The ego suppresses, represses, denies, displaces, externalizes, and projects conflicts onto the fear-of-being-fat complex. The pseudonormal part of the ego of the abstaining (restrictor) anorexic evidences many of the characteristics seen in compulsion neuroses. The pseudonormal part of the bulimic ego is an admixture of hysterical and compulsive traits.

Strober's conclusions (1981, 1983) about the differences between restrictors and bulimics correlate with my research. His type 1 and 2 anorexics, the restrictors, evidence "obsessionality," whereas his type 3 patients, the bulimics, present "a distinctive profile of low ego strength, impulsivity, proneness to addictive behaviors and more turbulent interpersonal dynamics."

Technique

In the technique of analysis or analytic psychotherapy, the first phase of treatment, the transference, is handled along the principles set forward by Kernberg (1975) and summarized by Boyer (1980) in regard to borderline cases:

1. The predominantly negative transference is systematically elabo-

rated only in the present without initial efforts directed toward full genetic interpretations.

2. The patient's typical defensive constellations are interpreted as they enter the transference (see discussion of particular defensive constellations below).

3. Limits are set in order to block acting out in the transference insofar as this is necessary to protect the neutrality of the therapist (but with many limitations; see below).

4. The less primitively determined aspects of the positive transference are not interpreted early since their presence enhances the development of the therapeutic and working alliance (only if we look at these alliances as part of the positive transference—see discussion of limiting transference above), although the primitive idealizations that reflect the splitting of "all good" from "all bad" object relations are systematically interpreted as part of the effort to work through those primitive defenses;

5. Interpretations are formulated so that the patient's distortions of the therapist's interventions and of present reality, especially the patient's perceptions during the hour, can be systematically clarified.

6. The highly distorted transference, at times psychotic in nature and reflecting fantastic internal object relations pertaining to early ego disturbances, is worked through first in order to reach the transferences related to actual childhood experiences.

The early interpretation of the denial of suicidal behavior (masochism) parallels the technique of Sperling (1978) and Hogan (1983) with psychosomatic patients and correlates with the therapeutic technique used in the therapy of schizophrenic, borderline, and character disorders by Boyer and Giovacchini (1980), Kernberg (1975), and Volkan (1976): (1) In the first phase of treatment these patients usually do not free associate, as also happens in the analysis of children and of patients with character disorders (Boyer and Giovacchini 1980); (2) the therapist takes an active stance, frequently using construction and reconstruction; (3) behavioral responses can be interpreted; (4) dreams have to be used in the context of the patient's psychodynamics; (5) first one interprets the masochism of these patients—their archaic superego and the guilt they experience in admitting any conflict; (6) next, one interprets defenses against facing masochistic behavior; then, when the ego is healthier, one interprets defenses against aggressive impulses; (7) such interpretations are inexact and frequently are not confirmed by the patient's associations; (8) for these patients who have an archaic, punitive superego and a relatively weak ego, the analyst provides auxiliary ego strength and a rational superego (Boyer 1980; Wilson, 1971, 1982, 1983a); (9) interpretations should be made in a firm, consistent manner (Boyer 1980); and (10) with such patients, the analyst needs to have authority.

Because anorexic patients in their projective indentifications can pick up almost imperceptible nuances in the tone of voice, facial expression, movements, and even feelings of the analyst, they provoke intense countertransference reactions (Sperling 1967; Wilson et al. 1983).

There is a special technique in the analysis of bulimic anorexia. The analyst must demonstrate to the patient the need for immediate gratification (the impulse disorder, i.e., the primary narcissism) early in treatment (Sperling 1967, 1978; Wilson et al. 1983). Thus the patient is shown that the symptoms of restrictor and bulimic anorexia are manifestations of a split-off impulsive part of the ego; that is, the fear-of-being-fat complex.[4]

It is important that the psychiatrist be in charge of the treatment process (Sperling 1978; Wilson et al. 1983). A split of transference with the medical specialist can vitiate treatment. Hospitalization should be reserved for true emergencies.

As with other psychosomatic symptoms, when bulimic anorexic symptoms subside, acting out increases. Patience is essential in the analysis of bulimic patients, whose habits, at their most primitive level, mask preverbal conflicts and traumas. Impulsive, psychotic, and psychosomatic patients, all of whom have preoedipal conflicts, have the means to communicate the impact and effects of their early preverbal traumas (Wilson 1968, 1971, 1981).

With habits, one has to be intuitive as to when to confront patients with their not bringing up the habit in therapy. One cannot ask them about it constantly or demand that they give up the habit. One should point out the reason for interrupting habits (e.g., to uncover fantasies and conflicts that are masked by the habit). Like obese patients, bulimic patients want and believe in magical control and want to stop the habit totally without analyzing it. The defensive purposes of habits, which mask suicidal and homicidal impulses and conflicts, have to be repeatedly interpreted. If the therapist does not actively interpret and confront patients with the meanings of their bulimic symptoms and habits that serve defensive purposes, the symptoms and habits will become more intense, while patients' treatment behavior will continue to be too pleasant and nice.

The Use of Antidepressant Medication

Because of the increasing number of reports of the use of antidepressants in the treatment of bulimic anorexics (Brotman, Herzog, and Woods 1984; Pope and Hudson 1982, 1984; Walsh, Stewart, Wright, Harrison, Roose, and Glassman 1982), I recently (Wilson 1985, 1983b) explored the psychodynamics and etiology of the bulimic anorexic's depression,[5] outlined our psychoanalytic technique with bulimics and documented the psychoanalytic resolution of depressed affects in the course of treatment, and described in detail the dangers, risks, and consequences of the use of medication. The treatment of bulimics has to be guided by the psychodynamic diagnosis of the individual case and the presenting clinical situation (Wilson et al. 1983). The presenting situation can be one of alcoholism, drug addiction, and/or a suicidal crisis. Obviously, if the patient is acutely suicidal, his life must be preserved, and if an antidepressant drug can alter the patient's behavior, it, like other medication and total parenteral nutrition, may have to be used. However, if analytic psychotherapy or analysis is feasible, the patient will have to be weaned from the drug to which he may have developed a psychological addiction.

Bulimic depression is caused by multiple preoedipal and oedipal conflicts. A crucial goal of the psychotherapy of bulimia is to strengthen the patient's ego so that she can face and tolerate both realistic and neurotic depression. Like the restrictor, the bulimic anorexic is obsessed with fantasies of remaining young forever and being free of any conflict, realistic or neurotic. They do not want to grow up (Wilson et al. 1983). They deny the conflicts they manifest, like their dependency on their parents or parent surrogates. They vehemently deny the masochistic nature of their symptoms and their character structure. It is the aim of the psychodynamic treatment to analyze their defenses against experiencing painful emotions, particularly depressed feelings. It is an advance in therapy when they become depressed and cry. To relieve depression by medication prevents the analysis of this most important aspect of their neurosis. Moreover, bulimic anorexics experience hyperactive states. In these anxiety conditions they gorge and vomit endlessly but also will disobey monoamine oxidase dietary restrictions, inducing dangerous side effects, and may ingest dangerous amounts of prescribed medication. Supervised cases attempted suicide with aspirin, acetaminophen, ipecac, imipramine, and amitriptyline. A colleague's case experienced a resolution of bulimic symptoms following the administration of phenelzine but developed a toxic manic psychosis, became noncommunicative, and acted out sexually. Dangerous overdosage with laxatives is a manifestation of the either/or nature of their ego functioning (Sperling 1978; Wilson et al. 1983). Bulimics, for example, resort to extremes of exercise to relieve anxiety and take off weight. Only a psychodynamic approach can change this neurotic behavior. Because of unresolved oral conflicts, the bulimic patient believes in magical solutions to problems, is intolerant of delay, and is ambivalent about such a lengthy learning process as analytic therapy. The temporary removal of symptoms can eventuate in premature termination of treatment.

The crucial therapeutic force is the transference neurosis. Patients must reexperience in the transference the dyadic relationship with the mother and understand depression and rage at not being able to control the therapist as they did the mother. Likewise, later in therapy, the triadic Oedipus complex emerges and can be analyzed in the transference neurosis. If the patient is on medication, the transference loses its intensity and the therapist's interpretations become diluted and intellectual. From the ego and psychodynamic point of view, a paradox emerges. Only those bulimics who are well motivated and have stronger egos can be medicated without the risk of alternate symptom development or acting out; however, it is just such healthier patients who have the most favorable psychotherapeutic prognosis.

In those situations where the use of medication, particularly antidepressants, is necessary, that is, medical crises or when patients cannot be motivated for psychotherapy, in treatment stalemates, or where cost and therapist availability are problems, the use of drugs is a trade-off with potentially disadvantageous consequences. Therapeutic stalemates can occur in cases of chronic bulimia where there has been a long-term resistance to insight and change in analytic therapy.

While medication in some intractable cases may facilitate therapy, we have found that, even in severe regressed states, knowledgeable interpretations have resolved the impasses. Before resorting to medication, one is well advised to try consultation and/or supervision. In cases seen in consultation and supervision, therapeutic impasses have been resolved by a deeper psychodynamic understanding, a review of the countertransference conflicts of the therapist, and an exploration of the often subtle treatment sabotage on the part of the parents, who frequently are unable to accept self-assertive behavior by the enmeshed bulimic anorexic. It must be kept in mind that at best medication may make the patient more amenable to dynamic therapy, but it cannot change the underlying impulsive, masochistic personality disorder.

Prognostic Differences in Restrictor and Bulimic Anorexics

Many bulimic anorexics, those who would diagnostically be termed neurotic, give an appearance of healthier (pseudonormal) ego functioning. Since they evidence an admixture of hysterical traits, their emotions are under less repression. They develop a seemingly good therapeutic alliance. Wilson (Wilson and Mintz 1982), as well as Bruch (1978), feels that the prognosis is poorer for the chronic bulimic. Hogan (1983) sees little difference (Wilson et al. 1983, pp. 147–148). In general, because of the lesser degree of acting out and the stronger ego, the prognosis would appear better for the restrictor anorexic; however, in some bulimic cases, where the symptoms are of recent development and limited to gorging and vomiting, the prognosis may be favorable because there is a readiness for the expression of affect. It is still felt by many analysts that the hysterical neurotic is easier to analyze than the compulsive neurotic. However, the degree of preoedipal psychopathology is the limiting factor in both the hysterical and compulsive neurotic and the bulimic and restrictor anorexic.

Ego Structure and Transference Interpretation

Therapeutic technique has to be adapted to the varying defenses of the ego. The bulimic patients utilize acting out, rationalization, denial, withholding, and lying more intensely and persistently than the restrictors. In many cases, once the restrictor's anorexic crisis subsides, the course of therapy is in some ways similar to that of a compulsive neurotic. There are, of course, many varieties of ego structure in anorexic patients. Technique varies with different patients and with the degree of regression encountered. Technique also varies according to the individual style and experience of the therapist. Most of my colleagues and I tend to see the patient face-to-face in the first dyadic phase of treatment. However, some restrictor and bulimic anorexics can be analyzed along more classical lines, with the couch used from the beginning (Wilson et al. 1983).

The technique of interpretation is determined by multiple factors, such as the transference and the quality of object relationships. A crucial consideration is the split in the anorexic's ego and the extent to which this split is comprehended by the self-observing functions of the patient's ego. The first phase of therapy involves making the healthier part of the patient's ego aware of the split-off, primitive, impulse-dominated part of the ego and its modes of functioning.

Typical defenses and character qualities of the bulimic anorexic are: (1) denial and splitting; (2) belief in magic; (3) feelings of omnipotence; (4) demand that things and people be all perfect—the alternative is to be worthless; (5) need to control; (6) displacement and projection of conflict; (7) ambivalence; (8) masochistic perfectionism that defends against conflicts, particularly those around aggression; (9) pathological ego ideal of beautiful peace and love; (10) fantasied perfect, conflict-free mother-child symbiosis.

Both the restrictor and bulimic anorexic make extensive use of the defense of projective identification (Bion 1956; Boyer and Giovacchini 1980; Carpinacci, Liberman, and Schlossberg 1963; Carter and Rinsley 1977; Cesio 1963, 1973; Giovacchini 1975; Grinberg 1972, 1976, 1979; Klein 1955; Ogden 1978; Perestrello 1963; Rosenfeld 1952; Rosenfeld and Mordo 1973; Searles 1965). The anorexic projects unacceptable aspects of the personality—impulses, self-images, superego introjects—onto other people, particularly the therapist, with a resulting identification based on these projected self-elements. The extreme psychotic-like denial of conflict of the anorexic is caused by primitive projective identification onto others of archaic destructive superego introjects.

Sperling (1978) noted that part of the anorexic's conflicts are conscious. Wilson et al. (1983) emphasize that conscious withholding, rationalization, distortion, and lying are characteristic defenses of the restrictor anorexic. The lying and stealing of bulimics are basically caused by a rebellion against their primitive archaic superego, which demands absolute perfection. It is necessary to repeatedly interpret the bulimic's projection of this archaic superego introject onto the therapist and other objects. This pseudopsychopathic behavior is analyzable (Hogan 1983).

A key to the therapy of bulimics is for the therapist to translate the anxiety aroused by the patients' self-destructive behavior into interpretations of their masochism. Thus the persistent interpretation of defenses, such as denial and rationalization, can bring them to accept responsibility for the sometimes irreversible tooth and gum damage they have caused and/or the life-threatening secondary effects of their bulimic habits, such as low potassium blood levels.

Thirst, Hunger, and Sand Symbolism in Anorexia Nervosa

The anorexic's defensive asceticism, stressed by Mogul (1980) and Risen (1982), is represented in the dreams of these patients by sand symbols. The analysis of sand symbols in the dreams of anorexics is of great importance. Spitz (1955) emphasized that infants feel thirst, but not hunger, in the hallucinatory state. In a recent paper, I (Wilson 1981) noted that sand can be used as a pregenital symbol in which repressed oral and anal conflicts are regressively represented. Sand symbolizes oral-phase thirst and/or the formless stool of the infant (diarrhea). Antithetically, it depicts a characteristic anorexic attitude, asceticism—the ability to do without mother's milk, to control impulse gratification.

Sand representations in dreams can symbolize aspects of conflicts and processes that are involved in addictions such as smoking, substance abuse, alcohol, or food—as in the eating disorders. Anorexic self-starvation and dehydration mask and express an Isakower-like phenomenon in that they induce a dry (thirsty) mouth.

For example, a bulimic anorexic who was becoming aware of the oral-phase meanings of her sand dreams reported the following clinical material when she was mourning the recent death of her mother. She had just paid the bill for her mother's funeral and had expressed weary resignation at paying her analytic bill. In her analysis she was trying to analyze three habits—vomiting, laxative taking, and cigarette smoking. She stated: "I have a dry mouth. Yesterday I was so thirsty I drank a quart of orange juice, but it did not help. For years while I have been anorexic I have been thirsty. I would just take a sip of water. When I am depressed I am more thirsty. I was crying yesterday; I miss my mother so much. Why couldn't I make everything up to her? Why did we have to fight so much?"

An interpretation was made that she not only wanted her mother's love but wished the analyst would love her, baby her, and give her gifts as her mother had done. This included not charging her for his services but giving them as a "present." The patient cried and said, "Yes, mother gave me so much—she'd say, 'My money is yours.' I used to try to refuse her gifts, which I did not need, but she made me take them."

The "Little Person" Phenomenon

Volkan (1976) described an anorexic patient with a split-off, archaic part of her ego—a "little person." He related this pathological ego structure to the "little man" phenomenon described by Kramer (1974) and Niederland (1956, 1965). In my experience, all psychosomatic patients, including anorexics, have a split-off, archaic primitive ego. A conscious manifestation of this split-off ego is represented by the fear-of-being-fat complex.

Susan, an impulsive anorexic high school student, brought in a series of dreams containing images of an innocent, wide-eyed little girl that reminded her of current sentimental oil paintings that depicted an innocent, raggedly dressed child with tears in her enormous eyes. Susan was beginning to understand that these paintings showed how she tried to come across to people and to the analyst. After these dreams were analyzed, she had a dream of a little prince whom she wanted to control. Analysis showed this little prince to be her "little person"—the archaic split-off ego. The little prince was narcissistic, omnipotent, and magical. That he was male was a reflection of her secret wish to be a boy. For her, males were aggressive and magical, while females were innocent, passive, and masochistic. The split-off part of her ego was filled with murderous rage and hatred.

Clinical Case Studies[6]

The analysis and psychotherapy of bulimic anorexics were recently described by Hogan, Mintz, Sperling, and myself (Wilson et al. 1983). I have worked analytically with nine bulimic cases, as well as seeing many more in consultation and supervision. Four cases who completed their treatment are illustrative. One adolescent, who alternately abstained, gorged, and vomited, resolved her conflicts in a year's analysis. She was neither amenorrheic nor dangerously underweight. The treatment prevented the development of phobic fear of being fat (anorexia nervosa). Both the second and third cases abstained, gorged, and vomited, but they did not use laxatives. Neither brought her weight down to dangerous levels. Diagnostically, they suffered from mixed neuroses with severe preoedipal conflicts. Both patients, unlike the typical abstaining anorexic, had an abundant psychosexual fantasy life and had masturbated in childhood. Doubts have been expressed to me by experienced analysts about the possibility of analyzing any bulimic. Cases that I have analyzed and supervised, however, have experienced a full resolution of their fear-of-being-fat body image and their obsession with being thin. Long-term follow-up studies in certain cases showed that they were able to face and master the conflicts of self-fulfillment in a career, pregnancy, childbirth, and motherhood. In my experience, if the bulimic anorexic process can be analyzed in statu nascendi, as in my first case, the prognosis is excellent. The difficulties encountered in the treatment of chronic bulimic anorexics are explicated in this chapter. Of course, statements about prognosis must be qualified by the psychodynamic diagnosis of the individual case and by the presenting situation. Obviously, if the addicted bulimic is seen when acutely alcoholic and/or under the influence of drugs, all the technical problems involved in the management and treatment of such cases confront the therapist.

CASE 1. A NINETEEN-YEAR-OLD BULIMIC

Nancy was a nineteen-year-old student who had been gorging and vomiting for the past five years. She was five feet four inches tall and currently weighed 115 pounds, although her weight varied between 160 and 98 pounds. She stated that, when she began gorging, she could gain thirty pounds in two weeks. She felt that she could not stop and would eat a gallon of ice cream, an entire chocolate cake, sandwiches, and almost everything in the refrigerator. She ate whatever she found on the shelves, including raw dough. Starving and vomiting resulted in an equally dramatic weight loss. Regular exercise, which included forty-five minutes of daily jogging, helped to maintain the weight loss. Menstrual periods were irregular but present.

The patient came from a fat-phobic, food-and-weight-conscious family. The father was a rigid, controlling engineer who would slap the patient when he became angry with her. The mother was obese, unable to maintain her own reasonable weight, but prone to make insulting remarks about the patient's weight gain. The patient stated that mother was so fanatic about the patient's weight that she would accuse her of still being fat when she weighed 115 pounds. Distortion in the mother's view of her child is not an uncommon finding. The patient had a sixteen-year-old acting-out sister who fought constantly with the parents. The patient noted urges to stuff the sister with food and experienced enjoyment watching the sister eat, "as if I was eating." Junk food was never allowed in the house. When the patient began gaining weight, the entire family found themselves on a diet because the mother limited the food brought into the house.

Early in the treatment the patient realized that when she was upset or depressed she began to eat. As she became increasingly preoccupied and disturbed with eating, her previous worries disappeared. She began to see that eating served to cover up anxieties. Her excessive attachment to the parents became apparent as she recounted dropping out of college in her first year because of stomach aches and feelings of depression. During her bouts of bulimia, the parents would never go out in the evenings. She saw that the gorging kept them close to her. As the months passed she became increasingly aware that she was unable to assert herself with either parent and that she harbored many feelings of resentment toward them. This anger was expressed indirectly against her father by not studying and against her mother by gaining weight. Weight gain was also unconsciously used to terminate relationships with boyfriends when feelings of closeness and sexuality became too threatening.

Analysis achieved a resolution to the patient's bulimic symptoms and insight into the underlying adolescent maturational conflicts.

In some bulimic cases, vomiting expressed fantasies about childbirth, as in the following case:

CASE 2. FEAR OF LOSING CONTROL AND OF A DISFIGURING PREGNANCY

The opposite of the wish to be ethereal was expressed by the dream of Wendy, another anorexic woman. In the dream, she was looking at her mother-in-law, who was dressed in a brassiere and panties. Someone referred to her as a fat pig. Her associations were that her mother-in-law was an overweight, sensual woman. The dream reminded her of how, at age five, she would watch, fascinated, as her mother dressed and undressed. A new baby had been born next door; she had adored the baby but had not understood how pregnancy or birth occurred. She felt that the "fat pig" represented her terror of losing all controls—particularly her fears of multiple pregnancies, of being blown up fat by pregnancy.

Wendy was another anorexic who gorged and vomited. She had long since realized that she was trying to get a magical pregnancy in her eating, that her full belly was a pregnancy, and that her vomiting was a giving-birth fantasy. There were many other meanings to this dream, an important one being her childhood idea that women had periodic seizures of uncontrollable sexual arousal like animals. Two conflicts were masked by the fear of being fat: a fear of losing all controls and a fear of a disfiguring multiple-birth pregnancy.

CASE 3. A SIXTEEN-YEAR-OLD BULIMIC

Thelma, a sixteen-year-old girl, was referred by her uncle. His daughter had been treated for anorexia a number of years earlier. Thelma was a bright, attractive girl who was quite unhappy. She stated that she had been gorging and vomiting for almost three years. She was five feet four and weighed 110 pounds, the correct weight for her height, but previously she had weighed 150 pounds. Overweight since childhood, she frequently had been mocked and had had few friends. In the seventh grade, she and her mother had gone to Weight Watchers, where Thelma lost thirty-five pounds. She had felt marvelous but eventually began to gain weight again.

In the beginning of high school, her friend had taught her how to vomit, and she had been eating and vomiting ever since. She could gorge and vomit up to twelve times a day. Sometimes the vomiting resulted in a sore throat, but she could not stop. Sometimes, when she overate, she felt so full that she could not go to sleep. After vomiting, she "felt like a new person." "When I don't throw up, I get frightened and I'm afraid that I'll get fat again. Why do I punish myself that way, as if I'm a terrible person? I always think that I could do a better job at whatever I'm doing, but all I ever do is vomit. I eat food the way an alcoholic drinks." The patient described eating as her way of avoiding things. Whenever she had school-work to do and did not feel like doing it, she went into the kitchen and ate.

Thelma was on a perpetual diet of salads, vegetables, cottage cheese, Jello, and tea. During her binging episodes, she would consume prodigious quantities of rich food—ice cream, soda, cereals, bread, cake, spaghetti, chocolate—until she felt that she would burst. Then she felt terrible, vomited, and felt guilty. The mother guessed that the patient's gorging cost the family fifty dollars a week more than the cost of her regular eating. The patient said that, during a bout of gorging, she would eat everything in sight, including any part of a dinner that was prepared for the evening. On one occasion, when her father and three brothers returned late from a ball game, the patient sneaked into the kitchen and nibbled away at their dinners until nothing was left. They all scolded her and she felt terrible. At other times, she would surreptitiously nibble away at their meals without getting caught. Gorging anorexics often eat the food of the individual toward whom they have aggressive feelings; eating the other person's food represents an attempt to identify with him or her. In contrast, the starving anorexic attempts to stuff the hated sibling or parent while continuing to starve herself. In this manner she expresses hostility toward the person, attempts to control him or her, and identifies with the aggressor.

Surprisingly, Thelma was very voluble in the first session. She spontaneously described the setting in which the vomiting began. Her father, an executive in a paper company, was transferred to a distant state just before the patient graduated from grammar school. He moved and found a house, and, after the June graduation, Thelma and the rest of the family joined him. Thelma was terribly distressed at the loss of all her friends and felt empty, lonely, and depressed. Her friend at a new high school was the one who suggested that she vomit when she felt full.

The productivity of the patient in the first session, which continued during treatment, was of special interest because of her two previous unsuccessful attempts at treatment. At age thirteen, she had seen a therapist who attempted to stop her gorging and vomiting and encouraged her to eat normally. When this did not work, the therapist became angry with her and threatened and scolded her, reminding her of her mother. After one month, the patient refused to continue. She stated that her second psychiatrist, also a man, stared at her and never said a word. He did tell her that she had problems that she would have to solve, but she felt that he was not helping her. Long periods of silence left the patient feeling increasingly uncomfortable. After three months, the patient refused to continue, and the therapist acknowledged to the parents that he could not help her because she would not cooperate.

Technically, it is advisable to be more active, talkative, and open with teenage patients than with adult patients. With anorexic patients, specifically, it is often helpful to interpret resistances and conflict earlier, especially when patients are on a rapid downhill course. With Thelma, active listening was sufficient to encourage her productions.

The parents, who were seen in the second visit, described her as a very

297

bright, sensitive child who easily felt rejected and had great difficulty reaching out to friends. Both parents were born and raised in the South and felt that it was important to be socially adept and to have friends, even though father clearly indicated that mother was socially ill at ease with people and quite isolated. Both acknowledged that Thelma had been an insecure, clinging child from the time she was able to walk. As a toddler, she had followed the mother all over the house, pulling at her dress. The youngest brother had been born when the patient was three, and after that, she became even more clinging and demanding. The mother had been hospitalized for two weeks for severe depression when Thelma was six. Both parents agreed that the patient had been very close to her mother and confided in her all the time up until high school. Then a dramatic change occurred, and mother and Thelma seemed to be at each other's throats all the time. The father said that the screaming was impossible, and he and the boys would clear out of the room when the arguments began to escalate. With some bitterness, the mother interjected that the father also knew how to scream and that he would not tolerate any independence on the part of the two older boys. The fighting between father and the oldest son became especially violent when father drank excessively, which he often did.

The initial interview with the parents quickly revealed that, although these parents loved their children and were obviously prepared to do whatever they could to help them, there was considerable turmoil in the household, including screaming, drinking, and physical punishment of the children.

In the third session, Thelma continued to describe her symptoms and behavior. She acknowledged an occasional loss of her menstrual period, but this was irregular rather than sustained. She had suffered from headaches in the back of her head, with occasional dizziness, for the past five years. She usually suffered in silence and rarely took medication. She clearly recognized that, when she fought with her mother or father, it was often followed by a headache that would last for hours. Her inability to face her mounting resentment was somatized into the headaches or displaced onto eating preoccupations.

While she was very angry at both parents' behavior, she was more furious with her mother. She felt that the mother was especially critical of her and would attack and belittle her every accomplishment. Thelma was an excellent science student and hoped to become a physician or get a doctorate in scientific research. Nevertheless, the mother would often tease her, telling her that she would not want to be her patient or that no university would ever hire her. The patient was especially incensed at the thought that the mother criticized her eating patterns but seemed to want her to be fat. She always bought her fattening foods. When Thelma weighed 110 pounds, the mother criticized her for being too fat. It seems that the mothers of gorging patients who have trouble with obesity may complain that they are too fat when they are normal, while the mothers of emaciated patients may complain that they are too thin when they are normal. Both sets of parents often have body image disturbances.

Thelma typically felt that she was both fat and ugly. When she ate, she felt fat in her stomach and thighs. Most anorexics are particularly concerned with the belly and thighs. Thelma also stated that her face, arms, wrists, fingers, back, and toes were fat. All these body parts have symbolic meanings.

In discussing the gorging in detail, the patient acknowledged that it seemed to happen when she was upset and that the upset feeling disappeared during the bulimic attack. It was pointed out that, if she could think about what upset her, she might not have to gorge. One month later, Thelma reported that she had gone for three weeks without gorging, until the previous night, when she had binged and vomited. Her mother yelled and screamed at her and hit her across the face when she defended her older brother's choice of a college. The mother became enraged, called her stupid, and told her to get out of the house. She ran upstairs sobbing, overwhelmed by the feeling that no one cared for her. Later that night she ate all the food in the ice box, felt stuffed, vomited, and then ate again and felt sick. The dorsum of her hand bled from the violent thrust into her throat. She admitted that the gorging episode had eliminated the previous depression and sense of panic. Instead, she hated herself for eating and vomiting. She had hated her mother and then felt guilty, but after the vomiting, she had felt "purged" and relieved. The vomiting seemed to serve both as a somatic eruption of anger and as a punishment.

Thelma remained in treatment and eventually was able to work out her problems.

A basic aspect of therapeutic technique is to repeatedly interpret to the patient the conflicts that are displaced and projected onto the bulimic habit. The following case material is illustrative:

CASE 4. DISPLACEMENT AND PROJECTION

On Easter weekend, Teresa, a thirty-year-old married anorexic patient, dreamed that she was gorging chocolates but could not vomit them up. Her associations were to a pregnant friend who might have a Caesarean section as the baby was in a breech position. She realized that vomiting meant giving birth through the mouth. She used to gorge until her stomach was swollen, which represented an oral pregnancy. She remembered that when she was eight years old she had seen a pregnant woman's big belly and had not understood what caused the swelling. At this stage of her analysis, Teresa had given up her gorging and vomiting, which dated back ten years. She had strong wishes to get her periods back and was gaining weight. Fantasies of oral pregnancy had appeared before but now were being worked through.

This dream was an indication of structural change. Her bulimic habits were becoming truly ego alien. Her ego was stronger; her superego less strict. Internalization of conflict resulted in a transitory symptom of a stiff neck, which had a multitude of meanings. In self-punishment, she could not move her head to gorge; it was painful. Interpretations of her disapproval of masculine self-assertiveness led to a clearing up of her neck symptom, at which point she exploded with anger at her analyst, husband, and father. It required many hours of analysis to work through these conflicts.

This dream reflects the analytic principle that, when patients dream of their symptoms, they are ready to give them up. The defense of displacement from below up is highlighted in this dream. This material illustrates the stage of analysis when the anorexic patient is able to free associate and when the Oedipus complex is being analyzed.

CASE 5. CHRONIC BULIMIA IN A TWENTY-EIGHT-YEAR-OLD WOMAN

Elaine, a twenty-eight-year-old woman, came for consultation after undergoing a long and expensive hospitalization with behavioral modification treatment that failed to resolve her anorexia. The history revealed chronic anorexia nervosa with symptoms of gorging, vomiting, and excessive use of laxatives dating back five years to the time of her father's death.

Elaine's family was of Irish-Catholic cultural background. The youngest of two girls, Elaine had been a model child, bright and precocious. As children, the daughters had differed markedly in appearance; Elaine's three-year-old sister had been blue-eyed, slender, and tall, whereas Elaine had been brown-eyed, chubby, and short. As an adult, Elaine thought of herself as "dumpy and fat," despite her awareness that men were very attracted to her. Photographs from her adolescence showed her to have been very attractive, with a sexy, almost voluptuous figure. Elaine, who was five feet two, always had envied her tall, slender sister. During her anorexia, she felt she looked beautiful at half her normal weight.

Elaine had been weaned from the breast at eighteen months and bowel trained before her second year. Throughout childhood, she had been so severely constipated that at times she had been given laxatives. Frequently, she would sit on the toilet and strain for up to half an hour. Walking, talking, and other motor functions had been normal. Severe nail-biting and cuticle chewing dated back to Elaine's earliest years. She had phobias of heights and closed spaces. During adolescence, when agitated, Elaine would bite her toenails and toe cuticles, which caused serious local toe infections. In late adolescence, because of intense shame at the appearance of her hands, she had stopped nail-biting, but she then became a chain-smoker. As an adult, she was very proud of her long, curved fingernails.

Elaine's mother was a sixty-year-old woman from a conservative Midwestern family who devoted her time to her husband, home, and daughters. She was in good health but was preoccupied with fears of being fat and was always going on and off diets, although she was actually never more than ten pounds overweight. She was a chain-smoker. Elaine's father had been an American success story—a man from an immigrant Irish-Catholic family who had built a small construction company into a successful statewide business. He had been a hardworking man who doted on his daughters but was away from the family much of the time because of his business. He had been in good health except for infrequent headaches, probably migraines. A chain-smoker, he had died of lung cancer during Elaine's twenty-second year after a year's illness and a painful period of hospitalization. He had been a stoical man who never complained and did not like or go to doctors. His cancer had been diagnosed after it had metastasized. Elaine had bitterly mourned her father and wished that it had been her mother instead. After her father's funeral she began dieting and in a period of three weeks lost one-third of her body weight. She then began an endless cycle of abstaining, vomiting, gorging, and excessive laxative use. For several months preceding the development of the anorexia she had hardly talked to her mother; after developing anorexic symptoms, she had become close to her mother again.

Elaine had done well in grade school and high school but had experienced extreme anxiety taking examinations. She was very sensitive to criticism and studied hard. In adolescence, she had shown musical ability and attended a two-year college, where she majored in music. Although she developed into a promising young pianist, she had felt "unreal" about a musical career and had taken a series of jobs largely at a secretarial level with the goal of becoming a business executive.

Elaine had not masturbated in childhood and was inhibited about sexual matters. She had been frightened by a vertical scar on the abdomen of her aunt, which she had been told was caused by an operation after her "aunt's insides fell out" because of childbirth. At age twelve, Elaine had her menarche, for which she was unprepared. In adolescence, she had crushes on boys, was popular, and had many dates. For several years, she had had intercourse with guilt and fear, using no contraceptives. She had been afraid to see a gynecologist and terrified of pregnancy, and she constantly watched her stomach for any swelling. She thought she would kill herself if she got pregnant.

In late adolescence, after she had "gotten the pill" from a gynecologist, she had not worried so much about her periods or pregnancy. A close adolescent friend had been a sexy, precociously mature, rebellious classmate who had already had intercourse at age twelve. The two girls had arranged double dates. Elaine frequently had disobeyed the family curfew rules and her father had criticized her for it. He also had disapproved of her first romance, which had led her to break it off.

She had enjoyed visits from her father at college. When he would take her out, "it was like a date." As a young woman, she had many boyfriends, several of whom wanted to marry her, but "something stopped me from marriage." Following her father's death, she had moved to another town, worked as a store manager, and had an affair with her boss, a young married man. She developed severe flu and had been nursed back to health by her boss's wife—a close friend of hers. On recovering her health, Elaine had moved back to her hometown.

Underneath Elaine's compliant, cooperative manner of relating to the analyst was the mistrust, suspicion, and hostility characteristic of patients who have undergone behavior modification therapy (Bruch 1974). After leaving the hospital, Elaine had become almost a recluse, living alone in her apartment, not looking for work, and seeing few people except for her mother, whom she talked to or saw daily. She spent most of her time fasting, gorging, vomiting, and taking laxatives. She said she would rather kill herself than go back into the hospital; she felt her lengthy and expensive hospitalizations had been "worthless and a rip-off." Her medical treatment was with an internist, who prescribed dietary supplements.

In therapy, gradually, the analyst acquainted Elaine with her masochism and interpreted her defenses against admitting to her anger toward, and mistrust of, her previous therapist, the hospital doctors, and him. She began to come out of isolation and consider work and socializing. Each of the following interpretations exemplifies a line of interpretation that was applied systematically as the defenses of the ego—denial, splitting, rationalization, belief in magic, acting in, and acting out—unfolded.

After the analyst's vacation break, Elaine said that she did not like his return, since during his absence she had done well at business school and had met a nice man who took her dancing. Away from sessions, she felt free; in her sessions, she felt strangled and hated treatment. The analyst interpreted her displacement; it was not the "treatment" she hated but him. She left the office visibly angry and did not come to her next session. In the subsequent hour, she talked of how much she wanted praise; she had not come to the last hour because she was angry at the analyst for not praising her. In the next session, she accused the analyst of being cold and machine-like. She associated to hysterical symptoms that had been precipitated by smoking pot, by receiving anesthesia at the dentist, and by dating certain aggressive men. The analyst interpreted her fear of emotions and her excessive need to control. During the next week she revealed that she was dating more, stating, "I don't like European men who flatter and wine and dine me, but plain down-to-earth American men don't ask me out." "Yesterday I came home so angry I was ready to jump out the window. Can I make an A grade? I hate myself. Nothing is ever good enough. I will never be satisfied. I do not know whom to hate more—you or the damn school." The analyst interpreted that she could face anger and did not have to get rid of it by not coming to sessions or by binging and vomiting. Elaine responded by saying that the longer she came to the analyst, the sicker she felt. She demanded that he change her hour because she "had to" go with her mother for their periodic visit to her senile maternal grandmother in a nursing home. The analyst asked Elaine why she had to go; perhaps her mother could go alone. Elaine became very upset and angry. The analyst pointed out that, if it was so important to her, she could ask mother to visit at another time that would not conflict with her session. Elaine snapped, "The plans are already made" and did not come for her session.

On her return, she talked of how useless it was to visit her grand-mother. She stated that once her mother had wet her panties (had been enuretic) in the car going to the nursing home. The analyst interpreted that Elaine had identified with her mother's extreme control. Elaine associated to mother's denial of all conflict; mother always had pretended that everything was all right, but it had not been. She was strict about manners and taught the children that yelling and getting angry were wrong. Control was the reigning word. Elaine had tried to be what her parents wanted, but it was not she.

In the next hour, Elaine bitterly criticized the analyst, saying that the analysis was psychological double-talk and that he did nothing for her. She had been anorexic for five years and so what? Near the end of the hour, she got up from the couch and went to the bathroom. She did not refer to her behavior in the next session but subsequently said that she had felt nauseated and had thrown up in the toilet. The analyst told her that it was he and what he had said that she had got rid of by vomiting. She replied that she was sick and tired of living, that she affected no one's life and had no reason to be alive. The analyst interpreted to her that, in order not to know of her anger toward her mother and him, she was trying to kill herself with her use of laxatives—no one knew the lethal dose of the laxative and no drug company would do experiments with humans such as those she was carrying out on herself. Elaine left, slamming the door to the waiting room.

In the next session, she said she had been to her internist, her lab tests were better, but her potassium was still low. The analyst interpreted to her some of her denial of suicidal behavior. He said that she vitiated her internist's careful diet advice and the absorption of food and medication by her habits, that she denied making him and the analyst medically concerned about her, and that neither the internist nor the analyst would be surprised if she became sick and forced hospitalization.

In the following hour, Elaine was silent for thirty minutes; the analyst interpreted to her her strict perfectionistic conscience, stating that she controlled speech to avoid conflict if she talked and that she vomited and took laxatives to avoid conflicts about being a woman and having a "figure." Elaine associated to having been a proficient ballet student— the best in her class. One day, she had had an anxiety attack and had given up dancing. At the end of the session, Elaine mentioned almost casually that her periods, which she had not had for years, had returned. The analyst's counterreaction was to feel that she was making more progress than she admitted to but that she was denying emotions and conflicts about her periods.

In a subsequent session, she was silent for twenty minutes, and her need to control was again interpreted. She then burst out: "The whole thing is mother. I am torturing her and can't stop. It is so stupid, I am getting back at her for all the things that were not her fault. I blame her for everything. I feel sorry for her, she is my victim. She doesn't know that I wind her around my little finger. I wonder if she does know. I tell her, don't give me things, but she does anyway. Everything ended when father died; he was the generator. Mother has done nothing since. You don't understand what I feel when I am cynical and bitter; everyone is divorced and bitter, few people are happy. If mother died, all my symptoms would clear up."

The interpretation was made that, by hanging on to her habits, she wished to control the analyst as well as her mother and that she preferred the humiliation of her habits to the anxiety, guilt, anger, and fear of her neurosis, which she thought she hid from people. Furthermore, her symptoms and neurosis would not magically clear up if her mother died.

Gradually, basic changes occurred in this patient's body image and in her attitudes toward her symptoms. Repeated interpretation of the unconscious reasons for inflicting such narcissistic mortification on herself was necessary (Eidelberg 1957, 1959). Elaine's acting out around time was intense: often, her response to an interpretation was to miss a session without even a phone call. I realized that part of her anger was about her previous treatment, but when it reached the extent of not coming for two successive sessions and not calling, I pointed out her denial of reality and avoidance of emotions and emphasized that I would not go on seeing her if she was not responsible for her hours. If she felt she could not come, she should call me. Her response was to devalue me by saying that I was paid anyway. I interpreted to her that she denied my interest in treating her. A second line of interpretation was that she treated me like food, which she unconsciously equated with the mother of the nursing phase. In the transference neurosis I became an addiction (Flarsheim 1975), and she expected me to be available to her always, no matter what she did. Her response was to cry and say I was throwing her out. I told her that she was blocking treatment and that I would refer her to another analyst, but that any experienced therapist would make the same request. Following this confrontation, Elaine stopped this aspect of her acting out.

As in any patient treated with a psychoanalytic method, the changes in Elaine resulted from the analysis of her ego's defenses against admitting to emotions and conflicts, particularly in the transference with the liberation of anxiety, anger, and depression in sessions. Although the relative strength or weakness of the ego is important, the relationship with the therapist is the most potent force in the reconstruction or construction of the ego, symptom resolution, and the achievement of healthy ego functioning.

Conclusions

There is a widespread application of psychoanalysis and analytic psychotherapy to the treatment of bulimia, and in either therapeutic modality the same psychodynamics and technique of treatment are utilized with modifications determined by the frequency of sessions.

A review of the extensive psychoanalytic literature shows that most psychoanalysts view bulimic anorexia nervosa as an emotional disturbance that emerges as a retreat from developing adult sexuality via a regression to the prepubertal relation to the parents. While agreeing with Sours (1980), Thoma (1967), Sperling (1978), and Wilson et al. (1983) that bulimic anorexics should be included under the diagnostic category of anorexia nervosa, I presented a number of new hypotheses about the psychodynamics and technique of treatment: (1) that restrictor or bulimic fat phobia should replace anorexia nervosa as a diagnostic term, as these patients do not suffer from a lack of appetite but the opposite, a struggle to avoid being overwhelmed by their impulses, including voraciousness; (2) while the underlying conflicts, their fear-of-being-fat complexes, are similar, the ego of the bulimic, unlike that of the restrictor, is defective in its impulse control capacities, so that it is periodically overwhelmed not only by impulses to gorge but by impulses of other kinds; (3) family psychodynamics that are viewed as etiologic were detailed. The bulimic family psychological profile, while similar to that of the restrictor anorexics, evidences a greater degree of neurotic conflict, addictive behavior, and divorce.

The technique of therapy advocated is intensive psychotherapy or analysis of the bulimic anorexic with conjoint therapy of the parents if necessary. In some cases the mother and/or the father need individual therapy to change their unhealthy relationship with their child. Five clinical cases were presented to illustrate new techniques of treatment that focus in the first phase of analysis on the dyadic transference, the failure to free associate, the patient's impulsivity, and her use of denial and projective identification. The importance of understanding sand symbolism in anorexia was emphasized as it reveals these patients' conflicts over thirst, impulse control, and asceticism. Early interpretation of the patient's impulse disorder is advocated. Acting out, rationalization, withholding, and lying are more frequent defenses of the bulimic anorexic. Most patients are seen face-to-face in the first dyadic phase of treatment. The therapist is in charge of treatment, with hospitalization reserved for true emergencies. Medication is contraindicated if psychotherapy or analysis is feasible. Our technique of treatment has similarities to the methods used by Boyer and Giovacchini (1980) and Kernberg (1975) in the analysis of patients with borderline and narcissistic disorders.

NOTES

1. I am particularly indebted to Drs. Otto Sperling, Ira Mintz, Cecilia Karol, Charles Hogan, Gerald Freiman, Anna Burton, Robert Grayson, and Leonard Barkin for their contributions.

2. A useful acronym for the profile is PRIDES: P = perfectionism; R = repression of emotion; I = infantilizing decision making; D = dieting and fears of being fat; E = sexual and toilet exhibitionism; S = the emotional selection of the child.

3. I am indebted to Dr. Howard Schwartz (1980), who restated my findings in a metapsychological framework that I have elaborated on in these formulations.

4. A useful acronym for the technique of interpretation in the initial phase of therapy is MAD: M = masochism; A = agression; D = dyadic transference.

5. Altshuler and Weiner seriously question the research methodology that links restrictor and bulimic anorexia nervosa to a family history of

depression. (K. A. Altshuler and M. F. Weiner. 1985. Anorexia nervosa and depression: a dissenting view. *American Journal of Psychiatry* 142[3]:328–332).

6. These clinical cases are drawn from C. P. Wilson, C. C. Hogan, and I. L. Mintz (1983) *Fear of Being Fat*. C. P. Wilson treated cases 2, 4, and 5. I. L. Mintz treated cases 1 and 3.

7. Each of the interpretations cited exemplifies a series or a line of interpretations that were applied systematically as the defenses of the ego (denial, rationalization, belief in magic, acting out) unfolded. At times, because of space limitations, there has been a condensation of multiple interpretations.

REFERENCES

Bion, W. R. 1956. Development of schizophrenic thought. *International Journal of Psycho-Analysis* 37:344–346.
Bliss, E. L., and Branch, C. H. H. 1960. *Anorexia Nervosa: Its History, Psychology, and Biology.* New York: Hoeber.
Blitzer, J. R.; Rollins, N.; and Blackwell, A. 1961. Children who starve themselves: anorexia nervosa. *Psychosomatic Medicine* 23:369–383.
Boyer, L. B. 1980. Work with a borderline patient. In L. B. Boyer and P. L. Giovacchini, eds. *Psychoanalytic Treatment of Schizophrenic, Borderline and Characterological Disorders.* New York: Aronson.
Boyer, L. B., and Giovacchini, P. L., eds. 1980. *Psychoanalytic Treatment of Schizophrenic, Borderline and Characterological Disorders.* New York: Aronson.
Brotman, A. W.; Herzog, D. B.; and Woods, S. W. 1984. Antidepressant treatment of bulimia: the relationship between binging and depressive symptomatology. *Journal of Clinical Psychiatry* 45(1): 7–8.
Bruch, H. 1962. Perceptual and conceptual disturbances in anorexia nervosa. *Psychosomatic Medicine* 24:187–194.
Bruch, H. 1965. Anorexia nervosa and its differential diagnosis. *Journal of Nervous and Mental Diseases* 141:555–566.
Bruch, H. 1970. Psychotherapy in primary anorexia nervosa. *Journal of Nervous and Mental Diseases* 150:51–67.
Bruch H. 1973. *Eating Disorders: Obesity, Anorexia Nervosa and the Person Within.* New York: Basic.
Bruch, H. 1974. Perils of behavior modification in the treatment of

anorexia nervosa. *Journal of the American Medical Association* 230:1409–1422.

Bruch, H. 1978. *The Golden Cage: The Enigma of Anorexia Nervosa.* Cambridge, Mass.: Harvard University Press.

Carpinacci, J. A.; Liberman, D.; and Schlossberg, N. 1963. Perturaciones de la communicacion y neurosis de contratransferencia. *Revista de Psicoanalisis* 20:63–69.

Carter, L., and Rinsley, D. B. 1977. Vicissitudes of "empathy" in a borderline patient. *International Revue of Psycho-Analysis* 4:317–326.

Ceaser, M. 1977. The role of maternal identification in four cases of anorexia nervosa. *Bulletin of the Menninger Clinic* 41(5): 475–487.

Cesio, F. R. 1963. La communicacion extraverbal en psicoanalisis: transferencia, contratransferencia e interpretacion. *Revista de psicoanalisis* 20:124–127.

Cesio, F. R. 1973. Los fundamentos de la contratransferencia: el yo ideal y las identificaciones directas. *Revista de Psicoanalisis* 30:5–16.

Crisp, A. H. 1965. Clinical and therapeutic aspects of anorexia nervosa: a study of 30 cases. *Journal of Psychosomatic Research* 9:67.

Crisp, A. H. 1968. Primary anorexia nervosa. *Gut* 9:370–372.

Dally, P. J. 1969. *Anorexia Nervosa.* New York: Grune & Stratton.

Deutsch, L. 1980. Psychosomatic medicine from a psychoanalytic viewpoint. *Journal of the American Psychoanalytic Association* 28:653–702.

Eidelberg, L. 1957. An introduction to the study of the narcissistic mortification. *Psychiatric Quarterly* 31:657–668.

Eidelberg, L. 1959. A second contribution to the study of the narcissistic mortification. *Psychiatric Quarterly* 33:636–646.

Falstein, E. L.; Feinstein, S. C.; and Judas, I. 1956. Anorexia nervosa in the male child. *American Journal of Orthopsychiatry* 26:751–772.

Fenichel, O. 1954. Anorexia. In *The Collected Papers of Otto Fenichel.* New York: Norton.

Flarsheim, A. 1975. The therapist's collusion with the patient's wish for suicide. In P. L. Giovacchini, A. Flarsheim, and L. B. Boyer, eds. *Tactics and Techniques in Psychoanalytic Therapy.* New York: Aronson.

Freud, A. 1945–1956. Indications for child analysis and other papers. *Writings of Anna Freud,* vol. 4. New York: International Universities Press, 1968.

Freud, S. 1918. From the history of an infantile neurosis. *Standard Edition* 17:7–122. London: Hogarth, 1955.

Freud, S. 1923. The ego and the id. *Standard Edition* 19:13–66. London: Hogarth, 1961.

Gero, G. 1953. An equivalent of depression: anorexia. In P. Greenacre, ed. *Affective Disorders: Psychoanalytic Contributions to Their Study.* New York: International Universities Press.

Gero, G. 1984. Book Review of J. Sours: *Starving to Death in a Sea of Objects: The Anorexia Nervosa Syndrome. Journal of the American Psychoanalytic Association* 32(1): 187–191.

Giovacchini, P. L. 1975. Self-projections in the narcissistic transference. *International Journal of Psychoanalytic Psychotherapy* 4:142–166.

Grinberg, L. 1972. *Practicas psicoanaliticas comparadas en las psicosis.* Buenos Aires: Paidos.

Grinberg, L. 1976. *Teoria de la identificacion.* Buenos Aires: Paidos.

Grinberg, L. 1979. Countertransference and projective counteridentification. *Contemporary Psychoanalysis* 15:226–247.

Halmi, K., and Falk, J. 1981. Common physiologic changes in anorexia nervosa. *International Journal of Eating Disorders* 1:28.

Hitchcock, J. 1984. Psychoanalytic treatment of restrictor anorexia nervosa. Psychosomatic Discussion Group. Meeting of the American Psychoanalytic Association, Philadelphia, May 2.

Hogan, C. C. 1983a. Anorexia versus bulimia. In C. P. Wilson, C. C. Hogan, and I. L. Mintz, eds. *Fear of Being Fat: The Treatment of Anorexia Nervosa and Bulimia.* New York: Aronson.

Hogan, C. C. 1983b. Psychoanalytic treatment of a bulimic anorexic woman. Psychosomatic Discussion Group. Meeting of the American Psychoanalytic Association, Philadelphia, April 27.

Jessner, L., and Abse, D. W. 1960. Regressive forces in anorexia nervosa. *British Journal of Medical Psychology* 33:301–311.

Karol, C. 1980. The role of primal scene and masochism in asthma. *International Journal of Psychoanalytic Psychotherapy* 8:577–592.

Kaufman, M. D., and Heiman, M., eds. 1964. *Evolution of Psychosomatic Concepts. Anorexia Nervosa: A Paradigm.* New York: International Universities Press.

Kernberg, O. F. 1975. *Borderline Conditions and Pathological Narcissism.* New York: Aronson.

Klein, M. 1955. On identification. In M. Klein, P. Heimann, and M. Money-Kyle, eds. *New Directions in Psychoanalysis.* London: Tavistock.

Kramer, S. 1974. A discussion of Sours's paper on "The anorexia syndrome." *International Journal of Psycho-Analysis* 55:577–579.

Lorand, S. 1943. Anorexia nervosa: report of a case. *Psychosomatic Medicine* 5:282–292.

Mahler, M. S. 1972. On the first three subphases of the separation-individuation process. *International Journal of Psycho-Analysis* 53:333–338.

Mahler, M. S., and Furer, M. 1968. *On Human Symbiosis and the Vicissitudes of Individuation*. New York: International Universities Press.

Masserman, J. H. 1941. Psychodynamics in anorexia nervosa and neurotic vomiting. *Psychoanalytic Quarterly* 10:211–242.

Masterson, J. 1977. Primary anorexia in the borderline adolescent—an object relations review. In P. Horticollis, ed. *Borderline Personality Disorders: The Concept, the Syndrome, the Patient*. New York: International Universities Press.

Mintz, I. L. 1980. Multideterminism in asthmatic disease. *International Journal of Psychoanalytic Psychotherapy* 8:593–600.

Mintz, I. L. 1982. Psychoanalytic treatment of a regressed restrictor anorexic. Psychosomatic Discussion Group. Meeting of the American Psychoanalytic Association, New York, December 15.

Mintz, I. L. 1983a. In C. P. Wilson, C. C. Hogan, and I. L. Mintz, eds. *Fear of Being Fat: The Treatment of Anorexia Nervosa and Bulimia*. New York: Aronson.

Mintz, I. L. 1983b. Anorexia nervosa and bulimia in males. In C. P. Wilson, C. C. Hogan, and I. L. Mintz, eds. *Fear of Being Fat: The Treatment of Anorexia Nervosa and Bulimia*. New York: Aronson.

Minuchin, S.; Rosman, B. L.; and Baker, L. 1978. *Psychosomatic Families: Anorexia Nervosa in Context*. Cambridge, Mass.: Harvard University Press.

Mogul, S. L. 1980. Asceticism and anorexia nervosa. *Psychoanalytic Study of the Child* 35:155–175.

Moulton, R. 1942. Psychosomatic study of anorexia nervosa including the use of vaginal smears. *Psychosomatic Medicine* 4:62–72.

Mushatt, C. 1975. Mind-body environment: toward understanding the impact of loss on psyche and soma. *Psychoanalytic Quarterly* 44:81–106.

Mushatt, C. 1982. Anorexia nervosa: a psychoanalytic commentary. *International Journal of Psychoanalytic Psychotherapy* 9:257–265.

Niederland, W. G. 1956. Clinical observations on the "little man" phenomenon. *Psychoanalytic Study of the Child* 11:381–395.

Niederland, W. G. 1965. Narcissistic ego impairment in patients with early physical malformations. *Psychoanalytic Study of the Child* 20:518–534.

Ogden, T. H. 1978. A developmental view of identifications resulting from maternal impingements. *International Journal of Psychoanalytic Psychotherapy* 7:486–506.

Perestrello, M. 1963. Um cao de intensa identifacao projetiva. *Journal Brasileiro de psiquiatria* 12:425–441.

Pope, H. G., and Hudson, J. I. 1982. Treatment of bulimia with antidepressants. *Psychopharmacology* 78:175–179.

Pope, H. G., and Hudson, J. I. 1984. *New Hope for Binge Eaters.* New York: Harper & Row.

Risen, S. E. 1982. The psychoanalytic treatment of an adolescent with anorexia nervosa. *Psychoanalytic Study of the Child* 37:433–459.

Rizzuto, A. M.; Petersen, R. K.; and Reed, M. 1981. The pathological sense of self in anorexia. *Psychiatric Clinics of North America* 4(3): 471–482.

Rosenfeld, D., and Mordo, E. 1973. Fusion, confusion, simbiosis e identificacion. *Revista de psicoanalisis* 30:413–423.

Rosenfeld, H. A. 1952. Notes on the psycho-analysis of the superego conflict of an acute schizophrenic patient. *International Journal of Psycho-Analysis* 33:111–131.

Schwartz, H. L. 1980. Discussion of C. P. Wilson's paper "The fear of being fat in female psychology." *Bulletin of the Psychoanalytic Association of New York* 17(1): 9.

Searles, H. F. 1965. *Collected Papers on Schizophrenia and Related Subjects.* New York: International Universities Press.

Selvini Palazzoli, M. 1961. Emaciation as magic means for the removal of anguish in anorexia mentalis. *Acta psychotherapica* 9:37–45.

Selvini Palazzoli, M. 1978. *Self-Starvation: From Individual to Family Therapy in the Treatment of Anorexia Nervosa.* New York: Aronson.

Sours, J. 1969. Anorexia nervosa: nosology, diagnosis, developmental patterns, and power-control dynamics. In G. Caplan and S. Lebovici, eds. *Adolescence: Psychosocial Perspectives.* New York: Basic.

Sours, J. 1980. *Starving to Death in a Sea of Objects: The Anorexia Nervosa Syndrome.* New York: Aronson.

Sperling, M. 1953. Food allergies and conversion hysteria. *Psychoanalytic Quarterly* 22:525–538.

Sperling, M. 1967. Transference neurosis in patients with psychosomatic disorders. *Psychoanalytic Quarterly* 36:342–355.

312

Sperling, M. 1968. Trichotillomania, trichophagy, and cyclic vomiting: a contribution to the psychopathology of female sexuality. *International Journal of Psycho-Analysis* 49:682–690.

Sperling, M. 1978. *Psychosomatic Disorders in Childhood*. New York: Aronson.

Spitz, R. A. 1955. The primal cavity: a contribution to the genesis of perception and its role for psychoanalytic theory. *Psychoanalytic Study of the Child* 10:215–240.

Strober, M. 1981. The significance of bulimia in juvenile anorexia nervosa: an exploration of possible etiologic factors. *International Journal of Eating Disorders* 1:28–43.

Strober, M. 1983. An empirically derived typology of anorexia nervosa. In P. L. Darby, P. E. Garfinkel, D. M. Garner, and D. V. Coscina, eds. *Anorexia Nervosa: Recent Developments*. New York: Liss.

Thoma, H. 1967. *Anorexia Nervosa*. New York: International Universities Press.

Volkan, V. D. 1976. *Primitive Internalized Object Relations: A Clinical Study of Schizophrenic, Borderline, and Narcissistic Patients*. New York: International Universities Press.

Waller, J. V.; Kaufman, M. R.; and Deutsch, F. 1940. Anorexia nervosa: a psychosomatic entity. *Psychosomatic Medicine* 2:3–16.

Walsh, B. J.; Stewart, J. W.; Wright, L.; Harrison, W.; Roose, S.; and Glassman, A. 1982. Treatment of bulimia with monoamine oxidase inhibitors. *American Journal of Psychiatry* 139:1629–1630.

Wilson, C. P. 1968. Psychosomatic asthma and acting out: a case of bronchial asthma that developed de novo in the terminal phase of analysis. *International Journal of Psycho-Analysis* 49:330–335.

Wilson, C. P. 1970. Theoretical and clinical considerations in the early phase of treatment of patients suffering from severe psychosomatic symptoms. *Bulletin of the Philadelphia Association of Psychoanalysis* 20:71–74.

Wilson, C. P. 1971. On the limits of the effectiveness of psychoanalysis: early ego and somatic disturbances. *Journal of the American Psychoanalytic Association* 19:552–564.

Wilson, C. P. 1973. The psychoanalytic treatment of hospitalized anorexia nervosa patients. Paper presented at the meeting of the Psychoanalytic Association of New York, November 19.

Wilson, C. P. 1974. The psychoanalysis of an adolescent anorexic girl. Discussion group on "Late Adolescence," S. Ritvo, Chairman. Meeting of the American Psychoanalytic Association. New York, December 12.

Wilson, C. P. 1980a. On the fear of being fat in female psychology and anorexia nervosa patients. *Bulletin of the Psychoanalytic Association of New York* 17:8–9.

Wilson, C. P. 1980b. Parental overstimulation in asthma. *International Journal of Psychoanalytic Psychotherapy* 8:601–621.

Wilson, C. P. 1980c. The family psychological profile of anorexia nervosa patients. *Journal of the Medical Society of New Jersey* 77:341–344.

Wilson, C. P. 1981. Sand symbolism: the primary dream representation of the Isakower phenomenon and of smoking addictions. In S. Orgel and B. D. Fine, eds. *Clinical Psychoanalysis*. New York: Aronson.

Wilson, C. P. 1982. The fear of being fat and anorexia nervosa. *International Journal of Psychoanalytic Psychotherapy* 9:233–255.

Wilson, C. P. 1983a. Fat phobia as a diagnostic term to replace a medical misnomer: "anorexia nervosa." American Academy of Child Psychiatry, G. Harper, M. D., Chairman. Tapes 96 and 97, by Instant Replay, 760 S. 23d Street, Arlington, Virginia 22202, October 25.

Wilson, C. P. 1985. The treatment of bulimic depression. Paper presented at Grand Rounds, Department of Psychiatry, St. Lukes Roosevelt Hospital, New York, March 6.

Wilson, C. P. 1983b. Psychodynamic and/or psychopharmacologic treatment of bulimic anorexia nervosa. In C. P. Wilson, C. C. Hogan, and I. L. Mintz, eds. *Fear of Being Fat: The Treatment of Anorexia Nervosa and Bulimia*. Revised ed. Riverside, N.J. Aronson, 1985.

Wilson, C. P.; Hogan, C. C.; and Mintz, I. L. 1983. *Fear of Being Fat: The Treatment of Anorexia Nervosa and Bulimia*. New York: Aronson.

Wilson, C. P., and Mintz, I. L. 1982. Abstaining and bulimic anorexics: two sides of the same coin. *Primary Care* 9:459–472.

Wurmser, L. 1980. Phobic core in the addictions and the paranoid process. *International Journal of Psychoanalytic Psychotherapy* 8:311–335.

LAURA LYNN HUMPHREY

The publication of this edited volume, devoted to the problem of bulimia at normal weight, attests to the growing concern about its alarming incidence and potentially chronic and devastating impact on the life of an adolescent or young adult. Both the clinical and empirical literature to date have focused on understanding the nature of bulimia within the individual, whether it be the psychodynamics, the behavioral topography, or the neuroendocrine substrate. Relatively little attention has been given to the familial processes that may contribute to the genesis and maintenance of the disorder. The intention of this chapter is to address familial components in bulimia.

Systemic Dynamics

Family systems theory of psychopathology views the identified patient's symptom as a homeostatic mechanism for maintaining balance and stability in the family. A family systems conceptualization of anorexia nervosa proposes that the disorder unifies the family in helping the sick child, maintains harmony, and avoids conflict in the marriage (Minuchin, Rosman, and Baker 1978; Palazzoli 1978). While there has not previously been a family systems model of bulimia per se, the Minuchin et al. and Palazzoli conceptualizations seem quite relevant to bulimia as well.

There are, though, some dramatic differences in the interactional patterns of these two types of families that also need to be incorporated into the functional interpretation of bulimia (cf. Garner, Garfinkel, and O'Shaughnessy 1983). Quite dissimilar to the anorexics', the bulimics' families do not appear to be the perfect, selfless family that avoids conflict at all cost. On the contrary, the families of bulimics do experience subjective distress and conflict in their relationships with one another (Johnson and Flach, in press; Ordman and Kirschenbaum, in press). The interaction patterns of bulimic families can also be overtly hostile, angry, and manipulative. Importantly, though, family members seem unable to express their negative feelings openly and directly; instead, they bicker, blame, and sulk about less central issues, sometimes endlessly, without ever being able to resolve the real conflict among them.

Thus, the bulimic provides a diversionary focus for both the enmeshed bickering and for the family's unified concern and help. This focus, negative and positive, on the bulimic child allows the family to avoid more dangerous, subterranean conflicts in the marriage. Typically, marital distress consists of a lack or loss of emotional intimacy, alcoholism, and/or depression. Such a pattern can be quite powerful in maintaining family stability even if the bulimic lives away from home because her parents can certainly continue to worry and argue together about her in her absence. Interestingly, the bulimic is often perceived as the "black sheep" of the family, despite her self-sacrifices for it. She is not so likely to be seen as the perfect daughter as is the anorexic.

Another related characteristic of the family system in bulimia is the transgenerational pattern of dysregulation and affective instability that are hallmarks in the bulimic herself (Goodsitt 1983; Hudson, Pope, Jonas, and Yurgelum-Todd 1983; Pyle, Mitchell, and Eckert 1981). Several recent studies have shown that both affective and self-regulatory disorders are also more common in parents of bulimics than in the general population. Carroll and Leon (1981) studied thirty-seven bulimics and found that their parents were often obese (29 percent mothers and 25 percent fathers) or alcoholic, especially fathers (49 percent). Similarly, other research groups have reported high incidences of affective disorder (44/251 in Hudson et al. study) and substance abuse (27/251 in Hudson et al., and 17/34 in Pyle et al. study) in the first-degree relatives of bulimics.

The parallels, then, between the central features of the bulimia itself and disturbances of affect and self-regulation in other members of the family are striking. In fact, the binge-purge cycle is itself a good interpersonal metaphor for the more family-wide problem of dysregulation and affective instability. Table 1 illustrates the similarities between the four primary components of the binge-purge cycle and the bulimic's psychological and family life. Each aspect of family relations, symbolized by the

TABLE 1
THE BINGE-PURGE CYCLE AS A METAPHOR FOR THE BULIMIC'S SELF AND FAMILY

Bulimic's cycle	Food cravings	Diet	Binge	Purge
Bulimic's self	Internal, unmet needs for nurturance and individuation	Strict and oppressive self-restraint and expectations	Loss of self-control, structure, and affective stability	Expression of hostility and frustration
Bulimic's family ...	Familywide needs for affection and autonomy	Interpersonal control and intrusion	Chaotic, unmodulated relations, and poor regulation and structure	Expulsion of conflict and negative affect, without focus, structure, or resolution

bulimic's cycle, will be presented separately in more detail. First, clinical observations and conceptualizations will be considered. Then any existing research support for these hypotheses will be summarized.

The Food or Nurturance Hypothesis

Just as the bulimic needs food, so the bulimic family needs emotional nurturance and empathy from one another; yet they too are unable to get enough. Family members are unable to meet one another's needs for affection and warmth or for acceptance of their separate identities, feelings, and experiences. Parents are usually quite well intentioned, even determined to give their children what they never had. Too often, though, the parents were also deprived of "good enough mothering" (Winnicott 1965), especially in support of their own individuation. Thus, they cannot provide a nurturing environment of easy affection and acceptance for their children, and everyone is left "hungry."

Some preliminary data exist to support this nurturance hypothesis. Ordman and Kirschenbaum (in press) compared the responses of twenty-five bulimic women with those of thirty-six normal controls on the Family Environment Scale (FES; Moos and Moos 1980) and on the Family Adaptibility and Cohesion Evaluation Scale (FACES; Olson, Bell, and Portner 1978). They found that bulimics reported significantly less cohesion in their families, on both scales, and also less expressiveness on the FES. Those two subscales reflect the degree of support and commitment family members feel toward one another as well as the extent to which

317

they can openly express their thoughts and feelings in the family. Another source of empirical support for the nurturance hypothesis derives from the fact that loss or separation from family are the most common precipitants to the onset of bulimia. Pyle et al. (1981) found that twenty-three of their thirty-four bulimics began binge-eating and vomiting after leaving home or losing a significant relationship.

A further source of evidence comes from a large-scale study of family processes in eating disorders that I am currently conducting. Analyses of interactions and ratings among the first fourteen bulimic family triads suggests that the entire family system is quite disturbed relative to controls. Utilizing Benjamin's (1974) Structural Analysis of Social Behavior (SASB) methodology, the bulimic families appear to be severely lacking in nurturance, comfort, and acceptance and support of autonomy in one another relative to normal families.

The Diet or Interpersonal Restriction Hypothesis

Since the bulimic family cannot fulfill its basic affectional and acceptance needs, like the bulimic herself, family members try to maintain a strict "diet." Their interpersonal diet consists of exerting rigid controls and protections over one another and by expecting superior performance in every aspect of life together. Typically, the bulimic's parents are quite watchful of her, highly controlling, and intrusive. There is usually a pattern of enmeshed relations, such as those described by Minuchin et al. (1978) in anorexic families. In bulimic families, though, the enmeshment can be hostile. It consists of both parents and daughter controlling or harshly controlling one another, while the other surrenders autonomy or resentfully submits. In addition, family members have high standards, even idealized ones, about how they each ought to be. The intergenerational boundaries can also be too rigid and impenetrable.

There are few published data to support this notion of an interpersonally restrictive diet in bulimic families. However, in an earlier paper I reported on the results of a sequential analysis of family interactions in bulimia (Humphrey 1983). In that study, an adolescent bulimic and her parents were videotaped while discussing separation issues. The results of that microanalysis, using Markov Chains and Benjamin's SASB coding of interactions, showed that both mother and father were highly intrusive and controlling toward their daughter, while she was ambivalent about taking autonomy. The bulimic was outwardly assertive, but she intro-jected her parents' harsh control and also treated herself oppressively. The study that is currently under way in my laboratory appears to be confirming these findings at the interfamilial level as well. In terms of the high expectations in the family's diet, Johnson and Flach (in press) found that their sample of bulimics had higher achievement orientation on the FES than did normal women. This finding seems somewhat supportive of the observed high standards in these families.

The Binge or Loss of Control Hypothesis

Despite the family's efforts to "diet," or restrict and control each other and themselves, their strong but unsatisfied needs for affection and acceptance compel them to keep striving. At times these drives and strivings can become so intense that they resemble the bulimic's binge. Family members may seek or demand immediate gratification or become impulsive and isolated. Their family boundaries can shift from hierarchi-cal rigidity to being too loose and ineffectual. Similarly, what is overly structured at one time may dissolve into virtual chaos at another. Perhaps most obviously, the affective expression among family members can be unmodulated and labile. Thus, the family's "binge" reflects a loss of self-regulation, effective relating, and an organizing structure to more basic needs and impulses.

Garner et al.'s (1983) study comparing bulimics to restricting anorexics and bulimic-anorexics is somewhat supportive of the concept of a family-wide emotional binge. They administered the Family Assessment Mea-sure (FAM) (Skinner, Santa-Barbara, and Steinhauer 1985) and found that both bulimic groups were significantly more disturbed in affective involvement and expression as compared to restricting anorexics and published norms. Further, data from several studies also suggest that alcohol abuse and obesity, perhaps both signs of dysregulation, are more frequent in the families of bulimics than in the general population (Car-roll and Leon 1981; Hudson et al. 1983; Pyle et al. 1981).

The Purge or Expelling of Hostility Hypothesis

The bulimic family's emotional "purge" consists of their overt expul-sion of tension, frustration, and anger. However, like the bulimic herself,

319

the family's expression is indirect, masked, and provides only temporary relief. Their anger is not often rageful and explosive but rather is one of continuous unresolved arguing, complaining, and belittling each other. In contrast to classical anorexics' families, conflict in these families is more overt and can be viciously hurtful and manipulative. The conflict often has no structure, no focus, no boundaries, and no end. Old injuries are considered fair game in an argument, then they may later be denied. This leaves the defendant with nothing to fight against. Family members do not accept responsibility for their feelings, and they cannot seem to negotiate about them openly. It is sometimes primitive conflict but is more often strategic, insidious, and enduring. Another way that conflict is expressed in these families is through hostile, indirect joking, followed by, "Can't you take a joke?" The bulimic daughter is herself a key figure in the family's well-rehearsed drama, sometimes allying with father against mother and sister, other times offering herself as a focus to divert the deeper conflict between her parents.

Several sources of existing data offer evidence for this set of observations. Both Johnson and Flach (in press) and Ordman and Kirschenbaum (in press) found that bulimics experience significantly greater conflict in their families than normal controls. Results from my observational study of bulimic families also seem to confirm these findings. There are greater hostility and conflict, both overt and covert, in the interactions of bulimic families relative to normal controls.

In sum, these families reflect a similar pattern of dysregulation and poor modulation of affect and impulses seen in the bulimic herself. All of the members of the family seem to need more acceptance of autonomy and nurturance (food) than they can get from one another. This emptiness leads them to react with overcontrol and restriction, interpersonally (diet). Their attempt to master these emotional deficits, however, does not really solve the problem, and periodically the other extreme emerges. The family will become chaotic, impulsive and labile (binge), or expel their hostility and frustration (purge) with one another. Thus, it is not difficult to imagine why the bulimic daughter introjects these patterns of poor self-regulation and self-care. These observations, however, are based primarily on clinical experience, with a paucity of empirical support. The following study was done in order to examine some of these patterns in bulimic and bulimic-anorexic families more directly.

LAURA LYNN HUMPHREY

A Comparison of Bulimic, Bulimic-Anorexic, and Normal Families

PURPOSE, SUBJECTS, AND METHODS

The purpose of this study was to examine differences in perceived family relations among those with bulimic, bulimic-anorexic, and normal teenage daughters. A total of fifty-four family triads, including father, mother, and daughter, participated in the study. There were fourteen bulimics' families, sixteen bulimic-anorexics', and twenty-four normal controls. Both sets of bulimic and anorexic patients had just begun treatment at the University of Wisconsin's Eating Disorders Program. They met their respective DSM-III criteria (*DSM-III 1980*) for bulimia, or anorexia nervosa with binge-eating and self-induced vomiting (sometimes also laxative abuse). The normal families were recruited through the University of Wisconsin's abnormal psychology class and the public high schools of Oregon and McFarland, Wisconsin. These families had no history of psychological problems in the immediate family. The average age of all three groups of daughters was approximately eighteen years (SD = two years).

Each of the families was asked to complete the Family Adaptibility and Cohesion Evaluation Scale (FACES) and the Family Environment Scale (FES) independent of one another. In a prior study (Humphrey, in press) both scales were factor analyzed and found to consist of eight orthogonal factors. The FACES comprised (1) involvement and support, (2) isolation and nondisclosure, (3) chaos, (4) boundaries, (5) detachment, (6) interdependence, (7) democracy, and (8) rules. Similarly, the FES comprised (1) order and organization, (2) involvement and support, (3) conflict, (4) moral and religious deemphasis, (5) isolation and nondisclosure, (6) intellectual deemphasis, (7) interdependence, and (8) recreational deemphasis.

Results

The data were analyzed using a series of six repeated measures analyses of variance (ANOVAs), with one between factor (three groups) and one within factor (eight factor scores). Each family member's responses were analyzed separately for the two scales. The three ANOVAs for fathers', mothers', and daughters' FACES ratings revealed highly significant main effects for factor (F's = 369.98–464.92, df = 7,357, P's < .0001), and, most important, for the factor × group interaction (F's = 6.71–9.47, df = 14,357, P's < .0001). The main effects for group were not significant. Results from the three ANOVAs for the FES ratings were also highly significant for factor (F's = 68.93, df = 7,357, P's < .0001) and for the factor × group interaction (F's = 4.82–5.91, df = 14,357, P's < .0001). Here too, there were no significant main effects for group.

Table 2 presents the results of the subsequent simple effects tests for each family member on both the FACES and the FES. These tests were then followed up by Newman-Keuls tests to analyze which groups differed on the significant factors (summarized in table 3). As the tables indicate, there were two major sets of findings. Families of bulimics and bulimic-anorexics were consistently more distressed than normal controls, and they were fairly comparable to one another. There was one

TABLE 2

F-Values from Simple Effects Tests Comparing Bulimic, Bulimic-Anorexic, and Normal Families on the FACES and FES Factors

	Fathers	Mothers	Daughters
FACES factors:			
Involvement	11.96****	8.99***	9.66***
Isolation	9.65***	5.04*	8.88***
Chaos	1.80	2.68	3.11
Boundaries	4.82*	4.78*	3.39*
Detachment	5.73**	4.86*	8.21***
Interdependence	2.14	.54	.91
Democracy	7.94***	.62	.56
Rules	1.21	.59	.61
FES factors:			
Organization	1.94	1.35	4.94*
Involvement	11.39***	9.74***	5.93***
Conflict	1.23	1.93	9.77***
Moral deemphasis	2.70	3.08	3.97*
Isolation	6.14***	8.80***	7.36***
Intellectual deemphasis	6.11***	8.27***	.52
Interdependence	1.28	.32	.68
Recreational deemphasis	.89	.44	.68

df = 2,51.
*P < .05.
**P < .01.
***P < .005.
****P < .0001.

TABLE 3

	Fathers	Mothers	Daughters
FACES factors:			
Involvement	B & BA < NC**	B & BA < NC**	B & BA < NC**
Isolation	B & BA > NC**	BA > NC**	B & BA > NC*
Boundaries	B & BA < NC*	BA < NC*	BA < NC*
Detachment	B & BA > NC*	BA > NC*	B & BA > NC**
Democracy	B & BA < NC*	. . .	. . .
FES factors:			
Organization	. . .	. . .	BA < B & NC**
Involvement	B & BA < NC**	B & BA < NC*	B & BA < NC*
Conflict	. . .	. . .	B & BA > NC**
Moral deemphasis	. . .	. . .	BA > NC*
Isolation	B & BA > NC*	BA > NC*	B & BA > NC**
Intellectual deemphasis	B & BA > NC*	B & BA > NC*	. . .

NOTE.—B = bulimic, BA = bulimic-anorexic, NC = normal control.
*$p < .05$.
**$p < .01$.

important exception to this pattern, however. Mothers of bulimics did not report nearly the level of dissatisfaction with family relations that their husbands and daughters, or their bulimic-anorexic counterparts, reported; in fact, these mothers of bulimics did not differ from normal mothers on most variables.

The second important set of findings addresses the specific pattern of differences among the family subtypes. Mothers, fathers, and daughters agreed that both bulimic and bulimic-anorexic families are less involved and supportive (on both the FACES and the FES) with one another than are normal families. Fathers and daughters also converged in their perceptions that both bulimic and bulimic-anorexic families are more isolated and nondisclosing (both scales), and detached (FACES), relative to controls. Similarly, mothers of bulimic anorexics agreed with their husbands and daughters about the isolation and detachment in the family, whereas bulimics' mothers did not. Moreover, both sets of bulimic parents perceived their families as less intellectually oriented (FES) than did normal controls.

Only the bulimic-anorexic families, all three members, reported significant problems with boundaries (FACES) relative to normal families. Less consistent, but still significant, differences were also found for:

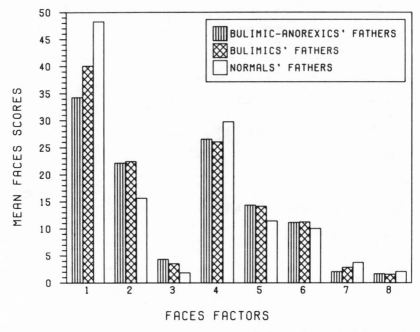

FIGURE 1. Group means for bulimic-anorexics', bulimics', and normals' fathers on the FACES.

democracy on the FACES, order and organization, conflict, and moral and religious deemphasis on the FES. Figures 1 and 2 illustrate the group means for fathers of bulimics, bulimic-anorexics, and normal controls on the FACES and the FES. Only results from fathers are depicted because they overlapped considerably with those of other family members, especially their daughters'. As the figures display, both groups of bulimics' fathers are more distressed than normal controls on five of eight FACES factors, and in three of eight FES factors, to approximately the same extent.

Discussion

Consistent with previous clinical and empirical findings, the present results indicate that both bulimic and bulimic-anorexic families report significantly more distress in their patterns of relating than did normal controls. Families of both bulimics and bulimic-anorexics experience less involvement and support, greater isolation and nondisclosure, and more

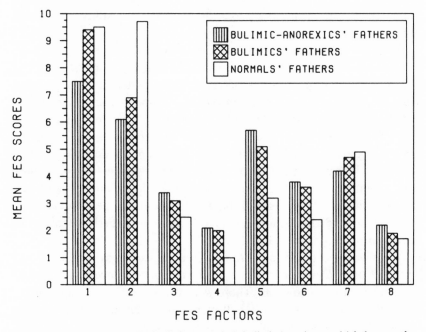

FIGURE 2. Group means for bulimic-anorexics', bulimics', and normals' fathers on the FES.

detachment, among family members relative to normal families. All three members of bulimic-anorexic families also reported poorer boundary differentiation among themselves as compared with normal controls. In bulimic-anorexic families, all three members converged in their perceptions of family relations. In contrast, only bulimics and their fathers experienced those families' detachment and nondisclosure, whereas bulimics' mothers did not. In bulimic families, all three members agreed only that there was a lack of support and involvement relative to control families.

Keeping such discrepancies in mind, though, we find that these results do support earlier clinical observations, especially the food or nurturance hypothesis. That hypothesis proposed that bulimic families experience a lack of affection and acceptance in family relations and feel emotionally distant. Such results also fit Ordman and Kirschenbaum's (in press) findings that bulimic daughters perceived their families as less supportive and expressive, and more conflictual, than did controls. In this study, however, only daughters perceived the interpersonal conflict among

325

family members. Thus, the purge, or expelling of hostility, hypothesis received only preliminary support.

It is interesting that fathers' and their bulimic daughters' experiences and/or reports of family life were so convergent with each other but so divergent from mothers' on both scales. Such a pattern may suggest that there is a father-daughter link in bulimia. It may be that their mutual problems with self-esteem and self-regulation are fueled by similar needs for emotional intimacy and similar dissatisfactions with the degree of isolation and nondisclosure in the family. Why mothers do not report this feeling of detachment and distance is intriguing. It could be that mothers are fulfilling more of their own needs through their daughters and husbands. Thus, until her husband and daughter confront their "addictions" and begin to individuate more, the mother may not experience threats to her own psychological self.

Another important finding from the present study was that families of bulimics and bulimic-anorexics reported comparable levels and types of distress relative to controls. There were two exceptions to this conclusion. First, bulimic-anorexic family members perceived greater problems with boundaries than did the other groups. This difference may reflect an even greater problem with roles and structure in bulimic-anorexic, as compared to bulimic, families. Second, mothers of bulimics responded to the questionnaires about family life in an anomalous pattern relative to their own husbands and daughters as well as to their bulimic-anorexic counterparts. It is somewhat surprising that there would be such a dramatic difference between mothers of normally weighted versus anorexic bulimics. This finding could reflect a more pervasive level of distress in the anorexic families, so that it disturbs all members more evenly. At least, this discrepancy suggests that the role of each parent may be unique in the various subtypes of eating disorders.

In many respects, though, the bulimic and bulimic-anorexic families appeared similarly distressed. Garner et al. (1983) also found a parallel between these two groups of bulimics (no other family members were included) relative to classical, restricting anorexics. In their study, too, both bulimic subtypes were more disturbed in the areas of affective expression and control. Relatedly, Strober and his colleagues (Strober 1981; Strober, Salkin, Burroughs, and Morrell 1981) found that families of bulimic-anorexics, as compared with restrictors, were less cohesive and organized and more negative and conflictual. In addition, fathers of bulimic-anorexics were more impulsive, were more likely to be alcoholic, and had poorer frustration tolerance relative to those of restrictors, whereas their mothers were more hostile and depressed than were those of their classical counterparts. Thus, the bulimic symptom constellation, more than the severe weight loss, may be associated with the negativistic relationship patterns found here and elsewhere in these families. However, even within the bulimic subtypes, there appear to be some important familial differences associated with each variant of the disorder.

Dyadic Dynamics

FATHER AND MOTHER

Findings from the foregoing study suggest that, in addition to the familywide patterns, there are also some unique dynamics present in various family dyads. There are even fewer existing data to delineate the dyadic relations in bulimic families, but some clinical observations may prove helpful. In the marital dyad, there is usually a marked absence of true emotional intimacy and deep, differentiated relating. The spouses often married each other with the (unconscious) hope of finding an idealized mother, only to be tragically disappointed when they discover that their partner needed as much from them. So a frequent solution to this profound disappointment is to reenact their own past in the marriage and to turn to their children for their affectional and self-esteem needs.

Often the marital relationship reflects the parents' unmet demands from their own childhood and aspects of their harsh or neglectful parental introjects. These family legacies combine with their current beliefs about how they ought to behave and feel as a devoted, self-sacrificing spouse and parent. Their roles are traditional ones, economically (sometimes) and interpersonally. The husband is the more overtly dominant one in the relationship, but his hidden feelings consist of inadequacy and dependency. The wife may appear to be quite submissive, and she usually feels helpless and ineffectual, but she maintains her own more covert control over her husband too. They give up on affection and turn to power as a means of attempting to get their deeper needs met.

FATHER AND DAUGHTER

The father-daughter relationship is also central and significant in bulimic families. In time, the fathers are often discovered to be alcoholic or depressed (Pyle et al. 1981) themselves. Thus, their daughters' addiction to food or drugs (Garner et al. 1983) may reflect more of an "addiction"

327

to their fathers than to the substances themselves. At the very least, their mutual addictions represent some link between father and daughter in the ways that they regulate their frustrations, impulses, and needs. This may be related to the earlier finding that fathers and daughters in bulimic families perceived their family relations so similarly.

Another striking aspect of the father-daughter relationship is that frequently they are much closer before adolescence begins. The bulimics will report poignant memories of the last time their father hugged them or complimented them, years earlier. Thus, the transition from "Daddy's little girl" to adolescent sexuality and separation is perhaps traumatic for them both. It may be that the fathers are alarmed by their own feelings and impulses in response to their daughters' sexual and emotional development. The daughter may even closely resemble his wife early in their relationship. Since the father himself has difficulty regulating his own tensions and impulses, he may respond to his daughter by abruptly and anxiously withdrawing his emotional closeness along with physical contact. This may also be related to why fathers exert such strict controls and standards over their daughters—that is, to control themselves indirectly.

MOTHER AND DAUGHTER

The mother-daughter relationship in eating disorders has received more attention in the literature than have other family dyads. My own clinical experience confirms recent conceptualizations of the nature of the mother-daughter relationship in bulimia (Sugarman and Kurash 1982) and similarly in anorexia nervosa (Bruch 1973; Masterson 1977; Palazzoli 1974; Sours 1974). On the basis of earlier work by Mahler (1968) and Winnicott (1965), current views suggest that the bulimic too has a developmental failure in separation-individuation primarily because the mother was unable to provide empathic mirroring, especially for efforts toward autonomy.

This failure to individuate is quite evident, in both mother and daughter, during family conferences that occur sixteen or thirty-six years following the original developmental arrest. Mothers expect their daughters to respond to the mothers' needs and vulnerabilities and to negate their own. When the bulimic does assert herself (ambivalently), mother is either hostile and/or controlling toward her. In the course of therapy, I find that mother's own mother was often harsh, demanding, and neglectful of her, as well. This led to her turning toward her bulimic daughter in the hope of getting mothered herself. Thus when the bulimic daughters try to differentiate, their mothers feel a desperate threat themselves and so tighten the hostile enmeshment.

Another aspect of the mother-daughter enmeshment is reflected by the mothers' own struggle with weight (Garner et al. 1983) and sometimes full-blown bulimia. Mother and daughter will at times report a greater closeness through their shared battles and indulgences with the loved and hated "food." There is also an obvious element of competition around who is thinner and who has better self-control. Interestingly, in those families where both mother and daughter have eating disorders, it is the mother who urges the daughter to seek help, but she accompanies daughter to the consultation. In this way mother too is cautiously asking for help herself, if only someone will listen.

SISTERS

Relatedly, sisters of bulimics seem to have an increased risk for developing an eating disorder themselves. There have been a number of sisters, including twins, at our clinic who developed their bulimia or anorexia when they first separated from each other and moved away from home. The sisters are extremely close and feel a tragic loss on separation. The shared bulimia can be a vital link to each other and a dangerous competition for love and acceptance.

Conclusions

This chapter has attempted to identify and characterize some of the disturbed processes and relations in bulimic families. From a family systems perspective, bulimia can be conceptualized as a homeostatic mechanism that enables the family to avert unacknowledged but perilous conflicts, especially in the marriage, and to maintain their enmeshment. It was also observed that there is often a transgenerational pattern of poor self-esteem, self-regulation, and affective instability. Thus, the bulimic cycle was proposed as a fitting metaphor for the proposed family-wide disturbances in interpersonal relations. All of the family members appear to be searching for the "food" of affection and autonomy, but, when they are left feeling "hungry," try to master that through a "diet" of restrictive, controlling relations. At times, though, their hunger for deep closeness with each other drives them to "binge" by losing control and structure over their needs and impulses. Family members will also "purge" themselves of their anger and frustration at times, either through open conflict or, more often, indirect sniping and bickering.

In addition to the clinical observations and review of existing research, this chapter included a new study comparing bulimic, bulimic-anorexic, and normal control families. The main findings from that study are that both subtypes of bulimic families reported *less* involvement and support, and *greater* detachment and nondisclosure among family members, relative to normal controls. The findings also suggested that different family dynamics may be associated with various subtypes of bulimia. Finally, this chapter has attempted to present some unique patterns of relating among different dyads in the family. For example, it examined the importance of the father-daughter link through their mutual addictions as well as the mother's search for her own mothering in her relationship with her daughter. Of course, all of these observations and findings are only preliminary at this point and subject to refinement and revision from new data as they evolve. Future research and theorizing will undoubtedly continue to clarify the familial contributions to this strange and dangerous disorder of adolescence.

NOTE

I am very grateful to Dan Kirschenbaum for his helpful suggestions on an earlier version of this chapter.

REFERENCES

Benjamin, L. S. 1974. Structural analysis of social behavior. *Psychological Review* 81:392–425.

Bruch, H. 1973. *Eating Disorders*. New York: Basic.

Carroll, K., and Leon, G. R. 1981. The bulimia-vomiting disorder within a generalized substance abuse pattern. Paper presented at the annual meeting for the Association for the Advancement of Behavior Therapy, Toronto, November.

Diagnostic and Statistical Manual of Mental Disorders, 3d ed. (*DSM-III*). 1980. Washington, D.C.: American Psychiatric Association.

Garner, D. M.; Garfinkel, P. E.; and O'Shaughnessy, M. 1983. Clinical and psychometric comparisons between bulimia in anorexia and bulimia in normal weight women. In *Understanding Anorexia Nervosa and Bulimia: Report of the Fourth Ross Conference on Medical Research.* Columbus, Ohio: Ross Laboratories.

Goodsitt, A. 1983. Self-regulatory disturbances in eating disorders. *International Journal of Eating Disorders* 2:51–60.

Hudson, J. I.; Pope, H. G.; Jonas, J. M.; and Yurgelun-Todd, D. 1983. Family history study of anorexia nervosa and bulimia. *British Journal of Psychiatry* 142:133–138.

Humphrey, L. L. 1983. A sequential analysis of family processes in anorexia and bulimia. In *Understanding Anorexia Nervosa and Bulimia: Report of the Fourth Ross Conference on Medical Research.* Columbus, Ohio: Ross Laboratories.

Humphrey, L. L. In press. Family relations in bulimic-anorexic and nondistressed families. *International Journal of Eating Disorders.*

Johnson, C., and Flach, R.A. In press. Family characteristics of bulimic and normal women: a comparative study. *American Journal of Psychiatry.*

Mahler, M. S. 1968. *On Human Symbiosis and the Vicissitudes of Individuation.* Vol. 1, *Infantile Psychosis.* New York: International Universities Press.

Masterson, J. F. 1977. Primary anorexia nervosa in the borderline adolescent: an object relations view. In P. Hartocollis, ed. *Borderline Personality Disorders.* New York: International Universities Press.

Minuchin, S.; Rosman, B. L.; and Baker, L. 1978. *Psychosomatic Families: Anorexia Nervosa in Context.* Cambridge, Mass.: Harvard University Press.

Moos, R., and Moos, B. S. 1980. *Family Environment Scale Manual.* Palo Alto, Calif.: Consulting Psychologists Press.

Olson, D. H.; Bell, R.; and Portner, J. 1978. *Family Adaptibility and Cohesion Evaluation Scale.* St. Paul, Minn.: Family Social Science, University of Minnesota.

Ordman, A. M., and Kirschenbaum, D. S. In press. Bulimia: assessment of eating, psychological adjustment and familial characteristics. *International Journal of Eating Disorders.*

Palazzoli, M. 1974. *Self-Starvation.* London: Chaucer.

Palazzoli, M. 1978. *Self-Starvation: From Individual to Family Therapy in the Treatment of Anorexia Nervosa.* New York: Aronson.

Pyle, R. L.; Mitchell, J. E.; and Eckert, E. D. 1981. Bulimia: a report of 34 cases. *Journal of Clinical Psychiatry* 42:60–64.

Skinner, H. A.; Santa-Barbara, J.; and Steinhauer, D. D. 1985. The family assessment measure. *Canadian Journal of Commmunity Mental Health*, in press.

Sours, J. A. 1974. The anorexia nervosa syndrome. *International Journal of Psycho-Analysis* 55:567–572.

Strober, M. 1981. The significance of bulimia in juvenile anorexia nervosa: an explanation of possible etiologic factors. *International Journal of Eating Disorders* 1:28–43.

Strober, M.; Salkin, B.; Burroughs, J.; and Morrell, W. 1981. Validity of the bulimia-restrictor distinction in anorexia nervosa. *Journal of Nervous and Mental Disease* 170:345–351.

Sugarman, A., and Kurash, C. 1982. The body as a transitional object in bulimia. *International Journal of Eating Disorders* 1:57–67.

Winnicott, D. W. 1965. *The Maturational Processes and the Facilitating Environment*. New York: International Universities Press.

18 A BEHAVIORAL APPROACH TO TREATMENT OF BULIMIA NERVOSA

HAROLD LEITENBERG AND JAMES C. ROSEN

In this chapter we will be addressing a subtype of bulimia, sometimes called bulimia nervosa (Russell 1979) or bulimarexia (Boskind-Lodahl 1978). There are three major defining criteria for bulimia nervosa: (1) complaints of uncontrollable binge-eating, with an emphasis placed on the word "complaints" because the definition of a binge-eating episode is purely subjective; (2) self-induced vomiting after binge-eating or after eating even minimal amounts of food considered fattening or "bad" or "too much"; (3) expressions of intense dread of weight gain or a change in bodily appearance, for example, stomach bulge or fatty thighs.

Patients with this eating disorder are distinguishable from individuals who binge-eat but who do not vomit, such as those men and women who alternate between deprivation diets and bouts of overeating (Polivy, Herman, Olmsted, and Jazwinski 1984). Although binge-eating with and without vomiting are both classified under "bulimia" in the *Diagnostic and Statistical Manual of Mental Disorders* (*DSM-III* 1980), there is good reason to consider these separately: they may have somewhat different etiologies, the course of the disorder may be different, the degree of associated pathology (both physical and psychological) is different, and the type of treatment that is likely to be effective may be different. It is also generally assumed that binge-eating coupled with vomiting is a more severe and recalcitrant disorder than binge-eating alone.

Because occasional episodes of binge-eating and vomiting are also observed in approximately 30 percent of anorexia nervosa patients (Gandour 1984) and because fear of weight gain is evident in both disorders, some very important distinctions between bulimia nervosa and anorexia are sometimes overlooked. For example: (1) bulimia nervosa refers to normal-weight individuals who generally do eat, whereas anorexia nervosa refers to emaciated individuals who are primarily engaged in self-starvation; (2) bulimia nervosa patients are usually trying to achieve some stereotyped and idealized conception of a perfect feminine and sexually attractive appearance—in fact, they have an exaggerated need to please and obtain approval from others in these areas, and in contrast, anorexic patients seem to be trying to prevent themselves from looking sexually attractive, and they are supposedly trying to reject or deny their adult sexuality; (3) bulimia nervosa patients tend to be older than anorexia nervosa patients (low twenties vs. low teens); (4) bulimia nervosa is a secretive disorder, whereas the signs of self-starvation in the anorexic are quite obvious and the center of attention by others; (5) bulimia nervosa patients are less likely than anorexia nervosa patients to minimize or deny their problem; and (6) bulimia nervosa patients feel their eating is out of control, whereas anorexic patients feel in perfect control.

Bulimia nervosa is a disorder primarily seem in females (easily over 90 percent), and although the exact incidence in the general population is still somewhat uncertain, recent surveys conducted in the United States (Clement and Hawkins 1980; Crowther, Chernyk, Hahn, Hedeen, and Zaynor 1983; Halmi, Falk, and Schwartz 1981; Stangler and Prinz 1980) and in England (Cooper and Fairburn 1983) suggest that approximately 3 percent of eighteen- to thirty-five-year-old adult women in these countries suffer from this disorder. These are individuals who binge-eat and vomit at least once a week. Most patients who appear in clinics do so much more often; several times a day every day of the week is not at all uncommon, and we have seen frequencies as high as ten times daily. Bulimia nervosa also appears to be a very chronic disorder as several reports indicate that an average of around five years elapses between its onset and the time therapy is sought (Johnson, Stuckey, Lewis, and Schwartz 1983). Although not life threatening like anorexia nervosa, it is still a disorder with serious psychological, social, and perhaps even physical consequences. In part because it elicits a great deal of self-disgust and fear of discovery and in part because it is such an all-consuming preoccupation, it often interferes with work and the establishment and maintenance of supportive interpersonal relationships (Clement and Hawkins 1980; Garner, Olmsted, and Polivy 1983; Spencer and Fremouw 1980). Depression is often associated with this disorder (Clement and Hawkins 1980; Garner et al. 1983; Hudson, Laffer, and

334

Pope 1982; Spencer and Fremouw 1980), and other substance-abuse problems are more common than in the general population (Mitchell and Pyle 1982). Theft of food from stores has also been reported in a number of bulimia nervosa patients. The short- and long-term medical consequences for normal-weight bulimia nervosa patients is still unknown. Some studies have reported abnormal electrolyte balance (Mitchell and Pyle 1982; Russell 1979), while others have not (Pyle, Mitchell, and Eckert 1981). Parotid gland swelling and dental problems resulting from acidic gastric secretions associated with vomiting have also been mentioned (Andrews 1982; Carni 1981; Russell 1979; Walsh, Craft, and Katz 1981).

As with most serious behavior disorders, there are many interlocking and converging pathways that undoubtedly contribute to the development and maintenance of bulimia nervosa. Figure 1 provides a framework for examining the complexity of these interacting influences. At the broadest level of analysis (see the lower right-hand corner) societal values are clearly implicated. In our current youth-fixated and relatively affluent times, there is tremendous pressure on women to be slim. Obviously this alone cannot account for bulimia nervosa, or otherwise all women, not just 3 percent, would be afflicted. However, if a woman for

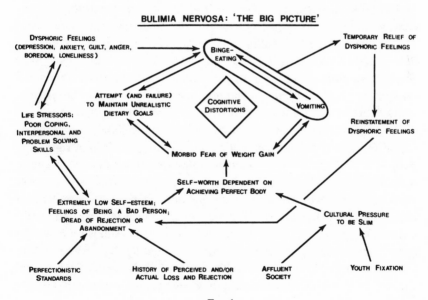

FIG. 1

whatever reason (see lower left-hand corner of fig. 1) also has extremely low self-esteem and strong fears of rejection, it is not difficult to see how she could develop the view that only a perfectly slim body will insure acceptance. She can easily believe that if her appearance is just right, no one will know how bad a person she really is. Hence self-worth becomes dependent on achieving a perfect body, with a resulting morbid fear of weight gain.

By itself, however, dread of weight gain cannot fully account for the vicious cycle of repetitive binge-eating and vomiting. In fact, one of the most obvious questions asked is: If bulimia nervosa patients are so terrified about weight gain, why would they ever binge-eat? The answer to this question brings us closer to the center of the web of figure 1 and probably represents the point where cognitive-behavior therapy has made its greatest contribution to the understanding and treatment of bulimia nervosa.

Until recently, conventional wisdom accounted for binge-eating in two different ways. These are both indicated in the left-hand portion of figure 1. The first factor pertains to the chain of low self-esteem, life stressors, poor coping skills, and the resulting host of dysphoric feelings that are evoked. One hypothesis is that many women who binge-eat do so in order to escape or "space out" or anesthetize, or self-nurture themselves against these negative feeling states. The second hypothesis that is often considered has to do with the unrealistically rigid and drastic diets these women attempt to adhere to in order to regulate their weight. When this fails, the patient gives up and binge-eats (Wardle and Beinart 1981). Such a pattern of binge-eating after dieting is analogous to the counterregulatory eating of chronic dieters who are temporarily forced to break their restraint in the laboratory (Herman and Polivy 1980).

According to both of these conceptions, binge-eating is triggered by either antecedent event, dysphoric feelings or lapses from a rigid diet. Although we agree that these factors are important, insufficient attention is being given to the central role of vomiting in this disorder. It is our hypothesis that women suffering from bulimia nervosa would never binge-eat unless they plan to vomit afterward. Once self-induced vomiting is learned, this becomes the driving force that sustains binge-eating rather than vice versa. Anticipation of vomiting, according to this hypothesis, frees bulimia nervosa patients from the normal inhibitions against binge-eating. If this hypothesis is correct, treatment initially needs to include a strong focus on eliminating vomiting.

Anxiety-Reduction Model of Bulimia Nervosa

There is great variation in the eating behavior of bulimia nervosa patients that precedes or triggers the desire to vomit. Studies of binge-eating behavior, which have reported subjects' food consumption prior to vomiting, estimate binge-eating episodes to be quite large, 3,415 calories (Mitchell, Pyle, and Eckert 1981), 4,800 calories (Johnson et al. 1983), and three to twenty-seven times the recommended daily caloric intake (Abraham and Beumont 1982).

Articles in the popular press have reported case histories of individuals with fantastic binge-eating episodes, up to 50,000 calories. These reports have relied on gross dietary intake recall rather than prospective detailed eating diaries, and consequently these estimates of binge-eating behavior are subject to distortion and error on the patient's part. It certainly is true that some individuals with bulimia nervosa do consume objectively large amounts of food or binge-eat before vomiting.

However, many bulimia nervosa patients also induce vomiting after a moderate food intake that would not be considered a binge in any objective sense but that the patient perceives as "too much" food, given rigid standards for an ideal or safe intake. For example, in a study of twenty of our patients who kept detailed eating diaries for three weeks, the average caloric intake of an eating episode, which they labeled as a binge and which preceded vomiting, was 1,458 calories, versus the non-binge, nonvomited eating episodes, which were 320 calories. Although binges and nonbinges were statistically different, there was considerable overlap in the caloric content of these two eating episodes. For example, 65 percent of the vomited binge-eating episodes were within the caloric range of eating episodes which the subject did not vomit and did not consider to be a binge. Further, only 8 percent of the vomited binge-eating episodes were close to the size of binge-eating episodes that previous reports estimated to be typical of bulimia nervosa patients. Instead of vomiting after binge-eating, many bulimia nervosa patients will vomit only after eating certain specific types of food, regardless of amount. They may be capable of consuming and not vomiting a large meal on one occasion. However, if on another occasion they eat even a small amount of a "forbidden" food, they will vomit. In our caloric analysis of eating records, for example, we compared the type of foods consumed in vomited binge-eating episodes versus the others. Out of nine categories of food (alchoholic beverages, nonalcoholic beverages, sauces-dressings-condiments, grains and cereals, snacks and desserts, fruits and vegetables, meat and protein, milk and other dairy products, and combination foods, e.g., casseroles), the distinguishing factor was the presence of snacks and desserts in the eating episode such as ice cream, cookies, candy, cake, potato chips, and nuts. Further, about one-third of the binge-eating episodes, which were accompanied by vomiting, were less than 600 calories or roughly the equivalent of eating four cookies or one ice-cream cone.

The point we wish to make here is that eating behavior in bulimia nervosa is quite varied. Not all bulimia nervosa patients actually binge-eat. The common element is that eating certain foods or certain amounts of food will elicit anxiety. Vomiting after eating momentarily reduces this anxiety. If the patient plans in advance to vomit after eating, she may be able to avoid the experience of anxiety completely. It could be argued that vomiting in bulimia nervosa serves an anxiety-reducing function similar to the anxiety-reducing rituals performed by individuals with obsessive-compulsive disorders such as compulsive hand washing and checking rituals. The bulimia nervosa patient is able to reduce anxiety about weight gain and to reduce other psychologically distressing experiences such as feeling full, feeling guilty, or feeling selfish by performing the vomiting ritual.

Three studies provide empirical support for the idea that the vomiting component of the eating-purge cycle is anxiety reducing. Johnson and Larson (1982) had bulimia nervosa patients rate their mood and eating-purging behavior every two hours throughout the day for one week. They found that vomiting relieved negative feelings of anger, inadequacy, and lack of control. Leitenberg, Gross, Peterson, and Rosen (1984) had bulimia nervosa patients eat a series of meals, which they ordinarily would vomit, such as five-course dinner, dinner serving of spaghetti, and candy bars. In therapy sessions, the patients were asked to push themselves to eat an amount of food that would elicit a strong urge to vomit, agreeing in advance that they would remain with the therapist and refrain from vomiting. In these instances, when the chain was broken and vomiting was blocked, eating was associated with a dramatic increase in anxiety.

In another study of the anxiety-reduction model of bulimia nervosa, we had bulimia nervosa subjects undergo a series of three standardized test meals (Rosen, Leitenberg, Fondacaro, Gross, and Willmuth 1985). Instead of pushing themselves to eat to the point they felt they had to vomit, as in the aforementioned study, these subjects were instructed to eat only as much food as they could comfortably "keep down" and to agree in advance that they would not vomit afterward. We were interested in how much food these subjects could consume when they had no plan to vomit afterward. The anxiety-reduction model would predict that bulimia nervosa patients would be unable to eat normal amounts of food when vomiting is prevented. To have some idea of what a normal amount of food is in these test situations, we compared the bulimia nervosa subjects with a matched sample of normal control subjects. The same three meals, five-course dinner, dinner serving of spaghetti, and three candy bars, were arranged on three separate days. The results were that the bulimia nervosa subjects ate a very small amount of food, 27, 15, and 12 percent respectively, while the normal controls consumed about 70 percent of the food in each of the three test meals. In addition, we compared the diaries of eating and vomiting behavior at home in bulimia nervosa patients who consumed an extremely small amount of food in the test meals with patients who consumed a relatively high amount of food. The "low eaters" had a much higher frequency of vomiting, sixteen vomiting episodes per week versus six for the "high eaters," and a much higher frequency of binge-eating, thirteen binge-eating episodes per week versus five for the "high eaters." In addition, the "low eaters" on average consumed about 2,800 calories per day that they vomited and the "high eaters" consumed about 450 calories per day that were vomited.

The results of these two studies indicate that women with bulimia nervosa will restrict their intake and not binge-eat or even eat "normal" amounts of certain high caloric or "frightening" foods when they do not plan to vomit afterward. This contrasts with their typical complaint of eating "too much" or binge-eating these foods when they do plan to vomit. Further, women with bulimia nervosa who eat very little or nothing in test meals when vomiting is prevented tended to consume much more at home when they are not constrained from vomiting. Bulimia nervosa patients who are not so restrictive in the absence of vomiting are less likely to overeat at home and do not vomit as often. These findings are consistent with the hypothesis that vomiting in bulimia nervosa is an anxiety-reducing behavior and that binge-eating is maintained by vomiting and not vice versa. The problem in bulimia nervosa is not that patients eat too much food. The problem is that they eat too little, that they do not let themselves eat enough of these foods when they do not vomit. Bulimia nervosa patients rarely, if ever, binge-eat unless they are planning to vomit afterward. If circumstances are such that they will not be able to vomit, they will not binge.

In contrast to bulimia nervosa, the classic obsessive-compulsive hand washers try to avoid initial contact with contaminating substances even though they know they can wash afterward. Why the difference? One possible explanation is that hand washing never completely resolves the dread of contamination, whereas the bulimia nervosa patient somehow seems to be more secure in the magical protection of vomiting. The faith that bulimia nervosa patients have in vomiting is evident by the misconceptions that they commonly hold. For example, they believe they completely rid themselves of their intake by vomiting even when vomiting is delayed for an hour or more after a binge begins. Also, they often believe that even if they ate normally, they still would gain a large amount of weight if they did not vomit. Another difference in avoidance behavior between the obsessive-compulsive and the bulimic is that there is no way for the bulimia nervosa patient to avoid the contaminant, food, unless she starves herself and becomes anorexic. Further, in the classic obsessive-compulsive there are no positive consequences of coming into contact with "dirt," "germs." In fact, there may be secondary gains associated with such avoidance; for example, control over spouse, rationalization for why they cannot deal effectively with the competitive pressures outside of the home. In contrast, binge-eating in bulimia nervosa does satisfy various psychological, gustatory, and physical needs. The fact that the bulimia nervosa patient will binge only if she can vomit afterward does not negate the pleasurable aspects of binge-eating or the contributions of other factors to binge-eating, for example, self-nurturance, boredom and loneliness, feelings of deprivation, depression, anxiety, guilt, and so on. These factors are probably as applicable, if not more so, to people suffering from bulimia nervosa as they are to people in the general population who occasionally binge but who do not vomit. However, in women suffering from bulimia nervosa, such distressing feelings are likely to be temporarily relieved only when binge-eating is coupled with vomiting afterward. These pleasurable aspects of binge-eating can be realized only if they are freed of anxiety by the anticipation of vomiting.

Once it has been established as an escape response, vomiting becomes the driving force that sustains binge-eating, not vice versa. In fact, in the typical progression of bulimia nervosa, once self-induced vomiting is learned, binge-eating usually becomes more severe and frequent (Abraham and Beumont 1982). Vomiting is so effective in relieving guilt and the fear of weight gain that it becomes increasingly unnecessary for the bulimia nervosa patient to resist her urges to binge-eat. Based on their sequential analysis of binge-eating, vomiting, and stress reduction, Johnson and Larson (1982) similarly suggested that vomiting rather than binge-eating may be the "primary mechanism for tension regulation" in bulimia nervosa and that vomiting comes to maintain binge-eating rather than the reverse.

In summary, according to this analysis binge-eating and self-induced vomiting in bulimia nervosa seem linked in a vicious cycle by anxiety. Vomiting is an escape response that is reinforced by the subsequent reduction in anxiety about weight and is analogous to anxiety-reducing compulsive behavior in obsessive-compulsive disorders. Binge-eating will usually occur only in anticipation of vomiting. Binge-eating becomes more severe as vomiting increases in frequency. In other words, binge-eating in bulmia nervosa is more a consequence of vomiting than vomiting is a consequence of binge-eating.

Exposure plus Response Prevention Treatment of Bulimia Nervosa

According to the anxiety-reduction model and in line with recent developments in behavioral treatment of obsessive-compulsive disorders (Foa and Steketee 1979) we have proposed an exposure plus response prevention model of treatment for bulimia nervosa. There are two basic ingredients of this treatment paradigm: (a) exposure to the feared stimulus in the presence of a therapist, that is, eating particular foods or amounts of foods; and (b) prevention of the habitual escape response, that is, vomiting. This approach is designed to gain control over the disorder by attacking the problem from the vomiting side rather than from the binge-eating side of the binge-eating-purging cycle. With repeated exposure to anxiety-provoking eating situations and without the opportunity to vomit, the patient will be forced to face her eating-related anxiety. The fears and other distressing feelings, which are elicited by this procedure, will eventually diminish or will be extinguished as the patient discovers either that the dreaded consequences do not materialize or that it is possible to control these feelings without recourse to vomiting.

This exposure plus response prevention treatment differs from other behavioral approaches to bulimia nervosa that seek to break up the binge-eating-vomiting cycle by gaining control of binge-eating. One alternative behavioral approach would be to help the patient avoid overeating by teaching her more effective interpersonal problem-solving strategies or stress management techniques that could reduce dysphoric feelings that are antecedent to binge-eating (Fairburn 1981; Kirkley, Schneider, Agras, and Bachman 1985; Mizes and Fleece 1984). Another behavioral approach would be to help the patient limit the amount of food she eats and avoid the pitfalls of an excessively restrictive diet. Scheduled mealtimes, reduction of food cues in the environment, scheduled alternative activities to coincide with high-risk times for binge-eating, and balanced diets are methods which have been used to prevent binge-eating episodes (Fairburn 1981; Grinc 1982; Johnson, Schlundt, Kelley, and Ruggiero 1984; Kirkley et al. 1985; Linden 1980; Mizes and Lohr 1983). In contrast to these behavior approaches, it is our hypothesis that vomiting, more than binge-eating, plays an important role in maintaining the behavior problems of bulimia nervosa and that, by being treated from the beginning with an emphasis on eliminating vomiting, the patient's binge-eating and restrictive dieting will give way in turn.

TREATMENT FORMAT AND RATIONALE FOR THE PATIENT

In the beginning phase of treatment, the sessions are scheduled on a frequent basis, for example, three sessions per week. Massed therapy sessions give the patient practice eating frightening foods without vomiting several times within a short period. This speeds the patient's learning about the effects of this change on her weight and eating behavior. Furthermore, in exposure plus response prevention treatment of obsessive-compulsive disorders, massed sessions have been shown to be more effective than less frequent sessions (Foa and Steketee 1979). The frequency of sessions should eventually be reduced in relation to the patient's improvement. In our previous studies the treatment schedule was standardized for research purposes. The patients participated in three sessions per week for six weeks before weekly sessions were scheduled. If we had been able to individualize this schedule, some people would undoubtedly benefit from a more gradual shift from multiple sessions a week to weekly sessions, to biweekly sessions, and so on. The therapy may be provided on either an individual or a group basis. In the treatment studies summarized below, the procedure was carried out on an individual basis. However, we have subsequently treated most of our research patients in a group format. At first glance there do not appear to be any significant disadvantages with this approach, and patients seem to benefit from the mutual feedback and support. However, we have not yet made a direct comparison of the group versus individual format to determine if one is more or less effective than the other.

The treatment rationale given to the patient during the initial sessions covers the following main points: she is told that binge-eating is being maintained by vomiting; that if she learns to gain control over vomiting, binge-eating will not be as likely to occur; that therapy sessions are designed to allow her to get in touch with the anxiety she experiences when eating; and that she will learn to overcome her anxiety without vomiting. This conceptualization often goes against most patients' theories of their disorder. Typically, patients argue that they would not vomit if only they did not binge-eat, that once they start eating, they cannot stop, and that therapy should help them to control their eating—not their vomiting. In essence, our response has been to tell the patient that our experience has been otherwise, that if she is not able to first learn to control her vomiting, she probably cannot learn to control her eating. We reiterate that if she did not plan to vomit, she would probably eat too little, not too much, but that we understand that this is hard for her to believe. Although it might take some time before the patient believes the treatment rationale, the education process should begin in the first session.

EXPOSURE PLUS RESPONSE PREVENTION PROCEDURE

During each treatment session, the patient is encouraged to eat an amount of food that causes a strong urge to vomit beyond the point where vomiting would ordinarily occur. The patient knows in advance that she will not be allowed to vomit and that the therapist will stay with her until the urge to vomit is under control. The patient is told that treatment would be most beneficial if vomiting did not occur within two and one-half hours after the end of any treatment session, so as to allow enough time for the anxiety to be reduced without recourse to vomiting, and that it is best to stay with the therapist until she feels she can safely leave without vomiting afterward. At the beginning of therapy, a two-hour session is usually needed for the patient to eat and gain control over the anxiety. Later sessions can be much shorter. The types of foods to be used in the therapy session are those which are found to be most anxiety provoking during the pretreatment evaluation. It is best to give the patient as much variety in food as possible, as long as the patient's choice will enable her to face some fear of eating. For example, under the category of snack food, a patient might need to alternate practicing with ice cream, brownies, granola, and tortilla chips if she usually vomits after eating each one. The amount of food to be brought in by the patient or presented to the patient in the therapy session should always be a "normal" amount or only slightly above the range most people could eat comfortably. It is not necessary for the patient to binge-eat in the session in order to become anxious. In the absence of vomiting, even small quantities of food are typically defined by patients as "too much" and provoke intense anxiety. You will recall that baseline consumption in test meals is very low (Rosen et al. 1985). Initially, the patient only needs to eat slightly more than she consumed in a baseline test of eating when vomiting is prevented. As therapy progresses, the patient should be encouraged to eat even more. However, it is also best to avoid extremely large amounts of food so that the patient does not use it as a standard for later consumption. Three pieces of pizza, a submarine sandwich, or three cups of macaroni and cheese will provide the patient with a sufficient range in amount with which to practice without being excessive. The order in which different foods are used depends on how much anxiety they provoke. The more frightening eating situations should be introduced after the patient has adapted to less frightening ones. One final guideline in regard to eating is that it may be better for the therapist not to eat with the patient during the session. To do otherwise could distract the patient from being aware of her feelings about eating and could influence the amount she eats.

COGNITIVE INTERVENTION

While the patient is eating and after she has finished, the therapist directs the patient's attention to the thoughts and sensations underlying the anxiety that is provoked by the exposure plus response prevention procedure. Typically the patient will verbalize various distorted cognitions or erroneous beliefs about food, eating, vomiting, weight, body image, and interpersonal relationships that sustain her anxiety after eating and her urge to vomit and will provoke further desires to binge-eat. These ideas are to be elicited by the therapist so they may be challenged during the therapy session. As therapy progresses and the patient has had repeated practice eating without vomiting, the therapist tries to help the patient make several important discoveries and reconceptualizations of her problem. Other investigators have also proposed that the vicious cycle of binge-eating and vomiting is sustained by irrational beliefs and that the patient will need to correct these beliefs in order to maintain control over her eating and vomiting behavior (Fairburn 1981; Grinc 1982; Loro 1984).

We believe there are some important differences in conducting cognitive modification in isolation, as is typically done, versus addressing these beliefs in the context of an in vivo exposure situation. First, the therapist may get a more accurate picture of the patient's erroneous beliefs while the patient is actually consuming the feared foods and is guided by the therapist to "get in touch" with these thoughts than is possible from a patient's recollection of maladaptive beliefs from eating experiences during the week prior to the session. Second, the exposure situation tends to be more affectively charged than merely talking about recent experiences. Under this circumstance, the thoughts that emerge may be more salient for the patient. Finally, challenges of these beliefs by the therapist may be facilitated by the patient having the opportunity to discover whether the erroneous predictions about herself when she eats and does not vomit come true. Although we believe a cognitive intervention is particularly effective during the exposure treatment, no direct comparison of a cognitive approach and exposure plus response prevention with or without a cognitive intervention has yet been conducted.

The specific concerns which are provoked during the exposure procedure will vary from session to session. The topics for discussion and intervention, however, typically consist of several recurring themes:

1. *Food and nutrition.*—The patient may believe that certain foods such as pasta or foods in general that are high in carbohydrates have no "nutritional" value and may even be harmful; that such foods lead to immediate and large weight gains and make one fat whereas other foods do not, even if the calories are the same; that certain foods are excessively high in calories, for example, a doughnut contains 800 calories; that when she eats these foods she is a bad, selfish, or gluttonous person and will appear so to other people.

2. *Weight.*—The patient may believe that minor fluctuations in intake of even 100 calories more than she thinks she should consume will immediately affect weight and that it is, therefore, necessary to stick to a rigid diet plan to maintain weight at a certain level; that if she ate

normally and did not vomit, she would gain an enormous amount of weight; that slight increases in weight are always due to eating "too much" as opposed to other factors, such as decreased exercise or fluid retention during the menstrual cycle. Many of these erroneous beliefs about food, nutrition, and weight may give way to proper nutritional information. The patient may discover that the anxiety she experiences after eating frightening foods is not as overwhelming as she first thought it would be and is capable of diminishing to tolerable levels even if she does not vomit.

3. *Physical appearance.*—The patient may believe that her weight is too high, even if she is in the thin normal range; that certain body parts (particularly stomach, thighs, and buttocks) are too large or bulge immediately after eating normal or even less than normal amounts of food; that slight weight fluctuations are noticeable; that by losing weight it will be possible to alter other physical characteristics, such as a large frame. In order to develop realistic perceptions of her weight and body size, the patient should be encouraged to accept feedback about her appearance, especially feedback from other women if she is being treated in a group setting, to reinterpret unpleasant physical sensations of weight gain or bloatedness to anxiety or even normal feelings of fullness after a meal, and to realize that such sensations will dissipate after digestion even if she does not vomit.

4. *Vomiting.*—The patient may believe that she has to vomit; that it will not be possible to tolerate certain feelings unless she vomits; that vomiting is all-protective, all-effective, for example, that vomiting after even long delays will prevent food eaten beforehand from being digested. In therapy sessions after a half-hour has gone by, we continually remind patients that the food "has gone its way" and vomiting now is too late.

5. *Binge-eating.*—The patient may believe that she has no control over her eating, that, once she takes one bite of a forbidden food, she has to continue to eat an excessive amount. We help the patient realize that in the absence of planned vomiting she does not have an uncontrollable craving to consume huge amounts of food. Instead, she has an obsessive craving to be slim, to eat as little as possible, to not gain weight. The patient will need to analyze the effects of not vomiting on her eating behavior in order to see that, in her own experience, binge-eating is more a consequence of vomiting than vice versa. Response prevention, which is carried out independently at home, away from the security and structure of the therapy session, is especially helpful in demonstrating to the

patient that she does not binge-eat if she does not plan to vomit and her problem is not that she eats "too much" but that she does not allow herself to eat enough without vomiting.

6. *Dieting.*—The patient may believe that she has to avoid eating certain foods because she has no control over her consumption of these or because even small amounts of these foods constitute being "bad" and "blowing" a healthy, normal diet. The patient should be encouraged to understand that her desire to maintain a strict diet in the absence of a need to lose weight and to eliminate certain foods from her diet will create biological pressure to overeat and psychological feelings of deprivation and a greater attraction to these foods. To permanently eliminate them from her diet is unrealistic and even harmful from the standpoint of preventing binge-eating and vomiting in the future. These foods should not be avoided but deliberately programmed into her diet so she can learn to eat these foods without "having to" vomit afterward. The patient's belief that in the absence of vomiting she will always "have to diet," for example, never eat more than 1,200 calories, in order to maintain a normal weight should be challenged by nutritional information and by having her sustain a "normal" caloric intake long enough to study the effect on her weight. Further, she should be encouraged to exercise rather than to restrain or vomit. In our previous studies, some patients who overcame bulimia nervosa did indeed gain several pounds but stayed within the normal range for weight. Others did not show any change in weight.

7. *Pressure to be thin.*—The patient may believe that she must stay thin or become even thinner if she is to be accepted in society, particularly by men. She should be helped to understand that the obsessive desire to achieve a "perfect" slim body usually stems from a complex mix of disturbed family relationships, low self-esteem and associated fears of rejection and abandonment, a variety of guilt feelings, and cultural values and stereotyped beliefs about appropriate feminine appearance and behavior. Interventions that can help the patient control the drive for thinness include: (*a*) support and encouragement to fight against the social pressure for thinness and the conception that if one is not exceedingly thin automatically means one is fat; (*b*) critical evaluation of the patient's current and ideal weights with respect to norms and her own weight history; (*c*) feedback that some physical characteristics which the patient disparages may in fact exist but that they are unalterable by weight loss, for example, "yes, you are big boned," "yes, your hips are

proportionately larger than your chest," "yes, your stomach has a round contour"; (d) encouragement to stop avoiding other situations, besides eating, that provoke anxiety about appearance such as wearing shorts, looking in the mirror, allowing a sexual mate to look at or touch certain body areas, and to face these situations without vomiting beforehand; (e) promotion of a longer-range view of factors affecting weight gain, that is, her appearance will not change overnight and her appearance does not change as a function of minor fluctuations of weight; and (f) assurance that her personality and worth as a person do not hinge on whether she loses or gains five pounds.

EXPOSURE PLUS RESPONSE PREVENTION AT HOME

The patient should be given recommendations about increasing intake and decreasing vomiting at home in order to promote transfer of the gains made during the treatment session to the patient's at-home eating behavior between treatment sessions. The timing and the nature of the recommendations for changing eating patterns at home should be individualized. Generally, the recommendations should be introduced when the patient has demonstrated improvement during the treatment sessions by reporting less anxiety and a lower urge to vomit after eating and by consuming a greater amount of food. The instructions should begin with avoidance behavior. The patient should practice eating a certain food or eating at a time of the day that has been avoided up to that time in treatment. For example, a patient who eats only in the late evening and who avoids breakfast and lunch may be asked to begin eating some small amounts of breakfast food on a regular basis without vomiting. After some reduction in avoidance of eating has occurred, a set of assignments to reduce the frequency of vomiting across the weeks should be provided. For example, "this week try not to vomit on one day of the week." It is often more effective to have the patient skip one day of vomiting instead of skipping several vomiting episodes in separate days of the week. This will give the patient a more accurate idea of what her daily dietary intake might be if she stopped vomiting. At the beginning of treatment most patients evaluate their day as being all "good" or all "bad" with respect to eating and vomiting. This all-or-nothing thinking might make it easier for the patient to not vomit for the entire day than to vomit only one time less on a given day. We also often eventually encourage mid-morning and

348

mid-afternoon snacks with "safe" foods (usually fruit) and, as mentioned earlier, for those individuals not already involved in any exercise we encourage exercise as well.

ASSESSMENT AND SELECTION OF PATIENTS FOR EXPOSURE PLUS RESPONSE PREVENTION

There are two essential eating behaviors that need to be determined in selecting and planning this treatment for patients with bulimia nervosa: (a) the foods which are avoided when vomiting is not possible; (b) the type and amount of food consumption that usually result in vomiting. The patient should keep a daily food diary and record all food and liquid intake. It is informative to have patients rate their anxiety for each eating episode and their urge to vomit, perhaps on a scale of 0–100. They should also record whether or not they considered an eating episode to be a binge and whether or not they vomited. These records should be collected for at least two weeks prior to treatment as well as throughout treatment to determine the patient's current pattern of eating, food avoidance, and vomiting.

In addition to the frequency of vomiting, it is important to determine which foods the patient will vomit after eating. Typically these foods include large meals, sweets, salty snacks, and other high-carbohydrate foods such as pasta or bread (Abraham and Beumont 1982; Basow and Schneck 1983; Mitchell et al. 1981). In order to extinguish fears of eating and weight gain, the foods to be used as stimuli in the exposure procedure must include those that elicit the greatest anxiety. These can be identified by observing which foods are usually if not always eaten before the patient vomits and which foods therefore are avoided unless vomiting is planned. Further, the patient should help to arrange the foods in a hierarchical order for their anxiety-provoking properties.

If the coupling of eating and vomiting is weak (if, e.g., there are no foods that regularly provoke vomiting and the frequency of vomiting is very low), it can be concluded that neither the anxiety nor the escape response is well developed. In this instance there are minimal fears to extinguish, and an alternative to an exposure plus response prevention therapy should be used.

There are at least two other patterns that may contradict the usefulness of the exposure plus response prevention paradigm. The first is the case of a patient who is literally unable to eat anything without vomiting afterward. Such a patient has too many opportunities to engage in the escape response (vomiting) outside of the therapy sessions in relation to her opportunities to practice eating without vomiting in the therapy sessions. It may be necessary in this instance to intensify the prevention of vomiting beyond what is possible with the outpatient approach described here by using instead a more controlled environment such as an inpatient setting. Further, this patient, who may be trying to avoid digesting any food, may have features that are more akin to anorexia nervosa. Accordingly, treatment approaches that are employed with anorexia nervosa patients with bulimia episodes could be used.

The second pattern for which exposure plus response prevention therapy may not be appropriate is the case of a patient who is very inconsistent—for example, sometimes she vomits a particular food or amount of food and other times the same food or amount of food is retained. The therapist should try to determine what conditions are associated with the episodes of eating that are followed by vomiting. For example, a particular patient sometimes vomits after eating potato chips but sometimes does not. She will keep potato chips down if she had not eaten much during the previous meals of the day. If she had been "good" and restrained her eating earlier, she may not feel so anxious about weight gain from potato chips. The likelihood of vomiting is influenced in part by that day's caloric preload. Another example is vomiting after eating a food when the patient anticipates having to eat a large meal later in the day. If she were not planning to eat again, she might not vomit. The exposure plus response prevention therapy might be viable in cases of inconsistent vomiting so long as a consistent set of "rules" for the decision to vomit, such as in these examples, can be ascertained. Further, to provoke anxiety during eating in the therapy session, it must also be possible to program these conditions, for example, a specific caloric intake before or after the session, into the treatment format.

Another assessment issue is whether or not vomiting is the only method of purging that the patient is using. In particular, is the patient primarily using laxatives rather than vomiting? A special characteristic of laxative use is that the purge is not completed for several hours after eating. In contrast, the more common method of purging, vomiting, can be performed immediately after eating. Do patients who use laxatives experience anxiety while they wait for the laxatives to take effect? Alternatively, do these patients feel so secure about the effects of laxatives on weight regulation that the delay of the purge is of no consequence to them? If the patient were prevented from using a laxative after eating in an exposure plus response prevention therapy session, how long would it be before anxiety was provoked? It might be that the duration of the exposure plus response prevention session would have to be greatly increased in order for the patient to experience anxiety. The effects on anxiety of using or being prevented from using laxatives have not been studied. To date, there is no report of exposure plus response prevention treatment in a case with laxative use as the sole purging behavior.

Empirical Support for Exposure plus Response Prevention Treatment of Bulimia Nervosa

In our first study (Rosen and Leitenberg 1982), we examined the effectiveness of this exposure plus response prevention treatment protocol using a multiple baseline design in which therapy sessions were provided in sequence for different food groups (typically full-course dinner, pasta dinner, and sweet snacks). The subject was a twenty-one-year-old female of normal weight who had had bulimia nervosa since age fifteen. At the beginning of treatment she was binge-eating and vomiting three times per day. Her baseline test meals showed that when planning to not vomit afterward she could eat about one-half of a multicourse dinner and small pizza and only one cookie. As each of the three food groups was treated in turn, the amount the subject could eat without vomiting increased, and her anxiety and urge to vomit decreased for only that particular food group. In posttreatment test meals she was able to eat the entire pizza, almost all of the large dinner, and five cookies, with minimal subjective discomfort. After eighteen sessions of exposure plus response prevention, her daily frequency of vomiting declined to 1.25. Another month and a half of treatment was provided during which time she did not practice eating in the therapy sessions but was instructed in a schedule of gradually decreased vomiting. At the end of this phase, she stopped vomiting completely. Only one episode of vomiting occurred during the ten months of follow-up. Without specific instructions to do so, the subject also stopped binge-eating.

In a second study (Leitenberg et al. 1984), we found further support for the anxiety-reduction model and exposure plus response prevention treatment. The subjects were one married and four single normal-weight females between the ages of twenty-one and thirty-five. The subjects had been suffering with bulimia nervosa for, respectively, 6, 6, 10, 3, and 1 years and the mean numbers of eating-vomiting episodes per day during a three-week baseline period were, respectively, 4, 1.2, 10, 1.6, and 1. Four of the subjects underwent eighteen exposure plus response prevention sessions with a schedule of three sessions per week. At the end of the experimental phase, three of these subjects continued to meet with the therapist in order to schedule further reductions of their vomiting at home. During these postexperimental sessions, the subjects no longer ate in front of the therapist. The fifth subject underwent twelve exposure plus response prevention sessions with a schedule of two sessions per week. The results of this study showed that, in the absence of the opportunity to vomit, food intake and associated thoughts and feelings about weight gain provoked anxiety. Also, in accord with behavioral treatments of other anxiety-based disorders, repeated exposure to feared stimuli (eating without vomiting) eventually led to both decreased anxiety while eating and an increased ability to eat more normal amounts of food. The specific findings were: (*a*) within treatment sessions while subjects were eating, self-reported anxiety and the urge to vomit increased; after subjects stopped eating, self-reported anxiety and the urge to vomit eventually declined even though subjects were not permitted to vomit; (*b*) across treatment sessions, the mean anxiety provoked by eating tended to decrease as did the mean urge to vomit; (*c*) across treatment sessions, the mean amount of calories consumed in therapy sessions tended to increase; (*d*) as treatment progressed, self-statements about eating problems (self-statements were analyzed from tape recordings of responses to probes to "think aloud and say whatever comes to mind") tended to become more positive and/or less negative; (*e*) reductions in anxiety and negative self-statements across successive sessions were not prerequisites for increased eating behavior or vice versa; (*f*) in four out of five subjects, binge-eating and vomiting at home at six-month follow-up were substantially reduced or entirely eliminated (two subjects stopped vomiting; one subject vomited one time each on nine days out of seventeen; one subject vomited four times one day out of seventeen; (*g*) finally, there were other positive effects of the treatment including improvements on the Eating Attitudes Test (Garner and Garfinkel 1979), Beck Depression Inventory (Beck, Ward, Mendelson, Mock, and Erbauch 1961), Lawson Social Self-Esteem Inventory (Lawson, Marshall, and McGrath 1979), and Rosenberg Self-Esteem Scale (Rosenberg 1979) even though the focus of treatment sessions was primarily on the binge-purge cycle rather than on these more global variables.

The exposure plus response prevention procedure has been evaluated by one other group of investigators (Johnson et al. 1984). In this study, exposure plus response prevention was compared with a behavior modification approach that is commonly employed with obese individuals who do not vomit but overeat. This latter treatment was designed to gain control of binge-eating, and it included scheduled meals, reduction of food cues in the environment, a balanced diet, and aerobic exercise. Only three out of six of their subjects completed the study. The results were: (a) one subject did not improve during six weekly sessions of exposure plus response prevention but stopped vomiting after a second treatment phase of six weekly sessions of behavior modification for binge-eating; (b) the second subject nearly stopped vomiting after six sessions of exposure plus response prevention but showed no further improvement with six subsequent sessions of other behavioral methods to control overeating; (c) the third subject started with behavior modification for overeating and showed a significant reduction of vomiting; during the second phase of six sessions of exposure plus response prevention the subject initially decreased her vomiting substantially but later increased vomiting somewhat. In sum, two out of three subjects improved during the exposure plus response prevention treatment phases and two subjects improved during the eating control treatment phases. There was no apparent advantage of one treatment over another. Although this study only minimally supported the exposure plus response prevention treatment paradigm, it is possible that the effectiveness of this approach with these subjects would have been greater had the investigators provided the subjects with more frequent sessions (more than once per week) over a longer period of time, as we have suggested.

Conclusions

We have tried to briefly summarize the essence of our anxiety-reduction model of bulimia nervosa, which places heavy stress on the maintaining role of vomiting in this disorder. Based on this analysis we have developed a treatment program that involves practice in eating without vomiting while the therapist concurrently explores with the patient anxiety-provoking feelings and thoughts under this exposure plus response prevention condition. Our initial series of studies with this approach has been promising. However, we have not yet completed a large-scale controlled evaluation. Thus, we are not in a position to say

353

that this is the most effective treatment paradigm available. Much more empirical development and evaluation are needed before any treatment paradigm can be said to be demonstrably the treatment of choice for this very serious and complex disorder. It might also be worth reiterating that we have been exclusively concerned in our research with normal-weight individuals who binge-eat and vomit. Also, our population has been restricted to adult women age eighteen to forty-five, usually living autonomously and far away from their parents, thus making family therapy approaches impractical, even though family issues are still often salient concerns.

REFERENCES

Abraham, S. F., and Beumont, P. J. V. 1982. How patients describe bulimia or binge-eating. *Psychological Medicine* 12:625–635.

Andrews, F. F. 1982. Dental erosion due to anorexia nervosa with bulimia. *British Dental Journal* 152:89–90.

Basow, S. A., and Schneck, R. 1983. Eating disorders among college women. Presented at Eastern Psychological Association.

Beck, A. T.; Ward, C. H.; Mendelson, M.; Mock, J.; and Erbauch, J. 1961. An inventory for measuring depression. *Archives of General Psychiatry* 4:53–63.

Boskind-Lodahl, M. 1978. The definition and treatment of bulimarexia in college women: a pilot study. *Journal of the American College Health Association* 27:84–97.

Carni, J. D. 1981. The teeth may tell: dealing with eating disorders in the dentist's office. *Journal of the Massachusetts Dental Society* 30:80–86.

Clement, P. F., and Hawkins, R. C. 1980. Pathways to bulimia: personality correlates, prevalence, and a conceptual model. Presented at Association for the Advancement of Behavior Therapy.

Cooper, P. J., and Fairburn, C. G. 1983. Binge-eating and self-induced vomiting in the community: a preliminary study. *British Journal of Psychiatry* 142:139–144.

Crowther, J. H.; Chernyk, B.; Hahn, M.; Hedeen, C.; and Zaynor, L. 1983. The prevalence of binge-eating and bulimia in a normal college population. Presented at Midwestern Psychological Association.

Diagnostic and Statistical Manual of Mental Disorders, 3d ed. (*DSM-III*). Washington, D.C.: American Psychiatric Association.

Fairburn, C. 1981. A cognitive behavioral approach to the treatment of bulimia. *Psychological Medicine* 11:707–711.

Foa, E. B., and Steketee, G. A. 1979. Obsessive-compulsives: conceptual issues and treatment interventions. In M. Hersen, R. M. Eisler, and P. M. Miller, eds. *Progress in Behavior Modification*. Vol. 8. New York: Academic Press.

Gandour, M. J. 1984. Bulimia: clinical description, assessment, etiology, and treatment. *International Journal of Eating Disorders* 3:3–38.

Garner, D. M., and Garfinkel, P. E. 1979. The Eating Attitudes Test: an index of the symptoms of anorexia nervosa. *Psychological Medicine* 9:273–279.

Garner, D. M.; Olmsted, M. P.; and Polivy, J. 1983. Development and validation of a multidimensional eating disorder inventory for anorexia nervosa and bulimia. *International Journal of Eating Disorders* 2:15–34.

Grinc, G. A. 1982. A cognitive-behavioral model for the treatment of chronic vomiting. *Journal of Behavioral Medicine* 5:135–141.

Halmi, K. A.; Falk, J. R.; and Schwartz, E. 1981. Binge-eating and vomiting: a survey of a college population. *Psychological Medicine* 11:697–706.

Herman, C. P., and Polivy, J. 1980. Restrained eating. In A. S. Stunkard, ed. *Obesity*. Philadelphia: Saunders.

Hudson, J. I.; Laffer, P. S.; and Pope, H. G. 1982. Bulimia related to affective disorder by history and response to the dexamethasone suppression test. *American Journal of Psychiatry* 139:685–687.

Johnson, C. L., and Larson, R. 1982. Bulimia: an analysis of moods and behavior. *Psychosomatic Medicine* 44:341–351.

Johnson, C. L.; Stuckey, M. K.; Lewis, L. D.; and Schwartz, D. M. 1983. Bulimia: a descriptive survey of 316 cases. *International Journal of Eating Disorders* 2:3–16.

Johnson, W. G.; Schlundt, D. G.; Kelley, M. L.; and Ruggiero, L. 1984. Exposure with response prevention and energy regulation in the treatment of bulimia. *International Journal of Eating Disorders* 3:37–46.

Kirkley, B. G.; Schneider, J. A.; Agras, W. S.; and Bachman, J. A. 1985. A comparison of two group treatments for bulimia. *Journal of Consulting and Clinical Psychology* 53:43–48.

Lang, P. J., and Lazovik, A. D. 1963. Experimental desensitization of a phobia. *Journal of Abnormal and Social Psychology* 69:519–525.

Lawson, J. S.; Marshall, W. L.; and McGrath, P. 1979. The Social Self-Esteem Inventory. *Educational and Psychological Measurement* 39:803–811.

Leitenberg, H.; Gross, J.; Peterson, J.; and Rosen, J. C. 1984. Analysis of an anxiety model and the process of change during exposure plus response prevention treatment of bulimia nervosa. *Behavior Therapy* 15:3–20.

Linden, W. 1980. Multi-component behavior therapy in a case of compulsive binge-eating followed by vomiting. *Journal of Behavior Therapy and Experimental Psychiatry* 11:297–300.

Loro, A. D. 1984. Binge-eating: a cognitive-behavioral treatment approach. In R. C. Hawkins, W. J. Fremouw, and P. F. Clements, eds. *The Binge-Purge Syndrome: Diagnosis, Treatment, and Research*. New York: Springer.

Mitchell, J. E., and Pyle, R. L. 1982. The bulimic syndrome in normal weight individuals: a review. *International Journal of Eating Disorders* 1:60–73.

Mitchell, J. E.; Pyle, R. L.; and Eckert, E. D. 1981. Frequency and duration of binge-eating episodes in patients with bulimia. *American Journal of Psychiatry* 136:835–836.

Mizes, J. S., and Fleece, E. L. 1984. On the use of progressive relaxation in the treatment of bulimia: a replication and extension. Presented at the Society of Behavioral Medicine.

Mizes, J. S., and Lohr, J. M. 1983. The treatment of bulimia (binge-eating and self-induced vomiting): a quasi-experimental investigation of the effects of stimulus narrowing, self-reinforcement, and self-control relaxation. *International Journal of Eating Disorders* 2:59–65.

Polivy, J.; Herman, C. P.; Olmsted, M. P.; and Jazwinski, C. 1984. Restraint and binge-eating. In R. C. Hawkins, W. J. Fremouw, and P. F. Clement, eds. *The Binge-Purge Syndrome: Diagnosis, Treatment and Research*. New York: Springer.

Pyle, R. L.; Mitchell, J. E.; and Eckert, E. D. 1981. Bulimia: a report of 34 cases. *Journal of Clinical Psychiatry* 42:60–64.

Rachman, S.; Hodgson, R.; and Marks, I. M. 1970. Treatment of chronic obsessive-compulsive neurosis. *Behavior Research and Therapy* 8:385–392.

Rosen, J. C., and Leitenberg, H. 1982. Bulimia nervosa: treatment with exposure and response prevention. *Behavior Therapy* 13:117–124.

Rosen, J. C.; Leitenberg, H.; Fondacaro, K. M.; Gross, J.; and Willmuth, M. In press. Standardized test meals in assessment of eating behavior in bulimia nervosa: consumption of feared foods when vomiting is prevented. *International Journal of Eating Disorders*.

Rosen, J. C.; Leitenberg, H.; Gross, J.; and Willmuth, M. In press. Standardized test meals in the assessment of bulimia nervosa. *Advances in Behaviour Research and Therapy*.

Rosenberg, M. 1979. *Conceiving the Self*. New York: Basic.

Russell, G. F. M. 1979. Bulimia nervosa: an ominous variant of anorexia nervosa. *Psychological Medicine* 9:429–448.

Spencer, J., and Fremouw, W. 1980. A broad band assessment of binge-eating among the nonobese. Presented at the Association for the Advancement of Behavior Therapy.

Stangler, R. S., and Printz, A. M. 1980. DSM-III: psychiatric diagnosis in a university population. *American Journal of Psychiatry* 137:937–940.

Taylor, C. B., and Agras, W. S. 1981. Assessment of phobia. In D. H. Barlow, ed. *Behavioral Assessment of Adult Disorders*. New York: Guilford.

Walsh, B. T.; Craft, C. B.; and Katz, J. L. 1981. Anorexia nervosa and salivary gland enlargement. *International Journal of Psychiatry and Medicine* 11:255–261.

Wardle, J., and Beinart, J. 1981. Binge eating: a theoretical review. *British Journal of Clinical Psychology* 20:97–109.

357

19 COGNITIVE THERAPY FOR
BULIMIA NERVOSA

DAVID M. GARNER

The use of the term bulimia to describe both a symptom and a syndrome has led to considerable confusion in the eating disorder literature. As a symptom, it simply refers to episodes of uncontrollable overeating; as a syndrome, it denotes a more distinct constellation of symptoms with significant psychological and physical morbidity. This chapter will follow the convention suggested by Russell (1979) by referring to the symptom as bulimia and to the syndrome as bulimia nervosa.

In an excellent historical review, Casper (1983) documented that bulimia appears to have been a rare symptom in anorexia nervosa throughout the past century but that since about 1940 it has become more common. She postulates that the gradual emergence of bulimia nervosa as a syndrome may be linked to the appearance of a desire for thinness as a pervasive cultural motive. In the past several years, there has been a growing recognition that bulimia is a common symptom affecting not only patients with anorexia nervosa (cf. Garfinkel and Garner 1982) but also those who present at a normal weight (Cooper and Fairburn 1983; Fairburn and Cooper 1984; Halmi, Falk, and Schwartz 1981; Pyle, Mitchell, Eckert, Halverson, Neuman, and Goff 1983) and with obesity (Edeleman 1981; Gormally, Black, Daston, and Rardin 1982; Loro and Orleans 1981). Some have argued that patients with bulimia occurring without a history of emaciation may be clearly distinguished from those with the bulimic subtype of anorexia nervosa (DSM-III 1980; Lacey 1982). Perhaps the distinction between bulimia with and without anorexia nervosa has been somewhat overstated, since both groups present with similar clinical and psychometric features (Fairburn and Cooper 1984; Garner, Garfinkel, and O'Shaughnessy 1983; Norman and Herzog 1983).

In the short time since its recognition as a clinical entity, bulimia nervosa has been conceptualized from a range of different theoretical vantage points. Explanations have been offered that emphasize early developmental events, family interactional patterns, specific personality traits, behavioral contingencies, biological determinants, and the social context of the disorder (Garner and Garfinkel 1985). Most of these formulations acknowledge the presence of distorted attitudes toward food, eating, weight, and the body. On standardized psychometric measures, bulimia nervosa patients report attitudes toward eating and body shape that are at least as aberrant as those observed in the restricting subtype of anorexia nervosa (Garner et al. 1983, 1985a; Garner and Olmsted 1984; Garner, Olmsted, Bohr, and Garfinkel 1982b; Garner, Olmsted, and Polivy 1983). Particularly salient beliefs that characterize both the bulimic and anorexic patients are a "morbid fear of fatness" (Russell 1979), dissatisfaction with body shape, and the inexorable conviction that strict control over body weight or thinness is necessary for happiness or well-being.

Fairburn (1981, 1983, 1985) has clearly articulated the details of a cognitive-behavioral treatment program for bulimia nervosa that is derived from methods used with obesity (Mahoney and Mahoney 1976). Three stages are distinguished in the treatment process (Fairburn 1983, 1985). Stage one lasts between four and six weeks and focuses on self-monitoring, a prescribed meal plan, information about sequelae, and self-control techniques. Conjoint interviews with family or friends are also advised. Stage two lasts approximately two months and involves the introduction of avoided foods, training in problem solving, and cognitive restructuring. Stage three consists of three or four meetings at two-week intervals at which earlier gains are consolidated.

Cognitive-behavioral methods have been employed in several recent case studies with bulimic patients. Grinc (1982) reported the successful treatment of a patient with a ten-year history of bulimia using self-monitoring, stimulus control, and cognitive restructuring. Long and Cordle (1982) describe successful treatment of two bulimic patients using cognitive restructuring combined with self-monitoring, behavioral self-control procedures, dietary education, and resocialization. A positive outcome was also reported by Linden (1980) in a similar multicomponent approach using cognitive methods. In an uncontrolled-outcome study of eleven bulimic patients, Fairburn (1981) reported a marked reduction of binging and vomiting following cognitive-behavioral intervention. Several other authors have advocated cognitive-behavioral interventions as part of broad-based programs combining approaches from various orientations (Boskind-White and White 1983; Johnson, Conners, and Stuckey 1983; Loro 1984; Mitchell, Hatsukami, Goff, Pyle, Eckert, and Davis 1985; Orleans and Barnett 1984; Roy-Bryne, Brenner, and Yager 1984). Loro (1984) identifies a number of cognitive distortions and dysfunctional attitudes that have been observed clinically in bulimic patients.

The cognitive and behavioral interventions proposed for bulimia nervosa are consistent with our recommendations for anorexia nervosa (Garner and Bemis 1982, 1985; Garner, Garfinkel, and Bemis 1982a). However, our emphasis has diverged somewhat from that of others since not all of our anorexic patients have the complication of bulimia. Our model has tended to focus on cognitive techniques aimed at reasoning errors, dysfunctional attitudes, and faulty assumptions that are characteristic of anorexia nervosa. It has been our experience that these also apply to most patients with bulimia, whether or not they are emaciated. Nevertheless, the differences between our methods and those that are more behaviorally oriented are of some note since they account for the contrasts in approaches. Whereas most cognitive-behavioral approaches to bulimia trace their origin to programs recommended for obesity, our principles have been derived primarily from the model described by Beck and his colleagues (Beck 1976; Beck, Rush, Shaw, and Emery 1979). These different historical roots have become less important with time since there has appeared to be a convergence in the methods advocated by various cognitive-behavioral theorists treating bulimia nervosa. The aim of the current review is to provide an overview of cognitive-behavioral therapy principles that have been advocated for this disorder.

The Vicious Cycle of Bulimia Nervosa

Factors that cause and then maintain the bulimic symptom pattern do not appear to be uniform across all individuals. Although many exhibit psychological disturbances that have been identified in anorexia nervosa, some cases of bulimia nervosa appear to be relatively free of primary psychopathology (Fairburn 1982; Lacey 1982; Russell 1979). Russell (1979) originally conceptualized bulimia nervosa as a self-perpetuating cycle involving an interaction between psychological and physiological mechanisms. Because of their relevance to cognitive and behavioral treatment principles, the following adapted and abbreviated versions of the principal aspects of Russell's (1979) model will be reviewed: (1) Shape dissatisfaction, usually (but not necessarily) accompanied by low self-esteem and in some cases by more severe personality disturbance, leads to an organized system of beliefs aimed at strict dieting and weight loss. (2) Weight loss and a sustained suboptimal weight produce physiological responses reflected by increased hunger, food preoccupations, and bouts of overeating, all of which are designed to return the organism to a "healthy weight" (Russell 1979) or a constitutionally determined "set point" for body weight (Nisbett 1972). (3) Cognitive and/or emotional factors determine whether binge-eating will be "triggered" or prevented; for example, even the slightest transgression from rigidly prescribed dieting leads to the conclusion that one might as well give in to the urge to eat since perfect self-control has been "blown" (Fairburn 1985; Garner et al. 1982a; Mahoney and Mahoney 1976; Orleans and Barnett 1984; Polivy, Herman, Olmsted, and Jazwinski 1984), and emotional distress may interfere with the cognitive self-control processes required to sustain dieting in the presence of intense hunger. (4) The reliance on self-induced vomiting perpetuates the disorder by keeping weight at a reduced level and by diminishing anxiety associated with consuming foods perceived as "fattening" (Garner et al. 1982a; Johnson and Brief 1983; Rosen and Leitenberg 1982, 1985; Russell 1979), while occasional self-induced vomiting may be maintained by positive contingencies such as attention from family members or by pleasurable sensations (Garner et al. 1982a; Stoller 1982).

These four sets of interacting mechanisms do not constitute the only factors contributing to this heterogeneous syndrome. They do not explain why some individuals who successfully manage to suppress their weight (restricting anorexia nervosa patients being the quintessential example) fail to develop the symptom of bulimia. Moreover, for some individuals, bulimia nervosa may be linked to an affective or neurological disorder (Hudson, Pope, Jonas, and Yurgelun-Todd 1983; Rau and Green 1984; Walsh, Stewart, Wright, Harrison, Roose, and Glassman 1982). However, it is proposed that the mechanisms mentioned account for the majority of cases and form the basis of the cognitive-behavioral treatment principles recommended for its management.

The Cognitive Model

The cognitive approach to understanding bulimia nervosa emphasizes how the symptom pattern logically derives from the faulty assumptive world of the patient. The bizarre eating patterns and the resolute refusal of adequate nourishment become plausible given the bulimic patient's conviction that dieting and weight control are absolutely essential for her happiness or well-being. The surplus meaning that has become attached to weight control also may provide a window into the patient's broader conceptual system, which is characterized by low self-esteem, depressive thinking, poor impulse control, perfectionism, and interpersonal fears. One advantage of a cognitive approach to bulimia nervosa is that it is not necessarily incompatible with other models that view the origin of the disorder from a wide variety of conceptual perspectives (cf. Garner and Garfinkel 1985). Some of these formulations emphasize events that are remote in time from the expression of symptoms, while others concentrate on events more proximal to the development of the disorder. Recently, several authors have accounted for the development and maintenance of bulimia nervosa by an analysis of functional relationships between antecedent events, positive reinforcers, and negative reinforcers (cf. Hawkins, Fremouw, and Clement 1984; Slade 1982). As with anorexia nervosa, much of the speculation regarding the pathogenesis of the bulimic symptom pattern conforms to a paradigm that presumes that behavior is maintained by reducing aversive consequences (i.e., a conditioned-avoidance model). Dieting is sustained because of its presumed efficacy in avoiding fatness. Vomiting and purgative abuse serve a similar role but also allow avoidance of the negative consequences of consuming large quantities of food. It is well recognized that avoidance behavior is resistant to extinction because it insulates the individual from recognizing when the aversive contingencies are no longer operating. However, the bulimic patient's behavior is motivated not simply by a fear of fatness and all that it might imply but also by cognitive self-reinforcement. The dietary restraint is often fueled by the gratification and sense of control or mastery that it provides. The tangible success at weight loss or simply the anticipation of rewards for weight reduction become powerful determinants of the bulimic's behavior. This same form of cognitive self-reinforcement has been credited with a major role in maintaining anorexia nervosa (Garner and Bemis 1982, 1985; Garner et al. 1982a; Slade 1982). Unpleasant sensations usually associated with hunger take on new meaning for the bulimic because they connote success at the much valued goal of weight control. Gastric emptiness becomes associated with virtue and mastery, while eating or fullness indicates weakness or lack of self-discipline. Encouraging the bulimic patient to discard this powerful system of cognitive self-reinforcement is one of the major obstacles in therapy. It has become deeply ingrained and is central to self-evaluation. In many cases it may be the singular or predominant frame of reference for bolstering an abysmal self-esteem. As Slade (1982) has indicated, these feelings are particularly potent when the individual experiences extreme dissatisfaction in other areas of her life. Noting that perfectionistic tendencies have also been associated with bulimia nervosa and anorexia nervosa, Slade postulates that the combination of perfectionism and general dissatisfaction are setting conditions for both disorders. They optimize the likelihood that the potential patient will turn to self-control in general and control over her body in particular as a means of consolation. It is not difficult to understand why an adolescent who is struggling with extreme feelings of ineffectiveness might embrace the idea that a thinner shape might lead to a greater sense of adequacy. The message that thinness is an assured pathway to beauty, success, and social competence is a consistent theme transmitted through the fashion and dieting industries (cf. Garner, Garfinkel, and Olmsted 1983; Garner, Rockert, Olmsted, Johnson, and Coscina 1985b; Wooley and Wooley 1982; Wooley, Wooley, and Dyrenforth 1979).

Thus, the simultaneous operations of positive and negative contingencies may account for bulimia nervosa's recalcitrance. What is important for the purposes here is that these contingencies may be covert or cognitive events. Cognitive therapy offers a variety of powerful clinical stategies that may be applied to distorted beliefs associated with eating and body shape as well as to those associated with a range of developmental, interpersonal, and self-attributional themes.

There are a number of distinctions between cognitive therapy and other approaches recommended for bulimia nervosa. In some cases, these differences relate only to philosophical and methodological points of emphasis, but in others the contrast extends to basic procedural issues. Drawing from other writers, Garner and Bemis (1985) have delineated a number of features that characterize the practice of cognitive therapy. These include: (1) reliance on conscious and preconscious experience rather than on unconscious motivation; (2) explicit emphasis on meaning and cognitions as mediating variables accounting for maladaptive feelings or emotions; (3) use of questioning as a major therapeutic device; (4) active and directive involvement on the part of the therapist; and (5) methodological allegiance to behavioral and scientific psychology in which theory is continually shaped by empirical findings. This involves a commitment to clear specification of treatment methods and objective assessment of changes in target behaviors.

Conventional cognitive therapy must be adopted in consideration of the following specific features of bulimia nervosa: (1) idiosyncratic beliefs related to food and weight; (2) the interaction between physical and psychological aspects of the disorder; (3) the patient's desire to retain certain focal symptoms; and (4) the prominence of fundamental self-concept deficits related to self-esteem and trust of internal state.

Two-Track Approach to Treatment

Throughout the course of therapy, we recommend that the therapist consciously adhere to a two-track approach to treatment. The first track pertains to the patient's current eating behavior and physical condition. The second track involves the more complex task of modifying misconceptions reflected in self-concept deficiencies, perfectionism, poor impulse regulation, depression, and disturbed family or other interpersonal relationships. Since themes on both tracks are characterized by reasoning errors, dysfunctional beliefs, and distorted underlying assumptions, they may be addressed using cognitive-behavioral therapy principles. A disproportionate emphasis on the first track is required early in the course of therapy, since other contributing factors may not be meaningfully assessed until the bulimic symptom pattern is brought under control. It is essential for the therapist to begin with a thorough understanding of methods for normalizing eating and weight. A first step in this process involves motivating the patient to discontinue potentially dangerous or ineffective weight-control practices.

Developing Motivation for Treatment

Several authors have suggested that bulimic patients' motivation to receive treatment may be contrasted with the resistance and denial typical of anorexia nervosa (Fairburn 1983; Fairburn and Cooper 1982; Lacey 1982). However, the bulimic's motivation may quickly fade with the recognition that the goals of treatment go beyond control of the

364

distressing symptoms of binging and vomiting. Bulimic patients are often as intransigent as their restricting anorexic counterparts in relinquishing ego-syntonic symptoms, such as dieting and, in many cases, the steadfast pursuit of a suboptimal weight (Russell 1979). Some patients are so resolved in their commitment to maintaining a suboptimal body weight that they admit that they would rather continue to struggle with bulimia, vomiting, and all of their pernicious consequences than gain weight. Although they do not articulate it as such, a minority of bulimic patients essentially request to be converted to what could be characterized as the restricting subtype of anorexia nervosa (i.e., submenstrual weight and rigidly controlled eating). The patient must gradually recognize that although her dieting behavior is functional in the sense that it provides short-term pleasure or a reliable means of self-rating, it has disastrous long-term consequences. Eating a wider range of foods and inhibiting the urge to vomit elicit intense anxiety for the patient with bulimia nervosa. Since therapy requires the patient to gradually engage in these behaviors and actually feel worse on the road to recovery, motivation must be elicited repeatedly during the course of treatment. Stringent dieting, retaining a suboptimal weight, avoiding fattening foods, and vomiting must be repeatedly redefined as inconsistent with the ultimate goal of recovery. The patient must be taught to examine the long-term implications of her behavior on a daily basis. A key ingredient in the patient's willingness to exchange the positive experiences of dietary and weight control for the promise of ultimate improvement is a trusting therapeutic relationship.

The Therapeutic Relationship

Various systems of psychotherapy have acknowledged the role of the therapeutic relationship in promoting change (cf. Frank 1973; Marmor 1976), and recent elaborations of cognitive therapy are no exception (Beck et al. 1979; Guidano and Liotti 1983; Mahoney 1974). In adapting the cognitive approach to patients with bulimia nervosa and anorexia nervosa, several authors have maintained that establishing a strong therapeutic alliance is a prerequisite for effective psychotherapy (Fairburn 1985; Garner and Bemis 1982, 1985; Garner et al. 1982a; Guidano and Liotti 1983). Garner and Bemis have emphasized that, beyond its vital role in facilitating motivation, a trusting relationship is necessary in cognitive therapy because this approach places a premium on assessment of cognition, affect, and behavior through self-reported, introspective data. Moreover, the relationship provides a conduit for examining distortions and misperceptions that the patient applies to her interpersonal world.

Psychoeducational Material

Providing the patient with advice regarding the physical consequences of bulimia, the biology of weight regulation, the consequences of dieting, and the social arguments against weight suppression is often helpful in enlisting motivation for change. Didactic instruction, which may be supplemented by written material (e.g., Garner et al. 1985b), has become an integral component of a growing number of approaches to bulimia nervosa and anorexia nervosa (Fairburn 1985; Garner et al. 1985b; Johnson et al. 1983; Mitchell et al. 1985; Wooley and Wooley 1985). Since it is directly aimed at attitude change, educational material is complementary to other cognitive strategies for modifying misconceptions about dieting, weight regulation, and nutrition.

Normalization of Eating and Weight

The process of psychotherapy is seriously influenced by chaotic eating patterns, vomiting, and rigorous dieting in that the physiological consequences of these behaviors exert a profound effect on cognitive and emotional functioning. Although specific strategies for dealing with distorted attitudes about eating and weight will be described later, there are a number of practical considerations in these areas that may be outlined as follows.

MINIMUM WEIGHT

Since patients with the symptom of bulimia are or may become emaciated, it must be understood that outpatient psychotherapy may proceed only if the patient's weight does not fall below a certain level (Bruch 1982; Selvini Palazzoli 1978) and the patient is not in imminent danger due to other complications (e.g., hypokalemia, cardiac irregularities). There are no absolute rules regarding the minimum weight level since it depends on the patient's overall health. In general, the patient's weight should be monitored regularly by a physician if it drops precipitously or if it approaches 75 percent of premorbid weight.

DETERMINING AN APPROPRIATE BODY WEIGHT

The vast number of research studies that illuminate the biological consequences of under- and overfeeding (cf. Garner et al. 1985b) may be used to convey to the patient the idea that body weight appears to be homeostatically regulated around a "set point" (Nisbett 1972). Significant deviations from this weight result in physiological compensations designed to return the organism to a state of equilibrium. Although there is considerable controversy surrounding the construct of set point, there is convincing evidence that it is a useful concept with sound empirical support (Keesey 1980; Mrosovsky and Powley 1977). Studies of body-weight regulation have clinical implications when determining an appropriate target weight for treatment. Although there has been a convention of setting a target weight of 90–100 percent of expected weight based on population norms, this may have disadvantages because the aggregate statistics on which norms are based do not provide particularly accurate estimates for individual patients. It seems plausible to assume that, like other physical attributes, "healthy" body weights (Russell 1979) are distributed normally in the population. Thus, it may be argued that many people who are heavier than average—or even obese—may not be suffering from an anomalous condition but instead are naturally overweight (Wooley et al. 1979). This is consistent with growing evidence that health risks associated with moderate obesity have been exaggerated (Bradley 1982; Fitzgerald 1981; Mann 1974; Sorlie, Gordon, and Kannel 1980; Wooley and Wooley 1979). Even if obesity does confer health risk, there is little evidence that dieting is an effective solution to the problem. Patients with a personal and family history of obesity may have to settle at a higher weight than they would prefer in order to reduce the biological pressure toward binge-eating.

The weight history of bulimic patients indicates not only that they are highly prone to obesity (and probably to a higher than average set point for body weight) but also that many of them have at one time lost as much body weight as anorexia nervosa patients yet have never been emaciated. This point is graphically illustrated by weight history data for two samples of bulimic women presented in table 1. Approximately one-third of our

TABLE 1

PERCENTAGES OF BULIMIA NERVOSA SUBJECTS FROM TORONTO AND OXFORD
SAMPLES IN DIFFERENT WEIGHT GROUPS

	% of Matched Population Mean Weight						
	75	75–85	86–100	101–115	115	Mean %	(SD)
Toronto Clinical Sample (N = 186):*							
Present Weight (%)............	0	14.5	54.3	27.4	4.3	96.4	(10.75)
Highest Adult Weight (%).......	0	0	18.9	47.6	33.5	113.0	(14.22)
Lowest Adult Weight (%).......	21.5	43.5	34.0	1.0	0	81.3	(10.27)
Desired Weight (%)†.........	3.4	37.7	53.7	5.1	0	87.4	(6.56)
Oxford Mail Survey Sample‡ (N = 601):							
Present Weight (%).........	1.0	10.5	54.0	29.2	5.5	97.2	(11.2)
Highest Weight Since Menarche (%).......	0.2	9.7	44.8	45.2	.2	116.2	(15.4)
Lowest Weight Since Menarche (%)	12.4	30.6	50.3	6.4	0	86.7	(10.1)
Desired Weight (%)	11.2	52.0	36.9	0	0	88.0	(7.0)

*Consecutive referrals between 1975 and 1985 to the Toronto General Hospital and the Clarke Institute of Psychiatry meeting weight criteria for "normal-weight bulimia" (bulimia nervosa) described by Garner, Garfinkel, and O'Shaughnessy (1985).

†N = 175.

‡Adapted from Fairburn and Cooper (1982).

patients and over 45 percent of Fairburn and Cooper's (1982) mail survey sample report a highest weight greater than 115 percent of the matched-population weight. The mean lowest adult weight is about 30 percent below the mean highest adult weight for the Oxford sample, and the contrast is even greater for the Toronto sample. The presenting weight for both samples is well below the mean highest weight. These data are similar to those of other clinical samples of bulimic patients (Abraham and Beumont 1982; Fairburn and Cooper 1984; Russell 1979) and may be distinguished from the more modest weight fluctuations in women not selected for eating disorders (Fairburn and Cooper 1984; Garner, Olm-sted, Polivy, Garfinkel 1984). These results indicate a close relationship between bulimia and anorexia nervosa. They contradict the common impression that "the distinguishing feature between the two disorders . . . is the extreme weight loss characteristic of anorexia nervosa but not bulimia" (Schlesier-Stroop 1984, p. 255). Table 1 also indicates that (1) a significant proportion of bulimic patients choose a "desired weight" that is consistent with anorexia nervosa and (2) those who prefer a more statistically normal weight may be no less unrealistic if they have a biological propensity for obesity.

The goals of treatment must not be defined exclusively in terms of self-control over binging and vomiting without emphasizing the likeli-hood that abnormal craving for food will persist as long as the patient remains at a suboptimal weight (Russell 1979). Certain therapeutic pro-grams that focus on exercise, self-control, and weight control (Johnson, Schlundt, Kelley, and Ruggiero 1984) may inadvertently provide jus-tification for the majority of bulimic patients who report a "desired weight" that is consistent with a diagnosis of anorexia nervosa (Fairburn and Cooper 1982; Russell 1979). Bulimic patients who prefer a statisti-cally normal weight may be no less unrealistic if they have a long-standing history of obesity.

An essential aspect of Russell's (1979) recommendations for treatment is that the bulimic patient be encouraged to achieve her premorbid "healthy" weight level. Similarly, we have begun recommending a goal weight range of within three to five pounds (which is as close as the patient can tolerate) of a weight 10 percent below her highest weight prior to the onset of the disorder. This is consistent with the observation that most bulimic patients report that this is the weight that existed prior to the onset of their disorder (Abraham and Beumont 1982). However, it is simply a guideline and may have to be accomplished very gradually or in stages. Moreover, it may have to be modified based on the patient's capacity for change. It must be emphasized that this does not mean that all patients are destined to remain at a weight that they find unacceptable. The patient may have to simply accept the possibility that her weight may have to be higher. Many patients actually maintain or lose weight when they cease dieting and vomiting and concurrently resolve that they are no longer willing to sacrifice personal health or comfort in the struggle for a lower weight.

MONITORING WEIGHT

Patients should be advised that once they refrain from vomiting or purgative abuse, they may gain a considerable amount of weight owing to "rebound" water retention (Fairburn 1982; Garner et al. 1985b). They should be reassured that this is not body fat and that it will "normalize" naturally if they are able to avoid vomiting and purgatives. Fairburn (1983, 1985) has recommended that patients weigh themselves on one particular morning each week. With patients who are extremely sensitive about weight changes, we recommend that patients discontinue weighing themselves at home and that they be weighed on a weekly basis by their therapist. Some patients prefer to be informed of their weight so that potential distress may be addressed in therapy; others who tend to become preoccupied with minute shifts in weight prefer to be "blind" to the weighings and to be informed only if there is a consistent trend up or down over several weeks.

MEAL PLANNING

Bulimic patients are invariably confused about what constitutes appropriate eating. Establishing precise guidelines for the quality, quantity, and spacing of meals is useful in helping patients tolerate guilt experienced when they deviate from symptomatic eating patterns. The patient should be encouraged to eat three meals and a snack each day and to record on self-monitoring sheets all food intake as well as incidents of bulimia or vomiting (Fairburn 1983, 1985; Garner et al. 1985b; Long and Cordle 1982; Loro 1984; Mitchell et al. 1985; Russell 1979). Patients should be encouraged to eat "mechanically," according to a predetermined plan, thereby minimizing the urge to "choose" dietetic foods at every opportunity.

Although the details of different meal planning methods vary somewhat, they all provide structure for the gradual development of appropriate eating patterns (Lacey 1985, Long and Cordle 1982; Loro 1984; Mitchell et al. 1985; Wooley and Wooley 1985). Structured eating and monitoring of food intake via detailed records may be gradually replaced by more natural eating behavior.

INTRODUCTION OF AVOIDED FOODS

Most long-standing inpatient programs for anorexia nervosa and bulimia nervosa have emphasized the value of encouraging patients to consume previously avoided foods in reasonable quantities (e.g., Crisp 1980; Russell 1979, 1981). These principles have been incorporated in outpatient treatment by using structured meal plans and the gradual introduction of foods that the patient craves but avoids except during binge-eating episodes (cf. Garner and Garfinkel 1985; Hawkins et al. 1984; Russell 1979). Patients should be presented with the evidence that dieting or rigid avoidance of desired foods may create the cognitive or physiological conditions that increase the probability of binge-eating (cf. Garner et al. 1985b; Mahoney and Mahoney 1976; Polivy et al. 1984; Wooley and Wooley 1985). The powerful urge to overeat certain foods usually subsides once they become a regular part of the meal plan and after weight has stabilized at an appropriate level.

In summary, while dealing with eating and weight in therapy may seem like a mundane, nonpsychological task, it is vital, for reasons beyond the obvious physical implications. The therapist's concern in these areas emphasizes the interdependence between mental and physical issues. Moreover, even the most resistant patients are willing to discuss the topic of food as part of an evaluation of their condition. The understanding shown by the therapist in this area often leads the patient to trust the therapist with more sensitive topics. Modifications in eating patterns should be presented as experiments that will provide the patient with data that may be used to evaluate various assumptions that determine her behavior. Resistance and fear of deviating from symptomatic behavior provide valuable opportunities to examine dysfunctional attitudes. Normalizing eating and weight through behavioral interventions is one of the primary vehicles for eliciting dysfunctional attitudes that may then be exposed to cognitive interventions.

371

STIMULUS CONTROL

It is widely recognized that binge-eating may be triggered by certain stressful circumstances, relationship conflicts, or negative feeling states (Abraham and Beumont 1982; Edeleman 1981; Fairburn 1981, 1983, 1985; Grinc 1982; Hawkins and Clement 1984; Johnson and Larson 1982; Lacey 1982; Loro and Orleans 1981; Orleans and Barnett 1984; Stunkard 1959). Various methods have been proposed for helping patients to (1) identify cues that elicit binging and then (2) either avoid them or develop more adaptive means of coping (Fairburn 1981, 1985; Grinc 1982; Orleans and Barnett 1984). Behavioral techniques may be supplemented by cognitive stimulus-control methods, such as thought stopping, guided imagery, delay, and distraction (cf. Orleans and Barnett 1984; Wilson 1984). Although emotional or situational factors may trigger binging or vomiting, it has been our opinion that this must be understood within the context of dieting or weight suppression. It could be predicted that bulimia would be an unlikely response among stressed or emotionally disturbed individuals who have not been dieting.

Medical Consultation and Hospitalization

Bulimia nervosa is a serious eating disorder with a significant risk of mortality or morbidity. Awareness of the complications of this disorder is a prerequisite for outpatient psychotherapy (Andersen 1984; Garfinkel and Garner 1982; Mitchell, Pyle, Eckert, Hatsukami, and Lentz 1983). Patients who are at a low weight, lose weight precipitously, induce vomiting, or abuse purgatives or other medications should be monitored frequently by a physician. Hospitalization may be required for renourishment, to control binging and vomiting, to assess or treat various physical complications, or to disengage the patient from an interpersonal system that is maintaining the disorder.

Reasoning Errors

Using Beck's (1976) taxonomy of logical errors in the thinking of depressed and phobic patients, we have described faulty thinking patterns that may be clinically observed in anorexia nervosa (Garner and Bemis 1982; Garner et al. 1982a). These forms of distorted thinking are also evident in many cases of bulimia nervosa. The following is a synopsis of the more common reasoning errors. The order of presentation does not reflect their relative prominence or sequence of appearance in psychotherapy.

DICHOTOMOUS REASONING

This thinking style involves thinking in extreme, absolute, or all-or-none terms and has been identified in the attitudes held by bulimic and anorexic patients toward food, eating, and weight (Fairburn 1983, 1985; Garner and Bemis 1982; Garner et al. 1982a; Loro 1984; Orleans and Barnett 1984; Polivy et al. 1984). The patient insists on dividing foods into good (calorie-sparing) and bad (fattening) categories. A one-pound weight gain may be equated with incipient obesity. Breaking a rigid eating routine produces panic because it means a complete loss of control. In bulimia nervosa, rigid attitudes and behaviors may not be restricted to food and weight but may extend to the pursuit of sports, careers, and school. It is most evident in the area of self-evaluation. Patients may evaluate themselves harshly and in extreme terms despite the fact that they may view others more realistically. The bulimic and anorexic patients often believe that such personal attributes as self-control, independence, self-confidence, and social ability must be completely and continually maintained. This leads to idealized and unattainable notions of happiness, contentment, and success.

PERSONALIZATION AND SELF-REFERENCE

This involves the egocentric interpretations of impersonal events or the overinterpretation of events relating to the self. Bulimic and anorexic patients frequently display the conviction that strangers or casual friends would notice if they gained a pound or ate a previously forbidden food. This style of thinking extends to other interpersonal situations in which the patient is unusually sensitive to disapproval from others. Given the enmeshed and overprotective family environment of many patients (Schwartz, Barrett, and Saba 1985), it is understandable how this thinking style could develop.

SUPERSTITIOUS THINKING

This error in reasoning is reflected in the belief in cause-effect relationships of noncontingent events. It is often reflected in magical thinking that is applied in the maintenance of eating or exercise rituals. Eating a small amount of a forbidden food may precipitate taking laxatives despite the knowledge that they do not result in malabsorption. Extreme anxiety is often experienced following a minute deviation from exercise rituals, because of the belief that some vague punishment will accrue. This is often unrelated to the calorie-burning effect of exercise, since patients will display great reluctance to perform even one less of a particular calisthenic after a standard has been set.

MAGNIFICATION

Magnification involves overestimation of the significance of undesirable consequent events. For the bulimic patient, the significance of small increases in weight is reliably overinterpreted. Moreover, momentary lapses in willpower are viewed as a precedent for consistently poor self-discipline. In a manner similar to that observed in depressed patients, the bulimic may magnify poor performances and minimize accomplishments in her self-evaluation.

SELECTIVE ABSTRACTION

This error in thinking is characterized by basing a conclusion on isolated details while ignoring contradictory or more salient evidence. This style of thinking is illustrated by the belief that thinness is the sole frame of reference for inferring self-worth. It is also represented by the reciprocal belief that fatness is a clear indication of incompetence. These beliefs persist in defiance of examples to the contrary.

OVERGENERALIZATION

Overgeneralization involves extracting a rule on the basis of one event and applying it to other dissimilar situations. Overgeneralization is evident in the inferences drawn about thinness. For example, a patient may conclude that weight loss is the secret to competence because someone she knows who is competent is also thin. Similarly, she may assume that because she was unhappy at a higher weight, weight gain will produce unhappiness. Overgeneralization is also evident in self-evaluations. A patient may infer that if she fails in one area, she is an abject failure as a person. Similarly, rejection by one person is viewed as a sign of social incompetence.

UNDERLYING ASSUMPTIONS

Beck et al. (1979) have described underlying or silent assumptions that organize and determine much of the depressed person's disturbed thinking. These may be distinguished from simple faulty beliefs in that underlying assumptions may not be readily identified or verbalized by the patient. The ideas that shape is a valid frame of reference for inferring self-worth or that family members are infallible are underlying assumptions that may be expressed by some bulimic patients. These assumptions may be central to the patient's personal identity. Directly challenging them is usually not advisable, since this may be interpreted as a personal attack and may elicit despair or rage that could seriously damage the otherwise therapeutic relationship (Garner and Bemis 1982). A particular class of underlying assumptions are relevant to self-concept deficits common in anorexia nervosa and bulimia.

SELF-CONCEPT DEFICITS

A detailed presentation of the cognitive basis for self-concept deficits in bulimia is beyond the focus of the current review and has been elaborated elsewhere (Garner and Bemis 1985; Garner et al. 1982a; Guidano and Liotti 1983). In earlier reports we have distinguished two components of self-concept: *self-esteem* and *self-awareness*. Whereas self-esteem relates to attribution of one's own value or worth, self-awareness has been defined as the ability to identify and accurately respond to inner experiences.

One guideline for modifying the bulimic patient's low self-esteem involves gradually assisting her in challenging the tendency to construe her self-worth in terms of idealized standards or by comparison with others. In therapy, more emphasis is placed on self-validation through the pursuit of self-defined goals and the experience of pleasure, rather than placing exclusive reliance on external performance standards. This is an idea that may be completely foreign to some patients. They are exceptionally outcome oriented and rarely experience pleasure from the process of engaging in an activity. Many are terrified or feel guilty at the

375

prospect of hedonic experience. This is often concealed by a supercilious facade of disinterest but almost invariably reflects a genuine incapacity in this area. An essential aspect of the later stages of cognitive therapy with bulimic patients is the gradual modification of the cognitive appraisal systems and underlying assumptions related to self-esteem.

A number of authors have suggested that bulimic patients often have difficulty accurately identifying and responding to affective cues or internal sensations such as hunger and satiety (Garner et al. 1982a; Goodsitt 1985; Gormally 1984; Johnson and Larson 1982; Loro 1984; Orleans and Barnett 1984; White and Boskind-White 1984; Wooley and Wooley 1985). These deficits in self-awareness have been best delineated by Bruch (1973), who has provided valuable clinical examples of patients' sense of "not knowing how they feel" (p. 338). We have described this inner confusion as being often related to distorted beliefs or assumptions about feelings or sensations arising in the body (Garner and Bemis 1985). They may relate to physiological needs or emotional states and may represent a conflict between the inner experience and the belief about its appropriateness, acceptability, justification, or legitimacy. The general principles for facilitating the development of self-awareness are similar to those for improving self-esteem and may be broken down into interrelated steps as follows: (1) identification of emotions, sensations, and thoughts; (2) identification of distorted attitudes about these experiences; (3) gradual correction of these erroneous convictions by cognitive methods (outlined below); (4) practice in responding to previously avoided experiences; and (5) reinforcement of the patient's independent expression of previously avoided emotions, sensations, and thoughts.

The bulimic patient's misperceptions, faulty reasoning, and erroneous beliefs about her body must be identified and labeled as such without undermining her confidence that she possesses the ability to think for herself. Thus, the treatment must proceed very gradually in correcting distortions and confirming authentic expressions of inner state, according to the methods outlined elsewhere (Garner and Bemis 1985; Garner et al. 1982a; Guidano and Liotti 1983).

Basic Cognitive Techniques

This section will describe specific interventions that have been derived from Beck and other cognitive theorists but adapted to anorexia nervosa (Garner and Bemis 1982, 1985; Garner et al. 1982a). As mentioned earlier, we view these techniques as equally applicable to patients with bulimia nervosa who have never been emaciated. The order of presentation does not reflect a particular sequence of application since cognitive methods may be interwoven and applied as errors in thinking emerge in therapy.

CHALLENGING BELIEFS THROUGH BEHAVIORAL EXERCISES

The interdependence of cognitive and behavioral change is so fundamental that it is somewhat misleading to consider them separately. Particularly in the areas of food and weight, behavior change is an important vehicle for modifying both attitudes and emotions. Patients must recognize that, for the same reason that it is fruitless to expect the elevator phobic to make progress by simply talking in the therapist's office, it is unrealistic to assume that food and weight fears can be overcome without approaching these phobic objects. Interweaving specific graded behavioral exercises with cognitive methods is a fundamental part of therapy for bulimia nervosa.

ARTICULATION OF BELIEFS

The mere articulation of beliefs may lead to belief change. One patient reported that hearing herself repeatedly verbalize her negative stereotype of obesity was an important factor in belief change because it was so inconsistent with her attitudes toward other minority groups.

OPERATIONALIZING BELIEFS

The precise or explicit definition of a construct that may have idiosyncratic meaning to the patient may lead to more realistic thinking. A patient's repeated observation that she reflexively defines a wide range of favorable attributes such as achievement, fulfillment, popularity, and competence in terms of weight status may gradually lead her to question the validity of these inferences.

DECENTERING

Evaluating a particular belief from a different perspective may lead to the development of more realistic attitudes. Despite "feeling fat," patients often evaluate others of a similar weight as "too thin." This recognition, along with other convergent observations made over the course of many months, may lead to the gradual erosion of unrealistic beliefs attached to one's own weight. Through other examples of de-centering during the course of therapy, patients often are able to appreciate that the standards for performance that they expect of themselves are far more stringent and unforgiving than those that they apply to others. The use of analogies and similes may provide another means of distancing the patient from her own distorted frame of reference. For example, one patient concluded that the reason that she was not satisfied by others complimenting her weight loss was that they were responding to a facade—that it was analogous to admiring the height of a short person wearing elevator shoes.

PALLIATIVE TECHNIQUES

When reasoning ability is impaired because of intense anxiety, patients may be taught the palliative techniques of "distraction" or "parroting" to suppress or override the urge to engage in destructive behavior (Garner and Bemis 1985). Both methods involve forcefully "changing the cognitive channel" rather than challenging beliefs with more sophisticated cognitive techniques. For example, patients who are overwhelmed with the urge to vomit after eating may interrupt the process by rehearsing prearranged coping phrases such as, "I need to have the food stay down to encourage the gradual return of normal satiety feelings." Going for a walk or talking to someone on the telephone immediately after eating may provide potent enough distraction to allay the urge to vomit after eating. It is important to bear in mind that these techniques presuppose the patient's general commitment to the goals of therapy.

DECATASTROPHIZING

Originally proposed by Ellis (1962), this technique may be used to challenge anxiety resulting from the arbitrary definition of negative consequences as intolerable despite evidence to the contrary. For example, the implicit assumption that performing one less sit-up would have disastrous consequences may be explored by the question, "What would be the worst thing that could really happen?"

CHALLENGING THE "SHOULDS"

The extreme thinking indicated by dichotomous reasoning, magnification, and overgeneralization is often reflected by the moralistic use of the
words *should, must,* or *ought* (Beck 1976; Ellis 1962; Horney 1950).
Many patients' internal imperatives about food, weight, and performance
in general are framed by these words, and detailed analysis usually
reveals the errors in reasoning.

PROSPECTIVE HYPOTHESIS TESTING

This technique is particularly well suited for use with behavioral exercises, since it involves generating specific predictors that may be tested by
experiments. For example, a patient may assume that reduced exercise
will have a major impact on weight. The consequences of a moratorium
on exercise may be evaluated objectively, and it can be used to disconfirm
the fear. If a client is self-conscious about eating a dessert because she
assumes others will view her as gluttonous, she might be encouraged to
conduct an informal poll to determine people's attitudes about dessert.
However, if experiments involve obtaining feedback from others, the
patient must be prepared in advance to interpret potential negative
results in a nondestructive manner.

REATTRIBUTION TECHNIQUES

Patients with anorexia nervosa and bulimia nervosa often misperceive
amounts of food eaten, hunger versus satiety, and their body size. They
then make self-defeating decisions based on their erroneous judgments.
Rather than directly modifying these refractory misperceptions, we have
recommended assisting patients in altering their interpretations of these
experiences (Garner and Bemis 1982, 1985; Garner and Garfinkel 1981;
Garner et al. 1982a). Since misperceptions in these areas are characteristic of anorexia nervosa and bulimia nervosa patients, it is helpful to
attribute them to the disorder with the recognition that subjective experience is unreliable in these cases. This approach is opposite to the general
therapeutic goal of promoting trust in the validity and reliability of
internal experiences; however, we have found that patients are so con-

fused about body shape and eating that perceptions in these areas must be temporarily replaced by nonself-defeating rules for conduct.

CHALLENGING CULTURAL VALUES REGARDING SHAPE

In the past several decades women have been victims of a rather tragic set of standards for physical appearance that have placed them under intense pressure to diet in order to meet the social expectations for thinness. It has been postulated that these and other cultural changes selectively affecting women have been responsible for the dramatic increases in both anorexia nervosa and bulimia nervosa (cf. Garner et al. 1983). Recent popular books (e.g., Bennett and Gurin 1982; Chernin 1981) and research studies (cf. Garner et al. 1985b) may be recommended as a cognitive approach to assist patients in challenging prevailing social norms that encourage women to diet in pursuit of a progressively more unrealistic standard of physical attractiveness.

Some of the more recent patients have appeared to become more entrenched in their disorder in response to a favorable social connotation that anorexia nervosa has acquired. Anorexia nervosa has been glamorized by the media's relentless association of it with positive attributes such as upper-class affiliation, intelligence, perfectionism, self-discipline, and fitness. It has been the topic of a full range of popular novels, television dramas, and accounts of heroic battles waged against it by media personalities. As mentioned earlier, many bulimic patients are emaciated, have had anorexia nervosa in the past, or have never been emaciated but have a not altogether unfavorable view of anorexia nervosa. Bruch (1985) has suggested that many bulimic patients have a desire to "share in the prestige of anorexia." In cases for whom this connection exists, the cognitive therapy must (1) encourage the patient to reattribute anorexia nervosa to failure rather than success and (2) focus on the self-concept deficits that have led to the patient's perverse identification with the illness.

The actual process of cognitive therapy closely conforms to that outlined by Beck and his colleagues (Beck 1976; Beck et al. 1979). Although the process is not simple or linear, it may be summarized by the following steps:

1. Teach the patient to monitor her own thinking or heighten awareness of her own thinking. This involves extracting the essential or

core aspects of particular dysfunctional beliefs. Beliefs must be articulated, clarified, and operationalized in order to determine their consequences.

2. Help the patient to recognize the connection between certain dysfunctional thoughts and maladaptive behaviors and emotions.
3. Examine with the patient the evidence for the validity of particular beliefs. The implications of certain attitudes or assumptions should be followed to their logical conclusion.
4. Teach the patient to gradually substitute more realistic and appropriate interpretations based on the evidence.
5. As the ultimate goal, seek to modify underlying assumptions that are fundamental determinants of specific dysfunctional beliefs.

Course and Duration of Treatment

Fairburn's (1981, 1983) approach tends to be time limited, lasting between four and six months with a different focus in his three stages. However, Fairburn (1983) does indicate that the duration of treatment must be tailored to the individual needs of the patient, with some requiring a more lengthy course. We have been impressed by the remarkable variability in the course and duration of treatment across patients with bulimia nervosa, which has led to our reluctance to specify uniform stages for the treatment process. For some patients, treatment is quite straightforward and largely limited to "track One" issues outlined earlier. Control of binging and vomiting is achieved with behavioral methods aimed at interrupting the process of dieting. The educational aspects of treatment are effective in discouraging vomiting and purgative abuse. The cognitive component is primarily restricted to modifying unrealistic attitudes about shape, with a major emphasis on challenging cultural values that have led to dieting. For these patients, treatment may be brief and highly successful. For others, many of whom have had a long history of anorexia nervosa, multiple treatment failures, and extremely chaotic eating patterns, the disorder may be complicated by profound psychosocial disturbances. Norman and Herzog (1984) have reported on a sample of bulimic patients who demonstrate a greater level of persistent social maladjustment than normal, alcoholic, and schizophrenic women. These patients may at some point require brief hospitalization, and the course of cognitive therapy is quite variable. Track One principles may have to be persistently applied over many months or reinstituted when eating patterns periodically deteriorate. Cognitive therapy must focus not only on intransigent assumptions related to eating and shape but also on self-concept deficits, depressive thinking, poor impulse control, and pervasive interpersonal fears. Although brief therapy should be the aim, some patients require cognitive therapy of longer duration.

Conclusions

Differences in patient populations may be a major factor accounting for conflicting opinions about treatment course and duration. As Long and Cordle (1982) have observed, optimistic reports have been based largely on college samples, in which severe psychological disturbance may be less typical (Boskind-Lodahl and White 1978; Coffman 1984; Linden 1980; Mizes and Lohr 1983; Rosen and Leitenberg 1982). Some treatment programs only admit patients who agree in advance to comply with the treatment protocol (Lacey 1982), which includes abstinence from vomiting (Mitchell et al. 1985). In contrast, less auspicious reports have come from centers that have developed a reputation in the professional community for treating bulimic patients with anorexia nervosa (Crisp 1980; Lucas, Duncan, and Piens 1976; Russell 1979). With the increased media coverage over the last several years, we have noticed that a larger proportion of our patients are self-referrals rather than professional referrals of cases who have experienced previous treatment failures.

Despite these cautions, we share the opinions of others who view attitude change as a prerequisite for complete recovery for most patients with bulimia and who consider cognitive-behavioral treatment as a valuable method for achieving this end. Preliminary reports have been encouraging and must be followed by more systematic evaluation of the active components in treatment, predictors of outcome, and durability of change.

NOTE

Accepted for publication, March 1985. I am indebted to Kelly Bemis and Victoria Mitchell for their contributions to this chapter. I also would like to acknowledge the continued support of Health and Welfare Canada, the Ontario Mental Health Foundation, and the Medical Research Council of Canada.

REFERENCES

Abraham, S. F., and Beumont, P. J. V. 1982. How patients describe bulimia or binge eating. *Psychological Medicine* 12:628–635.

Andersen, A. 1984. Anorexia nervosa and bulimia: biological and socio-cultural aspects. In J. R. Galler, ed. *Nutrition and Behavior.* New York: Plenum.

Beck, A. T. 1976. *Cognitive Therapy and the Emotional Disorders.* New York: International Universities Press.

Beck, A. T.; Rush, A. J.; Shaw, B. F.; and Emery, G. 1979. *Cognitive Therapy of Depression: A Treatment Manual.* New York: Guilford.

Bennett, W. B., and Gurin, J. 1982. *The Dieter's Dilemma: Eating Less and Weighing More.* New York: Basic.

Boskind-Lodahl, M., and White, W. C. 1978. The definition and treatment of bulimarexia in college women—a pilot study. *Journal of the American College Health Association* 2:27.

Boskind-White, M., and White, W. C. 1983. *Bulimarexia: The Binge/Purge Cycle.* New York: Norton.

Bradley, P. J. 1982. Is obesity an advantageous adaptation? *International Journal of Obesity* 6:43–52.

Bruch, H. 1973. *Eating Disorders: Obesity, Anorexia Nervosa and the Person Within.* New York: Basic.

Bruch, H. 1982. Anorexia nervosa: Therapy and theory. *American Journal of Psychiatry* 139:1531–1538.

Bruch, H. 1985. Four decades of eating disorders. In D. M. Garner and P. E. Garfinkel, eds. *Handbook of Psychotherapy for Anorexia Nervosa and Bulimia.* New York: Guilford.

Casper, R. C. 1983. On the emergence of bulimia nervosa as a syndrome: a historical view. *International Journal of Eating Disorders* 2:3–16.

Chernin, K. 1981. *The Obsession: Reflections on the Tyranny of Slenderness.* New York: Harper & Row.

Coffman, D. A. 1984. A clinically derived treatment model for the binge-purge syndrome. In R. C. Hawkins, W. J. Fremouw, and P. F. Clement, eds. *The Binge-Purge Syndrome: Diagnosis, Treatment and Research.* New York: Springer.

Cooper, P. J., and Fairburn, C. G. 1983. Binge-eating and self-induced vomiting in the community: a preliminary study. *British Journal of Psychiatry* 142:139–144.

Crisp, A. H. 1980. *Anorexia Nervosa: Let Me Be.* New York: Grune & Stratton.

Diagnostic and Statistical Manual of Mental Disorders, 3d ed. (*DSM-III*). 1980. Washington, D.C.: American Psychiatric Association.

Edeleman, B. 1981. Binge-eating in normal weight and overweight individuals. *Psychological Reports* 49:739–746.

Ellis, A. 1962. *Reason and Emotion in Psychotherapy.* New York: Stuart.

Fairburn, C. G. 1981. A cognitive-behavioral approach to the management of bulimia. *Psychological Medicine* 141:631–633.

Fairburn, C. G. 1982. *Binge-Eating and Bulimia Nervosa.* London: Smith, Kline, & French.

Fairburn, C. G. 1983. The place of a cognitive-behavioral approach in the management of bulimia. In P. L. Darby, P. E. Garfinkle, D. M. Garner, and D. V. Coscina, eds. *Anorexia Nervosa: Recent Developments.* New York: Liss.

Fairburn, C. G. 1985. Cognitive-behavioral treatment for bulimia. In D. M. Garner and P. E. Garfinkel, eds. *Handbook of Psychotherapy for Anorexia Nervosa and Bulimia.* New York: Guilford.

Fairburn, C. G., and Cooper, P. J. 1982. Self-induced vomiting and bulimia nervosa: an undetected problem. *British Medical Journal* 284:1153–1155.

Fairburn, C. G., and Cooper, P. J. 1984. The clinical features of bulimia nervosa. *British Journal of Psychiatry* 144:238–246.

Fitzgerald, F. T. 1981. The problem of obesity. *Annual Review of Medicine* 32:221–231.

Frank, J. D. 1973. *Persuasion and Healing.* Baltimore: Johns Hopkins University Press.

Garfinkel, P. E., and Garner, D. M. 1982. *Anorexia Nervosa: A Multidimensional Perspective.* New York: Brunner/Mazel. 1982.

Garner, D. M., and Bemis, K. M. 1982. A cognitive-behavioral approach to anorexia nervosa. *Cognitive Therapy and Research* 6:123–150.

Garner, D. M., and Bemis, K. M. 1985. Cognitive therapy for anorexia nervosa. In D. M. Garner and P. E. Garfinkel, eds. *Handbook of Psychotherapy for Anorexia Nervosa and Bulimia.* New York: Guilford.

Garner, D. M., and Garfinkel, P. E. 1981. Body image in anorexia nervosa: measurement, theory and clinical implications. *International Journal of Psychiatry in Medicine* 11:263–284.

Garner, D. M., and Garfinkel P. E. 1985. *Handbook of Psychotherapy for Anorexia Nervosa and Bulimia.* New York: Guilford.

Garner, D. M.; Garfinkel, P. E.; and Bemis, K. M. 1982a. A multi-dimensional psychotherapy for anorexia nervosa. *International Journal of Eating Disorders* 1:3–46.

Garner, D. M.; Garfinkel, P. E.; and Olmsted, M. P. 1983. An overview of the socio-cultural factors in the development of anorexia nervosa. In P. L. Darby, P. E. Garfinkel, D. M. Garner, and D. V. Coscina, eds. *Anorexia Nervosa: Recent Developments.* New York: Liss.

Garner, D. M.; Garfinkel, P. E.; and O'Shaughnessy, M. 1983. Clinical and psychometric comparison between bulimia in anorexia nervosa and bulimia in normal-weight women. In *Understanding Anorexia Nervosa and Bulimia: Report of the Fourth Ross Conference on Medical Research.* Columbus, Ohio: Ross Laboratories.

Garner, D. M.; Garfinkel, P. E.; and O'Shaughnessy, M. In press. The validity of the distinction between bulimia with and without anorexia nervosa. *American Journal of Psychiatry.*

Garner, D. M., and Olmsted, M. P. 1984. *The Eating Disorder Inventory Manual.* Odessa, Florida: Psychological Assessment Resources.

Garner, D. M.; Olmsted, M. P.; Bohr, Y.; and Garfinkel, P. E. 1982b. The eating attitudes test: psychometric features and clinical correlates. *Psychological Medicine* 12:871–878.

Garner, D. M.; Olmsted, M. P.; and Polivy, J. 1983. Development and validation of a multidimensional eating disorder inventory for anorexia nervosa and bulimia. *International Journal of Eating Disorders* 2:15–34.

Garner, D. M.; Olmsted, M. P.; Polivy, J.; and Garfinkel, P. E. 1984. Comparison between weight-preoccupied women and anorexia nervosa. *Psychosomatic Medicine* 46:255–266.

Garner, D. M.; Rockert, W.; Olmsted, M. P.; Johnson, C. L.; and Coscina, D. V. 1985b. Psychoeducational principles in the treatment of bulimia and anorexia nervosa. In D. M. Garner and P. E. Garfinkel, eds. *Handbook of Psychotherapy for Anorexia Nervosa and Bulimia.* New York: Guilford.

Goodsitt, A. 1985. Self-psychology and the treatment of anorexia nervosa. In D. M. Garner and P. E. Garfinkel, eds. *Handbook of Psychotherapy for Anorexia Nervosa and Bulimia.* New York: Guilford.

Gormally, J. 1984. The obese binge eater: diagnosis, etiology and clinical issues. In R. C. Hawkins, W. J. Fremouw, and P. F. Clement, eds. *The Binge-Purge Syndrome: Diagnosis, Treatment and Research.* New York: Springer.

Gormally, J.; Black, S.; Daston, S.; and Rardin, D. 1982. Assessment of binge eating severity among obese persons. *Addictive Behaviors* 7:47–55.

Grinc, G. A. 1982. A cognitive-behavioral model for the treatment of chronic vomiting. *Journal of Behavioral Medicine* 5:135–141.

Guidano, V. F., and Liotti, G. 1983. *Cognitive Processes and Emotional Disorders: A Structural Approach to Psychotherapy.* New York: Guilford.

Halmi, K. A.; Falk, J. R.; and Schwartz, E. 1981. Binge-eating and vomiting: a survey of a college population. *Psychological Medicine* 11:697–706.

Hawkins, R. C., and Clement, P. F. 1984. Binge eating: measurement problems and a conceptual model. In R. C. Hawkins, W. J. Fremouw, and P. F. Clement, eds. *The Binge-Purge Syndrome: Diagnosis, Treatment and Research.* New York: Springer.

Hawkins, R. C.; Fremouw, W. J.; and Clement, P. F. 1984. *The Binge-Purge Syndrome: Diagnosis, Treatment and Research.* New York: Springer.

Horney, K. 1950. *Neurosis and Human Growth: The Struggle Towards Self-Realization.* New York: Norton.

Hudson, J. I.; Pope, H. G.; Jonas, J. M.; and Yurgelun-Todd, D. 1983. Family history study of anorexia nervosa and bulimia. *British Journal of Psychiatry* 142:133–138.

Johnson, C. L.; Conners, M.; and Stuckey, M. 1983. Short-term group treatment for bulimia. *International Journal of Eating Disorders* 2:199–208.

Johnson, C. L., and Larson, R. 1982. Bulimia: an analysis of moods and behavior. *Psychosomatic Medicine* 44:333–345.

Johnson, W. G., and Brief, D. 1983. Bulimia. *Behavioral Medicine Update* 4:16–21.

Johnson, W. G.; Schlundt, D. G.; Kelley, M. L.; and Ruggiero, L. 1984. Exposure with response prevention and energy regulation in the treatment of bulimia. *International Journal of Eating Disorders* 3:37–46.

Keesey, R. E. 1980. A set point analysis of the regulation of body weight. In A. J. Stunkard, ed. *Obesity.* Philadelphia: Saunders.

Lacey, J. H. 1982. The bulimic syndrome at normal body weight—

reflections on pathogenesis and clinical features. *International Journal of Eating Disorders* 2:59–62.

Lacey, J. H. 1985. Time limited individual and group treatment for bulimia. In D. M. Garner and P. E. Garfinkel, eds. *Handbook of Psychotherapy for Anorexia Nervosa and Bulimia*. New York: Guilford.

Linden, W. 1980. Multicomponent behavior therapy in a case of compulsive binge-eating followed by vomiting. *Journal of Behavior Therapy and Experimental Psychiatry* 11:297–300.

Long, G. C., and Cordle, C. J. 1982. Psychological treatment of binge eating and self-induced vomiting. *British Journal of Medical Psychology* 55:139–145.

Loro, A. 1984. Binge eating: a cognitive-behavioral treatment approach. In R. C. Hawkins, W. J. Fremouw, and P. F. Clement, eds. *The Binge-Purge Syndrome: Diagnosis, Treatment and Research*. New York: Springer.

Loro, A., and Orleans, C. S. 1981. Binge eating in obesity: preliminary findings and guidelines for behavioral analysis and treatment. *Addictive Behaviors* 6:155–166.

Lucas, A. R.; Duncan, J. W.; and Piens, V. 1976. The treatment of anorexia nervosa. *American Journal of Psychiatry* 133:1034–1038.

Mahoney, M. J. 1974. *Cognitive and Behavior Modification*. Cambridge: Ballinger.

Mahoney, M. J., and Mahoney, K. 1976. *Permanent Weight Control*. New York: Norton.

Mann, G. V. 1974. The influence of obesity on health. *New England Journal of Medicine* 291:178–185.

Marmor, J. 1976. Common operational factors in diverse approaches to behavior change. In A. Burton, ed. *What Makes Behavior Change Possible*. New York: Brunner/Mazel.

Mitchell, J. E.; Hatsukami, D.; Goff, G.; Pyle, R. L.; Eckert, E. D.; and Davis, J. M. 1985. Intensive outpatient group treatment for bulimia. In D. M. Garner and P. E. Garfinkel, eds. *Handbook of Psychotherapy for Anorexia Nervosa and Bulimia*. New York: Guilford.

Mitchell, J. E.; Pyle, R. L.; Eckert, E. D.; Hatsukami, D.; and Lentz, R. 1983. Electrolyte and other physiological abnormalities in patients with bulimia. *Psychological Medicine* 13:273–278.

Mizes, J. S., and Lohr, J. M. 1983. The treatment of bulimia (binge eating and self-induced vomiting): a quasi-experimental investigation of the effects of stimulus narrowing, self-reinforcement and self-control relaxation. *International Journal of Eating Disorders* 2:59–65.

Mrosovsky, N., and Powley, T. L. 1977. Set points for body weight and fat. *Behavioral Biology* 20:205–223.

Nisbett, R. E. 1972. Eating behavior and obesity in men and animals. *Advances in Psychosomatic Medicine* 7:173–193.

Norman, D. K., and Herzog, D. B. 1983. Bulimia, anorexia nervosa and anorexia nervosa with bulimia: a comparative analysis of MMPI profiles. *International Journal of Eating Disorders* 2:43–52.

Norman, D. K., and Herzog, D. B. 1984. Persistent social maladjustment in bulimia: a one-year follow-up. *American Journal of Psychiatry* 143:444–446.

Orleans, C. S., and Barnett, L. R. 1984. Bulimarexia: guidelines for behavioral assessment and treatment. In R. C. Hawkins, W. J. Fremouw, and P. F. Clement, eds. *The Binge-Purge Syndrome: Diagnosis, Treatment and Research*. New York: Springer.

Polivy, J.; Herman, C. P.; Olmsted, M. P.; and Jazwinski, C. 1984. Restraint and binge eating. In R. C. Hawkins, W. J. Fremouw, and P. F. Clement, eds. *The Binge-Purge Syndrome: Diagnosis, Treatment and Research*. New York: Springer.

Pyle, R. L.; Mitchell, J. E.; Eckert, E.; Halverson, P.; Neuman, P.; and Goff, G. 1983. The incidence of bulimia in freshman college students. *International Journal of Eating Disorders* 2:75–85.

Rau, J. H., and Green, R. S. 1984. Neurological factors affecting binge eating: body over mind. In R. C. Hawkins, W. J. Fremouw, and P. F. Clement, eds. *The Binge-Purge Syndrome: Diagnosis, Treatment and Research*. New York: Springer.

Rosen, J., and Leitenberg, H. 1982. Bulimia nervosa: treatment with exposure and response prevention. *Behavior Therapy* 13:117–124.

Rosen, J., and Leitenberg. H. 1985. Exposure plus response prevention treatment of bulimia. In D. M. Garner and P. E. Garfinkel, eds. *Handbook of Psychotherapy for Anorexia Nervosa and Bulimia*. New York: Guilford.

Roy-Bryne, P.; Brenner, K.; and Yager, J. 1984. Group treatment for bulimia: a year's experience. *International Journal of Eating Disorders* 3:97–116.

Russell, G. F. M. 1979. Bulimia nervosa: an ominous variant of anorexia nervosa? *Psychological Medicine* 9:429–448.

Russell, G. F. M. 1981. The current treatment of anorexia nervosa. *British Journal of Psychiatry* 138:164–166.

Schlesier-Stroop, B. 1984. Bulimia: a review of the literature. *Psychological Bulletin* 95:247–257.

Schwartz, R. C.; Barrett, M. J.; and Saba, G. 1985. Family therapy for bulimia. In D. M. Garner and P. E. Garfinkel, eds. *Handbook of Psychotherapy for Anorexia Nervosa and Bulimia*. New York: Guilford.

Selvini-Palazzoli, M. 1978. *Self-Starvation: From Individual to Family Therapy in the Treatment of Anorexia Nervosa*. New York: Aronson.

Slade, P. D. 1982. Towards a functional analysis of anorexia nervosa and bulimia nervosa. *British Journal of Clinical Psychology*. 21:167–179.

Sorlie, P.; Gordon, T.; and Kannel, W. B. 1980. Body build and mortality: the Framingham study. *Journal of the American Medical Association* 243:1828–1831.

Stoller, J. 1982. Erotic vomiting. *Archives of Sexual Behavior* 11:361–365.

Stunkard, A. 1959. Obesity and the denial of hunger. *Psychosomatic Medicine* 21:281–289.

Walsh, B. T.; Stewart, J. W.; Wright, L.; Harrison, W.; Roose, S. P.; and Glassman, A. H. 1982. Treatment of bulimia with monoamine oxidase inhibitors. *American Journal of Psychiatry* 139:1629–1630.

White, W. C., and Boskind-White, M. 1984. An experimental behavioral treatment program for bulimarexic women. In R. C. Hawkins, W. Fremouw, and P. F. Clement, eds. *The Binge-Purge Syndrome: Diagnosis, Treatment and Research*. New York: Springer.

Wilson, G. T. 1984. Toward the understanding and treatment of binge eating. In R. C. Hawkins, W. Fremouw, and P. F. Clement, eds. *The Binge-Purge Syndrome: Diagnosis, Treatment and Research*. New York: Springer.

Wooley, O. W., and Wooley, S. C. 1982. The Beverly Hills eating disorder: the mass marketing of anorexia nervosa. *International Journal of Eating Disorders*. Editorial. 1:57–69.

Wooley, O. W.; Wooley, S. C.; and Dyrenforth, S. R. 1979. Obesity and women. II. A neglected feminist topic. *Women's Studies International Quarterly* 2:81–92.

Wooley, S. C., and Wooley, O. W. 1979. Obesity and women. I. A closer look at the facts. *Women's Studies International Quarterly* 2:67–79.

Wooley, S. C., and Wooley, O. W. 1985. Intensive outpatient and residential treatment for bulimia. In D. M. Garner and P. E. Garfinkel, eds. *Handbook of Psychotherapy for Anorexia Nervosa and Bulimia.* New York: Guilford.

KATHARINE N. DIXON

Although anorexia nervosa has been described as a clinical entity since 1873, literature references to bulimic symptoms in anorexia nervosa are sparse prior to 1960. Casper (1983) pointed out that Binswanger's (1944) study of Ellen West was the first documentation of bulimia nervosa. In the past decade and concurrent with the identification of bulimia as a syndrome separate from anorexia nervosa, published studies on bulimia have increased considerably in the medical literature. Since Boskind-Lodahl and Sirlin's (1977) article describing "bulimarexia" in a popular psychology magazine, increased reporting of bulimia has also occurred in the popular press. In conjunction with the proliferation of media information on bulimia, mental health professionals began to receive a growing number of requests for consultation and treatment from bulimic individuals, many of whom had been ill for several years with no prior treatment for bulimia. Indeed, a large survey of bulimic women with a mean illness duration of five years and five months (Johnson, Stuckey, Lewis, and Schwartz 1982) found that 56 percent of the sample had not sought professional help in spite of severe symptomatology and distress. Recent studies (Halmi, Falk, and Schwartz 1981; Stangler and Printz 1980) showing a high incidence of bulimic symptoms in college-age populations reflect the increasing numbers of individuals referred for these problems to university-associated mental health services.

Unfortunately, the availability of psychotherapists trained and experienced in the field of eating disorders has lagged significantly behind the rising requests and needs for treatment. The popularity of group therapy for bulimia has developed in part from the need for an efficient means to provide service to a large number of patients with the few available, experienced therapists.

A group approach is accepted and advocated in the treatment of a variety of specific disorders, including alcoholism and drug abuse. Regrettably, no primarily anecdotal reports are available regarding group treatment of anorexia nervosa. Polivy (1981) reported on six out of fourteen anorexia nervosa patients who benefited from group therapy as a treatment modality adjunctive to individual psychotherapy. The dropout rate in the group was high (57 percent), and objective outcome measures were not reported. Huerta (1982) reported his group experience using a supportive approach with over 100 anorectic outpatients with the goal being to avoid hospitalization. One-half of the group were restrictors and the other half had bulimic symptoms. No outcome measures were reported with this study. The group process with sixty-three hospitalized and postdischarge anorectic adolescents was described by Piazza, Carni, Kelly, and Plante (1983). Although the author felt the group experience was valuable to the anorectics' treatment program, no information was given on patient outcome or specific value of the group approach.

Several recent studies provide supporting evidence that group therapy is an effective adjunctive treatment modality for bulimia (table 1). However, these preliminary studies vary in treatment approach, duration, outcome measures, and often suffer from small sample size, making conclusions about the specific value of the group modality or techniques utilized difficult.

Group Types and Approaches

There are a variety of group types (self-help, patient oriented, parent, multifamily) and group approaches (educational, behavioral, supportive, psychodynamic) to bulimia. Kadis, Krasner, Weiner, and Winick (1974) have categorized group psychotherapy into three levels: repressive (behavioral, guidance, educational), ego-supportive (counseling, interactional), and evocative (psychoanalytic). Bulimic groups may operate at any of these levels, but they commonly incorporate a variety of techniques directed both toward changing the bulimic's here-and-now symptomatic behavior and restructuring conscious attitudes and interpersonal relationships. This eclectic approach arose from the clinical observation that traditional psychotherapy alone diminished distress but had little overall effect on the patient's symptoms and disability. Garfinkel and

Garner (1982) have documented the rationale for a multidimensional treatment approach for anorexia nervosa.

Anorexia nervosa treatment programs that focus largely on weight restoration contribute to chronicity and a high rate of recurrences unless meaningful psychotherapy is also provided. Likewise, any treatment plan for bulimia directed primarily toward remission of behavioral symptoms can be expected to contribute to a high residual effect of impaired relationships, affective disorder, and impulse-control difficulties, including alcohol abuse and other sequelae.

Peer self-help groups for anorexia nervosa and bulimia have gained momentum over the past decade. Such groups provide social support, encouragement, and information for members and relatives with shared concerns. Although self-help groups are usually leaderless or directed by a facilitator, professional participation frequently occurs in the role of consultant, board member, group facilitator, or trainer of facilitators. Ongoing professional involvement of a facilitator, however, may interfere with the group's autonomy and initiative and change the group's focus from support to providing therapy (Rubel 1984).

There is a scarcity of information on the use of parent groups in anorexia nervosa or bulimia, although family involvement in treatment, particularly with the adolescent patient, is known to be important for the patient's progress. Rose and Garfinkel (1980) reported on experience with ten parent pairs with an anorectic child for whom family therapy was contraindicated. Support, catharsis, and education were the main objectives, and parent and therapist evaluations indicated that the parent group was helpful in accomplishing these goals.

Goals of Group Psychotherapy

Group therapy with the bulimic patient will be successful only as part of a systematic and comprehensive treatment plan. The group type of approach necessarily depends on the treatment goals for the patient group. Treatment goals with bulimic patients commonly include eliminating binge-purging behaviors, normalizing eating and weight patterns and attitudes, improving stress management, and increasing the patient's awareness of the association between bulimic attitudes and behaviors and the chronic psychodynamic issues. Themes common to bulimia groups include need for others' approval, use of food as an avoidance of affect or

TABLE 1
STUDIES OF GROUP THERAPY FOR BULIMIA

Study	No. of Subjects	Approach	Study Interval	Session Length and Frequency
1. Boskind-Lodahl and White (1978)	13	Feminist	11 weeks	2 hours weekly; one 6-hour marathon
2. White and Boskind-White (1981)	14	Behavioral-experiential	5-day intensive program	5 hours daily
3. Lacey (1983)	30	Behavioral/insight	10 weeks	1½-hour group session preceded by ½-hour individual session weekly
4. Johnson et al. (1983)	10	Psycho-educational	9 weeks	12 2-hour sessions
5. Roy-Byrne et al. (1984)	9	Behavioral/insight/support	12 months	1½ hours weekly
6. Dixon and Kiecolt-Glaser (1984)	11	Behavioral/insight	10 weeks	1½ hours weekly

394

	Immediate Outcome	Long-Term Outcome	Other Measures
1. Boskind-Lodahl and White (1978).........	4 symptom free 6 improved 2 no change	Similar to Immediate	Body Cathexis Test 16 Personality Factor Questionnaire
2. White and Boskind-White (1978).........	No information	3 symptom free 7 improved 4 unchanged	California Psychological Inventory Body Cathexis Test
3. Lacey (1983)	24 symptom free	20 symptom free 8 improved 1 unchanged	Mood Analogue Scale
4. Johnson et al. (1983)	2 symptom free 7 improved	1 symptom free 8 improved 1 unchanged	Tennessee Self-Concept Scale Berndt Depression Inventory Eating Disorders Inventory Body Cathexis Test, Gambrill-Richey Assertion Inventory
5. Roy-Byrne et al. (1984)	3 symptom free 4 improved 2 unchanged	No information	None
6. Dixon and Kiecolt-Glaser (1984)	3 symptom free 8 improved	5 symptom free 6 improved	SCL-90 Marlowe-Crowne Social Desirability Scale, Eating Attitudes Test

395

irresponsible escape from otherwise overly responsible lives, fear of success misidentified as fear of failure, use of the eating symptoms in a hostile-dependent relationship with parents or other important figures, conflictual or mistrusting relationships with men and parents, a fat identity even though one is of normal weight or underweight, concerns of control and adequacy, procrastination, perfectionistic attitudes, and difficulties with impulse control (Dixon and Kiecolt-Glaser 1984; Roy-Byrne, Lee-Brenner, and Yager 1984).

Group emphasis placed on each of these goals or themes is often determined by the extent of work completed in these areas through the patients' prior individual psychotherapy or hospitalization. We found that the advent of our Eating Disorders Program and the increased availability of individual psychotherapists led to a shift of group emphasis from a behavioral focus on bulimic behaviors to a greater ego-supportive focus on the patient's intrapsychic and interpersonal issues. Our earlier treatment groups often incorporated a significant amount of work with behavioral techniques to correct the patient's dangerous binge-purging behaviors. However, less group time is consumed with work on behavioral techniques when patients have had prior exposure to these techniques in individual psychotherapy or in milieu therapy. Additionally, patients with individual psychotherapy experience generally are better prepared to use the group modality for work directed toward interpersonal and intrapsychic issues. On the other hand, a behaviorally focused group may be most beneficial to patients with extensive psychodynamically oriented, individual psychotherapy experience that did not include educational or behavioral techniques.

Selection of Group Members

The patient's suitability for group psychotherapy will depend on a number of factors, including the type of group, the patient's capacity for and motivation to change, prior psychotherapy experience, and existence of other psychiatric problems. Careful screening for admission to a group will enhance the therapeutic benefit to the patient, reduce the dropout rate, and increase the overall quality of the group.

Bulimic patients with coexisting psychiatric disorders or personality disturbances may make poor candidates for group therapy and should be carefully screened prior to inclusion in a group program. The schizophrenic's poor reality testing and mistrust may lead to deterioration in an active, insight-oriented group. While some patients may experience transient depression when discontinuing bulimic behaviors, the group process can aggravate symptoms and make significant behavioral change difficult for the severely depressed patient. The schizoid patient may be threatened by the activeness and emotional interaction of many bulimic groups. Firm limit setting will be necessary to enable the excessively talkative or hypomanic patient to remain in group. The extremely impulsive patient may be unable to use relationships or systematic behavior techniques constructively in a group setting. The chronic bulimic patient who is entrenched in her symptoms may drag the group down with her hopelessness and lack of progress. The hostility and shifting alliances of the borderline patient may interfere with her own and others' ability to use the group. Problems with alcohol and other substance abuse need to be resolved before beginning treatment in a bulimic group, except in instances in which the group is constituted of patients having dual problems of both bulimia and alcohol or other substance abuse.

Group Techniques

The methodology chosen for a group depends both on the purpose of the group and on theoretical orientation of the leader. That an integration of behavioral and dynamic approaches commonly occurs in bulimia groups is not surprising, given the multidimensional elements of the patient's disorder and general acceptance of the need for a comprehensive approach to eating disorders in general.

The most frequent behavioral techniques used in bulimia group-therapy studies include self-monitoring through daily diaries, goal setting or contracting, assertiveness training, and cognitive restructuring, with relaxation training and guided fantasy used less often (table 2). Emphasis on diary use varies, with one author (Lacey 1983) reporting that daily recording is required throughout the program while others (Dixon and Kiecolt-Glaser 1984; Johnson, Connors, and Stuckey 1983; Roy-Byrne et al. 1984) indicate that diary recording is used primarily during the initial phase of treatment, with optional continuation according to the patient's initiative or needs. Resistance and acting out are mentioned as problems associated with diary keeping in some patients. Johnson et al. (1983) noted that patients rated relaxation and assertiveness training as the least helpful group techniques.

Universality, altruism, catharsis, and insight are strong therapeutic

TABLE 2

Use of Behavioral and Cognitive Techniques

Study

Technique	Boskind-Lodahl and White (1978)	White and Boskind-White (1981)	Lacey (1983)	Johnson et al. (1983)	Roy-Byrne et al. (1983)	Dixon and Kiecolt-Glaser (1984)
Self-monitoring...........	+	0	+	+	+	+
Goal setting.............	+	+	+	+	+	+
Assertiveness training....	+	0	0	+	+	+
Relaxation training.......	0	0	0	+	0	0
Guided fantasy...........	+	0	0	0	0	0
Cognitive restructuring....	0	0	0	+	+	+

factors in groups for bulimic patients. However, the degree, depth, and origin of insight gained in a group setting are determined to a large extent by the group duration and other elements contributing to group cohesion. Short-term, time-limited groups, therefore, are more likely to owe a significant amount of "insight" to gaining an intellectual understanding of their symptoms and related difficulties. Only one study (Roy-Byrne et al. 1984) describes the therapeutic process of long-term group therapy with bulimic patients. The relative value of short-term versus long-term group therapy has not been demonstrated.

Premature Termination in Bulimic Groups

High dropout rates, tardiness, and erratic attendance have been mentioned as particular problems in bulimic groups (Dixon and Kiecolt-Glaser 1984; Johnson et al. 1983; Roy-Byrne et al. 1984). These difficulties are not unexpected in this population of patients whose histories tend to reflect long-standing problems with impulse control and self-responsibility. Normally, a group dropout rate of 10–35 percent can be expected, with the greatest risk of dropout occurring in the early weeks of group treatment (Yalom 1970). Of nineteen patients who attended groups described by Roy-Byrne et al. (1984), nine terminated early in treatment and two others left group prematurely after several months. Johnson et al. (1983) found that three of thirteen patients dropped out within the first three weeks of a nine-week program.

In our program, an early review (Dixon and Kiecolt-Glaser 1984) found that nineteen of thirty patients (63 percent) in an ongoing group that was open-ended for attendance terminated prematurely. Patients with a history of alcohol or other substance abuse were likely to drop out of group treatment early or make little change in their bulimic symptoms. In addition, premature terminators were characterized by higher scores on the Marlowe-Crowne Social Desirability Scale. The defensiveness, high need for approval, and difficulties with self-disclosure of such patients are liabilities in an open, goal-directed group.

Premature termination in group therapy may occur for various reasons, including inadequate pregroup preparation or screening of patients, patient resistance or unrealistic expectations, and therapist inexperience or leadership style. In an effort to reduce the high group-therapy dropout rate, we began to require all group candidates to have prior individual psychotherapy and be recommended by their individual psychotherapist as ready for group treatment. A subsequent review of thirty-nine patients (unpublished data) entering group therapy under these conditions revealed an overall dropout rate of 43.6 percent. However, it was noted that the dropout rate was only 20 percent (three of fifteen) for two therapy groups in which the majority (80 percent) of patients had the same psychotherapist for individual and group. Also, all prematurely terminating patients in these two groups left within the first six weeks, and two of the three dropouts had different individual and group therapists. A third group had twenty-four members over the course of a year, and of these 58 percent terminated prematurely. A notable feature of this high-dropout-rate group was that only 29 percent of the group members had the same psychotherapist for individual and group, in contrast to 80 percent having the same psychotherapists in the low-dropout-rate groups. Although all groups were open-ended for attendance, the two group-therapy groups having both a lower dropout rate and a higher percentage of patients with same individual and group therapists also had greater cohesiveness, more stable membership, and less absenteeism. The same therapist conducted the group with the high dropout rate and one of the low-dropout-rate groups.

Clearly, a pattern emerged, indicating that patients for whom the individual and group therapist were the same (combined psychotherapy) had a lower group dropout rate than did patients with different individual and group therapists (conjoint psychotherapy). Combined psychotherapy has been recommended for patients with personality disorders, including borderline and narcissistic disorders (Wong 1979), and, as such, may be preferable for the bulimic patient. Further, it could be expected that patients with a high need for approval and problems with self-disclosure would be less threatened in a group with stable membership and that the membership instability of the high-dropout-rate group may have been self-perpetuating. It is of interest that Lacey's (1983) study design used combined psychotherapy and apparently had a very low dropout rate over the ten-week treatment period.

Whether the premature termination rate in bulimic groups can indeed be positively influenced by placing the patient in a group led or co-led by the patient's individual therapist needs further investigation. Other variables associated with the bulimic patient's high risk for premature termination in psychotherapy need to be identified to assist the professional's selection and timing of treatment modalities.

Outcome of Group Therapy with Bulimics

Immediate and follow-up outcome data from reports of bulimia group-therapy patients is presented in table 1. Overall, of those patients whose immediate outcome is reported, 55 percent were free from bulimic symptoms and 38 percent improved at the end of the measurement interval. At follow-up, ranging from two months to two years, 43 percent were symptom free and 46 percent were improved. However, to what degree these results can be attributed to the group-therapy modality or to other treatment variables cannot be determined with currently available data. Several studies allowed introduction of other treatment modalities during the period of group therapy, and all studies allowed the introduction of new treatment variables during the follow-up interval. Furthermore, only two studies have used control (Lacey 1983) or comparison (Dixon and Kiecolt-Glaser 1984) groups in the research design.

Multiple measures of outcome are required for an accurate and comprehensive assessment of the specific benefits and value of a group-therapy modality. Measures used in bulimia group-therapy studies are shown in table 1. In summary, objective measures in the various studies indicate that, beyond change in eating behaviors and attitudes, patients may experience increased self-assurance, interpersonal adequacy and self-responsibility (Boskind-Lodahl and White 1978; White and Boskind-White 1981), a decrease in anger and in the associated increase in depression (Lacey 1983), a decreased drive for thinness and decreased bulimic tendencies along with increased introceptive awareness (Johnson et al. 1983), and decreased somatization, anxiety, and depression (Dixon and Kiecolt-Glaser 1984).

Conclusions

The global therapeutic effectiveness of group therapy for bulimia appears to receive positive support from the studies presently available. While a group-therapy approach may be an efficient and effective treatment intervention for many patients with bulimia, failure to prescribe group therapy appropriately and as part of a comprehensive treatment plan may contribute to patient and therapist frustration, inadequately reflect the actual value and effectiveness of the group-therapy modality, and result in inadequate treatment for the patient.

In view of the increasing use of group strategies in the treatment of bulimic patients, basic clinical and research questions need further investigation. What kinds of changes can be expected from a group-therapy approach to bulimia? What are the relative and specific values of individual versus group psychotherapy for the bulimic patient? What group techniques and approaches are beneficial and which are not beneficial with this population and subtypes of this population? What variables positively and negatively influence completion of group treatment? Which bulimic patients may not benefit or may show a negative effect with a group approach?

Clear descriptions of patient populations, including identification of coexisting psychiatric disorders, will help identify in research samples subgroups of patients who may or may not benefit from varying approaches. Standardized measures to assess changes in both bulimic symptoms and individual functioning are necessary for comparison of patient outcome across studies. Finally, replication of investigations using similar methods and populations in different settings are needed to validate findings applicable to the clinical approach to this diverse syndrome.

REFERENCES

Binswanger, L. 1944. Der Fall Ellen West. *Schweizer Archiv fur Neurologie und Psychiatrie* 54:69–117. (Binswanger, L. 1944. The case of Ellen West.) Reprinted in R. May, E. Angel, and H. Ellenberger, eds. *Existence.* 1958. New York: Basic.

Boskind-Lodahl, M., and Sirlin, J. 1977. The gorging-purging syndrome. *Psychology Today,* March 1977, pp. 50–52.

Boskind-Lodahl, M., and White, W. C. 1978. The definition and treatment of bulimarexia in college women—a pilot study. *Journal of the American College Health Association* 27:84–97.

Casper, R. C. 1983. On the emergence of bulimia nervosa as a syndrome. *International Journal of Eating Disorders* 2:3–16.

Dixon, K., and Kiecolt-Glaser, J. 1984. Group therapy for bulimia. *Hillside Journal of Clinical Psychiatry* 6:156–170.

Garfinkel, P. E., and Garner, D. M. 1982. *Anorexia Nervosa: A Multidimensional Perspective.* New York: Brunner/Mazel.

Halmi, K. A.; Falk, J. R.; and Schwartz, E. 1981. Binge-eating and vomiting: a survey of a college population. *Psychological Medicine* 11:697–706.

Huerta, E. 1982. Group therapy for anorexia nervosa patients. In M. Gross, ed. *Anorexia Nervosa*. Lexington, Mass.: Collamore.

Johnson, C.; Connors, J.; and Stuckey, M. 1983. Short-term group treatment of bulimia: a preliminary report. *International Journal of Eating Disorders* 2:199–208.

Johnson, C. L.; Stuckey, M. K.; Lewis, L. D.; and Schwartz, D. M. 1982. Bulimia: descriptive survey of 316 cases. *International Journal of Eating Disorders* 2:3–16.

Kadis, A. L.; Krasner, J.; Weiner, M. F.; and Winick, C. 1974. *Practicum of Group Psychotherapy*. New York: Harper & Row.

Katzman, M. A.; Wolchik, S. A.; and Braver, S. L. 1984. The prevalence of frequent binge-eating and bulimia in a nonclinical college sample. *International Journal of Eating Disorders* 3:53–62.

Lacey, J. H. 1983. Bulimia nervosa, binge-eating, and psychogenic vomiting: controlled treatment study and long-term outcome. *British Medical Journal* 286:1609–1613.

Piazza, E.; Carni, J. D.; Kelly, J.; and Plante, S. K. 1983. Group psychotherapy for anorexia nervosa. *Journal of the American Academy of Child Psychiatry* 22:276–278.

Polivy, J. 1981. Group therapy as an adjunctive treatment for anorexia nervosa. *Journal of Psychiatric Treatment and Evaluation* 3:279–283.

Pope, H. G.; Hudson, J. I.; Yurgelun-Todd, D.; and Hudson, M. S. 1984. Prevalence of anorexia nervosa and bulimia in three student populations. *International Journal of Eating Disorders* 3:45–51.

Rose, J., and Garfinkel, P. E. 1980. A parents' group in the management of anorexia nervosa. *Canadian Journal of Psychiatry* 25:228–233.

Roy-Byrne, P.; Lee-Brenner, K.; and Yager, J. 1984. Group therapy for bulimia: a year's experience. *International Journal of Eating Disorders* 3:97–116.

Rubel, J. 1984. The function of self-help groups in recovery from anorexia nervosa and bulimia. *The Psychiatric Clinics of North America* 7:381–393.

Stangler, R. S., and Printz, A. M. 1980. DSM-III: psychiatric diagnosis in a university population. *American Journal of Psychiatry* 137:937–940.

White, W. C., and Boskind-White, M. 1981. An experiential-behavioral approach to the treatment of bulimarexia. *Psychotherapy: Theory, Research and Practice* 18:501–507.

Wong, N. 1979. Clinical considerations in group treatment of narcissistic disorders. *International Journal of Group Psychotherapy* 29:325–33.

Yalom, I. 1970. *The Theory and Practice of Group Psychotherapy*. New York: Basic.

21 MEDICAL ASPECTS OF EATING DISORDERS

JAMES C. SHEININ

Anorexia nervosa, bulimia, and related eating disorders are a heterogeneous group of primary psychiatric disorders whose incidence has approached epidemic proportions in recent years (Bruch 1973; Vigersky 1977). Patients with eating disorders may have numerous secondary medical, hypothalamic, endocrine, metabolic, and nutritional abnormalities, some of which may be or may become severe enough to be life threatening. Further, it has been suggested that some of the psychologic abnormalities in patients with eating disorders may be secondary to starvation and undernutrition rather than intrinsic to the syndrome of anorexia nervosa (Bruch 1982). Response of the primary disorder to psychotherapy is associated with restoration of near-normal weight and reversal of the secondary medical, hypothalamic, endocrine, metabolic, and nutritional abnormalities. However, in addition, patients with bulimia may sustain irreversible damage to the gastrointestinal tract and the oral cavity as a result of emesis or laxative abuse.

Some general perspectives regarding the pathogenesis, incidence, severity, and evolution of the abnormalities seen in patients with anorexia, bulimia, and related eating disorders, and the adaptations to starvation, undernutrition, emesis or laxative or diuretic abuse will be provided. Subsequently, those specific abnormalities that are most significant for the diagnosis, evaluation, and management of patients with eating disorders and particularly patients with bulimia will be emphasized. This discussion is based on review of the literature cited and on unpublished observations in the medical, endocrine, and nutritional evaluation and management of over 250 patients with eating disorders.

General Perspectives

Anorexia nervosa has been appropriately described as starvation in the midst of plenty. Unlike people in other settings in which starvation and malnutrition occur, patients with anorexia nervosa have access to all foods and nutrients. They will selectively eat some things, albeit usually in meager quantities, and assiduously avoid others. Characteristically, they will eat little or no carbohydrate except as may be present in low-calorie fruits and vegetables, and little or no fat except as may be present in protein foods. However, their total caloric intake and relatively high protein intake further diminish protein breakdown and conserve lean body mass. The vitamin content of those foods they do eat, often supplemented by vitamin preparations, mitigates against vitamin deficiency in all but the most severe cases. Most patients with eating disorders are young and otherwise medically well. Many tolerate severe and protracted undernutrition, severe fluid and electrolyte depletion, and protracted emesis or inordinate laxative or diuretic abuse with minimal or no detectable clinical or laboratory abnormalities. When findings in older patients, patients with cardiac, gastrointestinal, neoplastic, or other systematic diseases and patients with protein-calorie malnutrition are extrapolated to patients with eating disorders (Harris 1983), the potential risks are exaggerated and exceed what is commonly observed.

The resilience of patients with anorexia nervosa further is facilitated by two prompt normal physiologic adaptations to starvation or to carbohydrate deprivation. (1) About 80–90 percent of the more active circulating thyroid hormone, triiodothyronine (T3), comes from extrathyroidal conversion of thyroxine (T4). Within days, peripheral conversion of T4 and T3 is inhibited, and T3 levels are decreased. In patients with anorexia nervosa, mean T3 levels usually are found to be about half those of normal controls (Boyar, Hellman, Roffwarg, Katz, Zumoff, O'Connor, Bradlow, and Fukushima 1977; Croxson and Ibbertson 1977; Miyai, Yamamoto, Azukiwa, Ishibashi, and Kumahara, 1975; Moshang, Parks, Baker, Vaidya, Utiger, Bongiovanni, and Snyder, 1975; Vigersky, Loriaux, Anderson, and Lipsett 1976). Findings such as cold intolerance, constipation, dry skin, bradycardia, carotenemia, hypercholesterolemia, and decreased basal metabolic rate provide further evidence for an apparent protective hypometabolic adaptation. (2) The needs of glucose-dependent tissues such as the central nervous system normally are met by food intake and by breakdown of liver glycogen to glucose. Within hours of starvation, glycogen stores are depleted and glucose can be provided only by gluconeogenesis from the amino acid constituents of proteins. Within days, stimulation of lipolysis and ketogenesis provides ketones at levels high enough to be utilized by the central nervous system as an alternate fuel (Cahill, Herrara, Morgan, Soeldner, Steinke, Levy, Reichard, and Kipnis 1966). Glucose requirements and protein breakdown are diminished, and lean body mass is conserved.

For young women, a reasonable general guideline for ideal body weight would be 100 pounds for five feet plus five pounds for each additional inch in height. Patients with eating disorders who are less than 20 percent below ideal body weight almost always are asymptomatic and have no clinical or laboratory abnormalities except as discussed below. Patients between 20 and 40 percent below ideal body weight begin to have clinical and laboratory abnormalities, which frequently are life threatening. Patients 40 percent or more below ideal body weight usually are symptomatic and have clinical and laboratory abnormalities that almost invariably are life threatening. Among other variables that may affect the incidence and severity of the abnormalities, there are the percent weight loss from premorbid weight, the rate of weight loss, the total weight loss, the duration of undernutrition, and the susceptibility of the individual patient.

There are two specific exceptions. (1) Amenorrhea may occur before or concurrent with onset of weight loss in up to one-third of patients with anorexia nervosa and may persist following normalization of weight. These patients (Boyar, Katz, Finkelstein, Kapen, Weiner, Weitzman, and Hellman 1974) exhibit an immature twenty-four-hour pattern of luteinizing hormone (LH) secretion characteristic of prepubertal or pubertal girls, a physiologic as well as psychologic regression from adulthood to childhood. (2) Significant and sometimes life-threatening clinical and laboratory abnormalities caused by emesis or laxative or diuretic abuse may occur in normal-weight or overweight patients with bulimia.

Findings reported as individual values, range of values or percent abnormal values, comparison of findings from different reports, and observation of large numbers of patients indicate that the incidence and severity of clinical and laboratory abnormalities among patients are extremely variable. It should be emphasized that laboratory evaluation usually provides the initial evidence for these abnormalities.

The use of weight as the sole or primary criterion for assessment of medical and nutritional status has several significant limitations. (1) The patient has an overriding concern about weight and is extremely fearful of, threatened by, and resistant to weight gain. (2) Despite repeated explanations and reassurance, the patient almost invariably reacts adversely to the rapid and sizable weight gain that is associated with refeeding edema or cessation of purging (a quart of fluid weighs two pounds). (3) The patient can readily manipulate weight before weigh-ins by eating, drinking, wearing heavy clothing, or loading clothing with heavy objects. (4) There may be little or no correlation between the absolute weight or the percentage below ideal or premorbid body weight and the presence, severity, and evolution of clinical and laboratory abnormalities. However, it must be emphasized to the patient with undernutrition that weight gain is a prerequisite for improvement of medical and nutritional status.

Hypothalamic, Endocrine, and Metabolic Abnormalities

Substantial alterations of thyroid status in patients with anorexia nervosa have been reported (Boyar et al. 1977; Brown, Garfinkel, Jeuniewic, Moldofsky, and Stancer 1977; Casper and Frohman 1982; Croxson and Ibbertson 1977; Hurd, Palumbo, and Gharib 1977; Miyai et al. 1975; Moshang et al. 1975; Vigersky, Anderson, Thompson, and Loriaux 1976; Warren and Vande Wiele 1973). The protective hypometabolic adaptation of decreased peripheral conversion of T4 to T3 and the resultant marked diminution in T3 levels previously have been described. Total T4 levels (T4 is normally 99.96 percent bound to plasma proteins) usually have been found to be lower than in normal controls but within the normal range. However, dialyzable free T4 levels, felt to be the most sensitive parameter of thyroid function, have been found to be normal. That there is hypothalamic dysfunction or a protective hypothalamic hypometabolic adaptation has been suggested by the findings of normal basal pituitary thyroid-stimulating hormone (TSH) levels and quantitatively normal and temporally normal or delayed response of TSH to hypothalamic thyrotropin–releasing hormone (TRH). In addition to the clinical and laboratory findings previously described, other hypothyroid-like alterations in glucocorticoid and androgen metabolism have been reported in patients with anorexia nervosa (Boyar et al. 1977; Bradlow, Boyar, O'Connor, Zumoff, and Hellman 1976).

These perturbations in hypothalamic-pituitary-thyroid status may be seen in patients with other forms of caloric deprivation, with various severe nonthyroidal illnesses, with certain medications, and after major surgery (Wartofsky and Burman 1982), and have been dubbed the "euthyroid sick syndrome."

The physiologic regression of the twenty-four-hour pattern of LH secretion to a prepubertal or pubertal pattern previously has been described. Basal LH and follicle-stimulating hormone (FSH) levels have been found to be low (Beumont, George, Pimstone, and Vinik 1976; Brown et. al. 1977; Hurd et al. 1977; Sherman, Halmi, and Zamudio 1975; Vigersky et al. 1976; Warren and Vande Wiele 1973). The FSH and LH responses to gonadotropin-releasing hormone (GnRH) have been reported to be normal, blunted, temporally delayed, and discordant. As would be anticipated in amenorrheic women with low FSH and LH levels, plasma estradiol levels are low.

Although a critical body weight has been suggested as a prerequisite for maintenance or onset of menses (Frisch and McArthur 1974), the clinical observation that women often become amenorrheic with little or no antecedent weight loss and may remain amenorrheic for months after restoration of a normal or near-normal weight suggests that factors other than weight are involved in the pathogenesis of amenorrhea in patients with anorexia nervosa. Stress-induced amenorrhea ("hypothalamic amenorrhea") in otherwise normal young women has long been recognized. That vigorous physical activity may be associated with delayed menarche and amenorrhea has been described more recently (Frisch, Gotz-Welbergen, McArthur, Albright, Witschi, Bullen, Birnholz, Reed, and Hermann 1981; Frisch, Wyshak, and Vincent 1980; Warren 1980), but the significance is uncertain since comparable vigorous physical activity ("obligatory" running) has been suggested to be an analogue of anorexia nervosa (Yates, Leehey, and Shisslak 1983). Finally, simple weight loss to about 20 percent below ideal body weight in nonanorexic women has been associated with amenorrhea and altered basal and post-GnRH, FSH, and LH levels (Vigersky, Anderson, Thompson, and Loriaux 1977).

Basal plasma cortisol levels have been found to be normal or elevated (Boyar et al. 1977; Brown et al. 1977; Casper, Chatterton, and Davis 1979; Walsh, Katz, Levin, Kream, Fukushima, Weiner, and Zumoff 1981; Hurd et al. 1977; Vigersky et al. 1976; Warren and Vande Wiele 1973). Diurnal variation of plasma cortisol levels has been found to be normal or absent. Prolongation of the half-life of cortisol and decreased metabolic clearance rate of cortisol were thought to be responsible for the increased twenty-four-hour mean cortisol level. Subsequently, the cortisol production rate, initially thought to be normal, was found to be elevated in proportion to body mass. Dexamethasone suppression of plasma cortisol levels has been found to be impaired in patients with anorexia nervosa more than 20 percent below ideal body weight (Doerr, Fichter, Pirke, and Lund 1980; Gerner and Gwirtsman 1981) and in patients with bulimia as well (Hudson, Pope, Jonas, Laffer, Hudson, and Melby 1983). Bulimia was considered to be related to affective disorders and to be responsive to therapy with tricyclic antidepressants (Pope, Hudson, Jonas, and Yurgelen-Todd 1983). However, the clinical utility of the dexamethasone suppression test for psychiatric diagnosis and management has not been supported by recent critical evaluation (Health and Public Policy Committee, American College of Physicians 1984; Hirschfield, Koslow, and Kupfer 1983).

The mean plasma concentration of the adrenal androgen dehydroisoandrosterone (DHA) recently was found to be similar to that of preadrenarcheal children. Like the immature twenty-four-hour pattern of LH secretion, this represents another endocrine regression from adulthood to childhood (Zumoff, Walsh, Katz, Levin, Rosenfeld, Kream, and Weiner 1983).

Basal growth hormone (GH) levels have been found to be normal or increased (Vigersky et al. 1976; Brown et al. 1977; Hurd et al. 1977). An inverse relation between basal GH levels and dietary intake and a direct relation between basal GH levels and severity of weight loss have been noted. Both GH and cortisol are protective counterregulatory hormones that stimulate gluconeogenesis in response to the threat of hypoglycemia. The presence of normal or elevated GH and cortisol levels readily distinguishes anorexia nervosa from hypopituitarism. Further, hypopituitarism now is known to be rarely associated with undernutrition.

Evidence for partial central diabetes insipidus (DI) using the fluid deprivation test with subsequent administration of exogenous antidiuretic hormone (ADH) has been reported in one study (Vigersky et al. 1976) but not confirmed in another (Fohlin 1977). The distinction between DI and primary or psychogenic polydipsia may be difficult to make using the fluid deprivation test, and patients with anorexia nervosa frequently hoard and consume large amounts of noncaloric fluids. Abnormal levels of plasma and cerebrospinal fluid arginine vasopressin recently were described in patients with anorexia nervosa, but the causes and consequences were not determined (Gold, Kaye, Robertson, and Ebert 1983). In addition, impaired concentration of urine in patients with bulimia may result from nephrogenic DI induced by hypokalemic nephropathy (Cohen 1979).

It is of interest that qualitatively similar but quantitatively less dramatic perturbations in hypothalamic and endocrine status have been found in nonanorexic women with secondary amenorrhea associated with simple weight loss (Vigersky et al. 1977).

Frequent mild to moderate and occasional marked fasting hypoglycemia is seen in patients with anorexia nervosa and apparently is asymptomatic. The adaptive stimulation of lipolysis and ketogenesis, which provides ketone bodies as an alternate fuel and diminishes glucose requirements, and the stimulation of gluconeogenesis by GH and cortisol previously have been described. It has been found that total fasting for seventy-two hours in normal women results in similarly marked and asymptomatic hypoglycemia (Merimee and Tyson 1974). It remains to be established that these observations diminish the clinical significance of hypoglycemia in patients with anorexia nervosa. Accordingly, it seems prudent to be concerned about moderate to marked fasting hypoglycemia in these patients.

The association of hypercholesterolemia with anorexia nervosa is not commonly recognized but has been clearly demonstrated (Crisp, Blendix, and Pawan 1968; Klinefelter 1965; Mordasini, Klose, and Greten 1978). The elevation of total cholesterol was found to be related to an increase in low-density lipoprotein (LDL) cholesterol and to be reversible in patients who regained their original weight and began to menstruate. Yet patients with anorexia nervosa may have normal or low cholesterol levels as well. The relative contributions of the protective hypometabolic adaptation of diminished peripheral conversion of T4 to T3 and of diet to the hypercholesterolemia and hypercarotenemia (Pops and Schwabe 1968; Robboy, Sato, and Schwabe 1974) of anorexia nervosa are not fully established.

Medical and Nutritional Abnormalities

Alterations in fluid status are common in patients with eating disorders. Starvation or carbohydrate deprivation as well as emesis or laxative or diuretic abuse gives rise to fluid depletion. Refeeding or cessation of purging are associated with fluid repletion and retention and sometimes with dramatic edema. The effect of the accompanying rapid weight gain may be devastating to patients with eating disorders. Initial laboratory evaluation in patients with fluid depletion and decreased plasma volume frequently provides falsely high values, particularly for blood count and serum proteins. With fluid repletion and retention, laboratory values may fall precipitously, sometimes to falsely low levels. In such patients, some short-term weight loss usually is associated with ultimate restoration of normal fluid balance.

Patients with anorexia nervosa frequently have mild anemia and moderate to severe leukopenia with neutropenia or lymphopenia (Bowers and Eckert 1978; Kay and Stricker 1983; Mant and Faragher 1972; Warren and Vande Wiele 1973). Thrombocytopenia has been found to be mild, infrequent, and asymptomatic. The deficiency in all hematologic cellular elements appears to be a result of reversible bone marrow hypoplasia with increased gelatinous acid mucopolysaccharide ground substance in the marrow. Sporadic cases of decreased granulocyte bactericidal activity and hypocomplementemia have been described in patients with anorexia nervosa and may contribute to increased susceptibility to infection. In addition, significant lymphopenia may affect immune competence (Blackburn and Thornton 1979). However, clinical observations do not support an increased susceptibility to infection, even in those patients with leukopenia, neutropenia, or lymphopenia.

Levels of serum proteins measured in routine multichannel automated chemistry profiles, that is, total protein and albumin, often are normal in patients with anorexia nervosa. When present, significant hypoalbuminemia indicates severe or protracted undernutrition. However, because of its shorter half-life of six to eight days, serum transferrin levels, measured directly or calculated from measurement of total iron-binding capacity (TIBC), reflect significant protein deficiency much earlier than total protein or albumin levels (Blackburn and Thronton 1979). Transferrin levels almost always are low in patients initially presenting with anorexia nervosa and may be as low as half of normal values in patients with severe or protracted undernutrition.

Life-threatening potassium depletion and hypokalemia may occur as a result of emesis or laxative or diuretic abuse. Potent diuretics, such as thiazides and furosemide, induce potassium depletion by increasing renal excretion of potassium as well as sodium. The potassium concentration of gastric fluid is relatively low, so only a small portion of the potassium depletion in patients with protracted emesis is a result of gastric potassium loss. However, loss of gastric fluid hydrochloric acid gives rise to metabolic alkalosis, and most of the potassium depletion in patients with protracted emesis is a result of increased renal potassium loss associated with chronic metabolic alkalosis. On the other hand, potassium depletion in patients with laxative abuse is a direct result of significant intestinal potassium losses in chronic diarrhea (Cohen 1979).

Small to moderate potassium loss usually is asymptomatic. Symptoms of moderate to severe potassium depletion and hypokalemia include skeletal and smooth muscle weakness and paralysis, cardiac arrhythmias and conduction abnormalities, and hypokalemic nephropathy, which may give rise to nephrogenic DI. When hypokalemia becomes significant and mandates treatment has been a subject of recent debate (Harrington, Isner, and Kassirer 1982; Kaplan 1984). Even patients with emesis or laxative or diuretic abuse who have significant hypokalemia often have no symptoms or electrocardiographic abnormalities. Surreptitious emesis or laxative or diuretic abuse may simulate Bartter's syndrome, a rare syndrome characterized by hypokalemic alkalosis, hyperaldosteronism, and hyperplasia of the renal juxtaglomerular apparatus. Differentiation from Bartter's syndrome may be made by measurement of serum or urinary laxative or diuretic levels and urinary chloride levels (Veldhuis, Bardin, and Demers 1979).

Renal function as measured by BUN and creatinine is affected by protein intake and catabolism and by fluid status as well as by intrinsic renal function in patients with eating disorders. With normal fluid status and renal function, BUN, creatinine, and uric acid levels are normal or low. With significant fluid depletion, almost always associated with emesis or laxative or diuretic abuse, hypovolemia results in prerenal azotemia, with BUN disproportionately more elevated than creatinine. Renal excretion of uric acid and of calcium may be compromised, and hyperuricemia and hypercalcemia may ensue.

Orthostatic hypotension often is seen in patients with eating disorders. While reduction of plasma volume and significant electrolyte imbalance such as occurs in patients with emesis or laxative or diuretic abuse are known to induce orthostatic hypotension, the pathogenesis of orthostatic hypotension in patients with anorexia nervosa who have not purged is uncertain (Schatz 1984).

A variety of electrocardiographic changes have been observed in patients with eating disorders (Gottdiener, Gross, Henry, Borer, and Ebert 1978; Isner, Roberts, Yagar, and Heymsfield 1983; Thurston and Marks

413

1974; Warren and Vande Wiele 1973), some of which may be related to undernutrition, hypometabolic adaptation, and hypokalemia. The pathogenesis and significance of frequently seen nonspecific and occasionally seen ischemic-like ST segment and T wave contour changes are uncertain. Arrhythmias and conduction abnormalities have caused the greatest concern. Prolongation of the QT interval has been observed and recently was reported in an abstract (Isner et al. 1983) to be associated with the sudden death of three patients with anorexia nervosa. However, such ominous findings are most uncommon in these patients.

Gastrointestinal symptoms and evidence for gastrointestinal dysfunction abnormalities are extremely common in patients with eating disorders. Symptoms and abnormalities may be related to undernutrition, hypometabolic adaptation, decreased food intake, binge-eating, emesis, laxative abuse, and hypokalemia. Irreversible damage to the gastrointestinal tract and to the oral cavity may ensue. Abnormal liver function tests, SGOT (AST) and SGPT (ALT) disproportionately more than GGTP are seen not uncommonly and presumably reflect hepatocellular injury as a result of moderate to severe undernutrition. Elevated serum amylase levels have been attributed to pancreatitis. However, salivary gland enlargement is seen occasionally in patients with bulimia and is associated with elevated serum amylase levels (Levin, Falko, Dixon, Gallup, and Saunders 1980). The pathogenesis of the sialopathy is uncertain, but elevated serum amylase levels in untreated patients with eating disorders are more likely a result of sialopathy rather than of pancreatitis. Characteristic dental deterioration has been observed in patients with eating disorders (Hurst, Lacey, and Crisp 1977). Dissolution of tooth enamel and altered caries response may occur as a result of emesis, abnormal diet, and alteration in the quality and composition of saliva.

Specific Aspects of Bulimia

Bulimia often occurs as part of the syndrome of anorexia nervosa with attendant undernutrition, and bulimia occurs in the absence of anorexia nervosa and undernutrition as well. In the latter instance, which has been defined as a separate psychiatric syndrome, the hypothalamic, endocrine, metabolic, and nutritional abnormalities seen in patients with anorexia nervosa are conspicuously absent. In patients with bulimia alone, amenorrhea, a sine qua non of anorexia nervosa, is rare and usually is transient. Although impaired suppression of plasma cortisol levels by dexamethasone has been found in some patients with bulimia and some with anorexia nervosa, the clinical significance of this finding is uncertain.

As in patients with undernutrition, the clinical and laboratory abnormalities seen in patients with bulimia are extremely variable and are affected by the frequency, extent, and duration of the bulimic behavior(s) and the susceptibility of the individual patient. Laboratory evaluation typically provides the initial evidence for these abnormalities. Life-threatening abnormalities in patients with bulimia may occur irrespective of nutritional status. It is likely that patients previously compromised by starvation and undernutrition may be more susceptible to the consequences of bulimic behavior. However, as the nutritional status and the appearance of patients with bulimia alone do not readily suggest the presence of an eating disorder, bulimic behavior and its consequences may be severe and protracted before the presence of an eating disorder is recognized.

Specific clinical and laboratory abnormalities that are consequences of emesis, laxative or diuretic abuse, binge-eating, or episodic starvation are due to either (1) direct or indirect effects of fluid and electrolyte depletion or of fluid retention, or (2) direct effects on the oral cavity, the salivary glands, and the gastrointestinal tract.

Sophisticated examination and laboratory evaluation will readily identify the presence and the sequelae of bulimia. Unexplained fluid depletion, orthostatic hypotension, electrolyte abnormalities, or edema may indicate the presence of bulimia. Surreptitious bulimic behavior must be distinguished from other disorders associated with hypokalemic alkalosis, particularly Bartter's syndrome. The presence of other clinical and laboratory stigmata of bulimia as well as the findings of the special studies previously described will unmask the surreptitious bulimic.

Cardiac arrhythmias and conduction abnormalities and skeletal and smooth muscle weakness and paralysis induced by severe potassium depletion are the most likely life-threatening sequelae of bulimic behavior. Marked fluid and electrolyte depletion may result in orthostatic hypotension, prerenal azotemia, impaired excretion of calcium and uric acid, and hypercalcemia and hyperuricemia. Hemoconcentration and hemodilution, respectively, may falsely raise or lower certain laboratory values that need be interpreted accordingly. Unexplained fluid depletion, orthostatic hypotension, electrolyte abnormalities, or edema may indicate the presence of bulimia.

The presence of bulimia also is suggested by findings of dental de-

415

terioration or unexplained salivary gland enlargement. In addition to the characteristic gastrointestinal symptoms found in patients with eating disorders, patients with bulimia may sustain irreversible damage to the oral cavity or the gastrointestinal tract as a result of emesis or laxative abuse. However, as previously emphasized, it is remarkable how well most patients with eating disorders tolerate fluid and electrolyte depletion, emesis, and laxative or diuretic abuse, and how uncommonly life-threatening abnormalities are observed.

Conclusions

Patients with anorexia nervosa, bulimia, and related eating disorders have numerous secondary medical, hypothalamic, endocrine, metabolic, and nutritional abnormalities, some of which may be or may become severe enough to be life threatening. Some general perspectives regarding the pathogenesis, incidence, severity, and evolution of the abnormalities seen in these patients and the adaptations that facilitate their resilience to starvation, undernutrition, emesis, and laxative or diuretic abuse have been provided. Specific abnormalities that are most significant for the diagnosis, evaluation, and management of patients with eating disorders and particularly patients with bulimia have been emphasized.

NOTE

With the foreknowledge and approval of Drs. Sherman C. Feinstein and Barton J. Blinder, I was asked to write this chapter after agreement had been made to publish portions of the manuscript in a textbook, *Modern Concepts of the Eating Disorders: Research, Diagnosis, Treatment*, edited by Barton J. Blinder et al. and to be published by SP Medical and Scientific Books (Spectrum Publications).

REFERENCES

Beumont, P. J. V.; George, G. C. W.; Pimstone, B. L.; and Vinik, A. I. 1976. Body weight and the pituitary response to hypothalamic releasing hormones in patients with anorexia nervosa. *Journal of Clinical Endocrinological Metabolism* 43:487–496.
Blackburn, G. L., and Thornton, P. A. 1979. Nutritional assessment of

the hospitalized patient. *Medical Clinics of North America* 63:1103–1115.

Bowers, T. K., and Eckert, E. 1978. Leukopenia in anorexia nervosa: lack of increased risk of infection. *Archives of Internal Medicine* 138:1520–1523.

Boyar, R. M.; Hellman, L. D.; Roffwarg, H.; Katz, J.; Zumoff, B.; O'Connor, J.; Bradlow, L.; and Fukushima, D. K. 1977. Cortisol secretion and metabolism in anorexia nervosa. *New England Journal of Medicine* 296:190–193.

Boyar, R. M.; Katz, J.; Finkelstein, J. W.; Kapen, S.; Weiner, H.; Weitzman, E. D.; and Hellman, L. 1974. Anorexia nervosa: immaturity of the 24-hour luteinizing hormone secretory pattern. *New England Journal of Medicine* 291:861–865.

Bradlow, H. L.; Boyar, R. M.; O'Connor, J.; Zumoff, B.; and Hellman, L. 1976. Hypothyroid-like alterations in testosterone metabolism in anorexia nervosa. *Journal of Clinical Endocrinology and Metabolism* 43:571–574.

Brown, G. M.; Garfinkel, P. G.; Jeuniewic, N.; Moldofsky, H.; and Stancer, H. C. 1977. Endocrine profiles in anorexia nervosa. In R. A. Vigersky, ed. *Anorexia Nervosa*. New York: Raven.

Bruch, H. 1973. *Eating Disorders*. New York: Basic.

Bruch, H. 1982. Anorexia nervosa: therapy and theory. *American Journal of Psychiatry* 139:1531–1538.

Cahill, G. F.; Herrera, M. G.; Morgan, A. P.; Soeldner, J. S.; Steinke, J.; Levy, P. L.; Reichard, G. A., Jr.; and Kipnis, D. M. 1966. Hormone-fuel interrelationships during fasting. *Journal of Clinical Investigation* 45:1751–1769.

Casper, R. C.; Chatterton, R. T., Jr.; and Davis, J. M. 1979. Alterations in serum cortisol and its binding characteristics in anorexia. *Journal of Clinical Endocrinology and Metabolism* 49:406–411.

Casper, R. C., and Frohman, L. A. 1982. Delayed TSH release in anorexia nervosa following injection of thyrotropin-releasing hormone. *Psychoneuroendocrinology* 7:59–68.

Cohen, J. J. 1979. Disorders of potassium balance. *Hospital Practice* 14:119.

Crisp, A. H.; Blendix, L. M.; and Pawan, G. L. S. 1968. Aspects of fat metabolism in anorexia nervosa. *Metabolism* 17:1109–1117.

Croxson, M. S., and Ibbertson, H. K. 1977. Low serum triiododthyronine and hypothyroidism in anorexia nervosa. *Journal of Clinical Endocrinology and Metabolism* 44:167–174.

Doerr, P.; Fichter, M.; Pirke, K. M.; and Lund, R. 1980. Relationship between weight gain and hypothalamic function in patients with anorexia nervosa. *Journal of Steroid Biochemistry* 13:529–537.

Fohlin, L. 1977. Body composition, cardiovascular and renal function in adolescent patients with anorexia nervosa. *Acta paediatrica scandinavia* (Suppl.) 268:1–20.

Frisch, R. L.; Gotz-Welbergen, A. V.; McArthur, J. W.; Albright, T.; Witschi, J.; Bullen, B.; Birnholz, J.; Reed, R. B.; and Hermann, H. 1981. Delayed menarche and amenorrhea of college athletes in relation to age of onset of training. *Journal of the American Medical Association* 246:1559–1563.

Frisch, R. L., and McArthur, J. W. 1974. Menstrual cycles: fatness as a determinant of minimum weight for height necessary for their maintenance or onset. *Science* 185:949–951.

Frisch, R. L.; Wyshak, G.; and Vincent, L. 1980. Delayed menarche and amenorrhea in ballet dancers. *New England Journal of Medicine* 303:17–19.

Gerner, R. H., and Gwirtsman, H. E. 1981. Abnormalities of dexamethasone suppression test and urinary MHPG in anorexia nervosa. *American Journal of Psychiatry* 138:650–653.

Gold, P. W.; Kaye, W.; Robertson, G. L.; and Ebert, M. 1983. Abnormalities in plasma and cerebrospinal-fluid arginine vasopressin in patients with anorexia nervosa. *New England Journal of Medicine* 308:1117–1123.

Gottdiener, J. S.; Gross, H. A.; Henry, W. L.; Borer, J. S.; and Ebert, M. H. 1978. Effects of self-induced starvation on cardiac size and function in anorexia nervosa. *Circulation* 58:425–433.

Harrington, J. T.; Isner, J. M.; and Kassirer, J. P. 1982. Our national obsession with potassium. *American Journal of Medicine* 73:155–159.

Harris, R. T. 1983. Bulimarexia and related serious eating disorders with medical complications. *Annals of Internal Medicine* 99:800–807.

Health and Public Policy Committee, American College of Physicians. 1984. The dexamethasone suppression test for the detection, diagnosis and management of depression. *Annals of Internal Medicine* 100:307–308.

Hirschfield, R. M. A.; Koslow, S. H.; and Kupfer, D. J. 1983. The clinical utility of the dexamethasone suppression test in psychiatry. *Journal of the American Medical Association* 250:2172–2174.

Hudson, J. I.; Pope, H. B., Jr.; Jonas, J. M.; Laffler, P. S.; Hudson, M. S.; and Melby, J. C. 1983. Hypothalamic-pituitary-adrenal axis hyperactivity in bulimia. *Psychiatric Research* 8:111–117.

Hurd, H. P., II; Palumbo, P. J.; and Gharib, H. 1977. Hypothalamic-endocrine dysfunction in anorexia nervosa. *Mayo Clinic Proceedings* 52:711–716.

Hurst, P. S.; Lacey, J. H.; and Crisp, A. H. 1977. Teeth, vomiting and diet: a study of the dental characteristics of seventeen anorexia nervosa patients. *Postgraduate Medical Journal* 53:298–305.

Isner, J. M.; Roberts, W. C.; Yagar, J.; and Heymsfield, S. 1983. Sudden death in anorexia nervosa: role of Q-T interval prolongation. *Circulation* 68 (Suppl. 30): 426.

Kaplan, N. M. 1984. Our appropriate concern about hypokalemia. *American Journal of Medicine* 771:1–4.

Kay, J., and Stricker, R. 1983. Hematologic and immunologic abnormalities in anorexia nervosa. *Southern Medical Journal* 6:1008–1010.

Klinefelter, H. 1965. Hypercholesterolemia in anorexia nervosa. *Journal of Clinical Endocrinology* 25:1520–1521.

Levin, P. A.; Falko, J. M.; Dixon, K.; Gallup, E. M.; and Saunders, W. 1980. Benign parotid enlargement in bulimia. *Annals of Internal Medicine* 93:827–829.

Mant, M.J., and Faragher, B. S. 1972. The haematology of anorexia nervosa. *British Journal of Haematology* 23:737–749.

Merimee, T. J., and Tyson, J. E. 1974. Stabilization of plasma glucose during fasting. *New England Journal of Medicine* 291:1275–1278.

Miyai, K.; Yamamoto, T.; Azukizawa, M.; Ishibashi, K.; and Kumahara, Y. 1975. Serum thyroid hormones and thyrotropin in anorexia nervosa. *Journal of Clinical Endocrinology and Metabolism* 40:334–338.

Mordasini, R.; Klose, G.; and Greten, H. 1978. Secondary type II hyperlipoproteinemia in patients with anorexia nervosa. *Metabolism* 27:71–79.

Moshang, T., Jr.; Parks, J. S.; Baker, L.; Vaidya, V.; Utiger, R. D.; Bongiovanni, A. M.; and Snyder, P. J. 1975. Low serum triiodothyronine in patients with anorexia nervosa. *Journal of Clinical Endocrinology and Metabolism* 40:470–473.

Pope, H. G., Jr.; Hudson, J. I.; Jonas, J. M.; and Yurgelun–Todd, M. S. 1983. Bulimia treated with imipramine: a placebo-controlled double blind study. *American Journal of Psychiatry* 140:554–558.

Pops, M. A., and Schwabe, A. D. 1968. Hypercarotenemia in anorexia nervosa. *Journal of the American Medical Association* 205:553–554.

Robboy, M. S.; Sato, A. S.; and Schwabe, A. D. 1974. The hypercarotenemia in anorexia nervosa: a comparison of vitamin A and carotene levels in various forms of menstrual dysfunction and cachexia. *American Journal of Clinical Nutrition* 27:362–367.

Schatz, I. J. 1984. Orthostatic hypotension. I. Functional and neurogenic causes. *Archives of Internal Medicine* 144:773–777.

Sherman, B. M.; Halmi, K. A.; and Zamudio, R. 1975. LH and FSH response to gonadotropin-releasing hormone in anorexia nervosa: effect of nutritional rehabilitation. *Journal of Clinical Endocrinology and Metabolism* 41:135–142.

Thurston, J., and Marks, P. 1974. Electrocardiographic abnormalities in patients with anorexia nervosa. *British Heart Journal* 36:719–723.

Veldhuis, J. D.; Bardin, C. W.; and Demers, L. M. 1979. Metabolic mimicry of Bartter's syndrome by covert vomiting: utility of urinary chloride determination. *American Journal of Medicine* 66:361–363.

Vigersky, R. A. 1973. *Anorexia Nervosa*. New York: Raven.

Vigersky, R. A.; Anderson, A. E.; Thompson, R. H.; and Loriaux, D. L. 1977. Hypothalamic dysfunction in secondary amenorrhea associated with simple weight loss. *New England Journal of Medicine* 297:1141–1145.

Vigersky, R. A.; Loriaux, D. L.; Anderson, A. E.; and Lipsett, M. B. 1976. Anorexia nervosa: behavioural and hypothalamic aspects. *Clinics in Endocrinology and Metabolism* 5:517–535.

Walsh, B. T.; Katz, J. L.; Levin, J.; Kream, J.; Fukushima, D. K.; Weiner, H.; and Zumoff, B. 1981. The production rate of cortisol declines during recovery from anorexia nervosa. *Journal of Clinical Endocrinology and Metabolism* 53:203–205.

Warren, M. P. 1980. The effects of exercise on pubertal progression and reproductive function in girls. *Journal of Clinical Endocrinology and Metabolism* 51:1150–1157.

Warren, M. P., and Vande Wiele, R. L. 1973. Clinical and metabolic features of anorexia nervosa. *American Journal of Obstetrics and Gynecology* 117:435.

Wartofsky, L., and Burman, K. D. 1982. Alterations in thyroid function in patients with systemic illness: the "euthyroid sick syndrome." *Endocrine Reviews* 3:164–217.

Yates, A.; Leehey, K.; and Shisslak, C. M. 1983. Running—an analogue of anorexia? *New England Journal of Medicine* 308:251–155.

Zumoff, B.; Walsh, B. T.; Katz, J. L.; Levin, J.; Rosenfeld, R. S.; Kream, J.; and Weiner, H. 1983. Subnormal plasma dehydroisoandrosterone to cortisol ratio in anorexia nervosa: a second hormonal parameter of ontogenic regression. *Journal of Clinical Endocrinology and Metabolism* 56:668–672.

ENRIQUE J. FRIEDMAN

As a newly defined clinical entity (*DSM-III* 1980), bulimia is still more of an enigma than anorexia from the neuroendocrinological point of view. Neuroendocrinological studies of anorexia, first defined as a clinical entity in 1694, are multiple. In recent years studies in the area of bulimia have begun to shed some light on the potentially severe metabolic changes that take place with purging. Some of the studies suggest that anorexia and bulimia have a common pathophysiological matrix, namely, that both syndromes reflect a hypothalamic-pituitary-adrenal dysfunction and impairment. Gwirtsman, Byrne, Yager, and Gerner (1983) found in a study of eighteen bulimics, eight of ten (80 percent) showed blunted thyrotropin-releasing hormone (TRH) tests.

In a recent unpublished study Friedman, Gerner, Stolar, and Kramer (1984) demonstrated that the bulimic who practices emesis as a means of weight reduction presents a different abnormal endocrinological picture than the laxative-abuser group. This study was conducted with a group of thirty-seven normal-weight bulimic female patients, age range twenty-two plus or minus six with ideal body weight range. The average purging was one to three purges per day for emetics and two to three times weekly for laxative takers. The authors found that the emetic group showed a lower level of luteinizing hormone (LH) and follicle-stimulant hormone (FSH) compared with the laxative group, who showed high normal levels of such hormones. The more severe the binging and purging, the lower the value of FSH and LH. Such low values were accompanied by either amenorrhea or oligomenorrhea. In the same study, the investigators found that the emetic group showed a high level of growth hormone compared with very low levels of such hormone in the laxative-taker,

TABLE 1
NORMAL-WEIGHT BULIMIC ($N=7$)

	Laxative Group ($N=30$)	Emetic Group ($N=7$)
Prolactin	Low	High
Growth hormone	Low	High
Follicle-stimulant hormone	High (normal)	Low
Luteinizing hormone	High (normal)	Low

bulimic group. Prolactin levels were higher in the latter group than in the former (table 1).

The authors hypothesized that the emetic group, through their purging mechanism (emesis), were reactivating dopamine receptors present at the level of the trigger zone (TZ) of the vomiting center in the medulla. In turn, dopamine would enhance the production of growth hormone, while it would suppress the release of gonadotropin (LH and FSH) as well as prolactin. Dopamine and prolactin interact by suppressing each other. High levels of dopamine will correspond with low levels of prolactin and vice versa. The following diagram (fig. 1) illustrates the interaction of some of the brain neurotransmitters and their hormonal influence. Similar studies have been conducted extensively in anorexia nervosa. Low gonadotropin levels are a distinct pattern of anorexia (Beumont, Carr, and Gelder 1973; Brown, Garfinkel, Jeuniewic, Moldofsky, and Stancer 1977; Frisch and McArthur 1974; Hurd, Palumbo, and Gharib 1977).

In anorexia, low levels of LH and FSH are attributed to low weight, which in turn contributes to the decrease of body fat content. Apparently, under normal circumstances, the female body requires a minimum of 22 percent fat content to produce menses (Frisch and McArthur 1974).

	NE	DA	END	5HT	ACH	GABA
LH-FSH	↑	↓	↓	↓	↑	↑
GH	↑	↑	↑	↑	→	↑↓
PRL	↓	↓	↑	↳	↑	↑↓
ACTH	↓	↓	↓	↑	↑↓	↓
TSH	↑	↓	↓	↳	→	→

Fig. 1.—Neurotransmitters regulation of anterior pituitary hormones. Key: NE = norepinephrine; DA = dopamine; END = endorphin; 5HT = serotonin; ACH = acetylcholine; GAMA = gamma-aminobutyric acid; LH = luteinizing hormone; FSH = follicle-stimulant hormone; GH = growth hormone; PRL = prolactin; ACTH = adrenocorticotrophin; TSH = thyrotropin-stimulating hormone.

423

According to these authors, a decreased body weight of 10–15 percent is associated with cessation of menses. Obviously such a hypothesis cannot be applied to normal-weight bulimics (NWB), yet they show low gonadotropin levels. In the Friedman et al. (1984) studies, 61 percent of the normal-weight, bulimic, emetic group showed low LH levels, while 69 percent of the same group showed low FSH levels. The findings in anorexia were the opposite; LH levels are lower than FSH levels. The explanation for this phenomenon can be made on the basis that the ovarian-negative-feedback mechanism in bulimia may be intact, while in anorexia it is impaired because of ovarian failure. Further studies should be done in bulimia to elucidate such an enigma, namely, the measuring of estrogen and estradiol in patients affected by such illnesses. Elevated levels of resting growth hormone have been reported in patients suffering from anorexia nervosa by Brown et al. (1977), Casper, Davis, and Pandey (1977), and Garfinkel, Brown, Stancer, and Moldofsky (1975).

While, in anorexia, low gonadotropin levels are attributed to low weight and low body fat content, elevated growth hormone seems to be a consequence of starvation. Seemingly, the preceding hypothesis cannot be applied to normal-weight bulimics. In contrast with the variations of prolactin levels among bulimic subtypes described in the Friedman and Gerner studies, a series of studies in anorexia have reported normal resting prolactin levels (1984). In the area of the pituitary-thyroid function, the TSH resting levels in approximately ten bulimic patients showed a normal level (E. Friedman, unpublished studies, 1984). Such findings coincide with similar studies done on anorexia by Beumont, George, Pimstone, and Vinik (1976). The area of pituitary-adrenal regulation in bulimia presents a distinct and interesting picture. Gwirtsman et al. (1983) reported normal levels of morning cortisol in normal-weight bulimics. These findings are in contrast with similar findings in anorexia where early morning cortisol levels were found to be elevated by Alvarez, Dimas, Castro, Rossman, VanderLaan, and VanderLaan (1972) and Brown et al. (1977). In anorexia a correlation was established between resting plasma morning cortisol and plasma thyroxine, possibly caused by abnormality in plasma-binding globulin. Such a connection was not established in bulimics.

Nonsuppression in the dexamethasone test (DST) was reported by Gwirtsman et al. (1983) in 67 percent of bulimics ($N = 18$) as well as by Hudson, Pope, Jonas, Laffler, Hudson, and Melby (1983). The studies of thirty-seven bulimics by Friedman et al. (1984) showed similar findings;

approximately 69 percent of their bulimic samples ($N = 37$) showed non-suppression.

The controversy about the high percentage of bulimics is centered in the specificity of the test and the significance of such findings. Are we talking about hyperactivity of the HPO axis caused by stress, starvation, metabolic changes, or affective disorder? The answer is not yet clear.

It has been proposed that, with high carbohydrate consumption, the metabolism of the latter may be affected. Glucose tolerance tests carried out in ten bulimic patients by Friedman seemed to fall within normal limits. Similar results were arrived at by Gwirtsman (personal communication). However, low normal levels of fasting glucose are found in the great majority of bulimics. The same findings applied to anorexics and both cases may be due to poor nutrition and starvation. Similar findings were reported by Kaye and Gwirtsman (1984) on normal-weight bulimics. These authors also found that blood glucose levels dropped considerably after purging (by emesis), reaching hypoglycemic levels (less than sixty milligrams per 100 milliliters). The same investigators also found that normal-weight bulimics showed normal levels of insulin compared with control groups, but abstinent, normal-weight bulimics had a significant decrease in plasma insulin during purging periods. These findings may be consistent with insulin supersensitivity, which is also found in anorexia nervosa. This metabolic picture is characterized by subnormal levels of glucose accompanied by low levels of insulin and heightened responsiveness to injected insulin. In patients with anorexia nervosa the concentration of insulin receptors is elevated and may well contribute to the heightened sensitivity to insulin. Refeeding restores insulin sensitivity, plasma insulin, and receptors.

Both anorectic and bulimic insulin hypersensitivity may be phenomena present resulting from continuous or intermittent starvation. The opposite of insulin sensitivity is the insulin resistance that has been also described in anorexia but not as yet in bulimia. This picture is composed of high levels of insulin and reduced response to insulin injection as well as low levels of insulin receptors. Such findings are also observed in obesity and acromegaly.

Conclusions

We have presented a parallel neuroendocrinological picture between anorexia and bulimia to emphasize the possible pathophysiological similarity of both clinical entities. We have discussed findings that affect the hypothalamic-pituitary-thyroid-adrenal axis in bulimics as well as anorexics. Neuroendocrinological investigation in bulimia is still new. One area that should be studied is the influence of different neurotransmitters at the level of the hypothalamus. The status of insulin receptors as well as glucose receptors in the hypothalamic level also needs further research. The influence of gut hormones such as cholecystokinin (CCK) and bombesin, and the mechanism that regulates the interaction of all the hormone and neurotransmitters for feeding processes, need further extensive clarification.

The understanding of the physiology and interaction of the hypothalamus as a possible regulator of feeding and its interaction with pituitary hormones as well as brain neurotransmitters will shed a great deal of light on the problem of eating disorders.

REFERENCES

Alvarez, L. C.; Dimas, C. O.; Castro, A.; Rossman, L. G.; VanderLaan, E. F.; and VanderLaan, W. P. 1972. Growth hormone in malnutrition. *Journal of Clinical Endocrinology and Metabolism* 43:400–409.

Aro, A.; Lamberg, B. A.; and Pelkonen, R. 1975. Letter: Dysfunction of the hypothalamic-pituitary axis in anorexia nervosa. *New England Journal of Medicine* 292:594–595.

Beumont, P. J. V.; Carr, P. J.; and Gelder, M. G. 1973. Plasma levels of luteinizing hormone and of immunoactive estrogen (estradiol) in anorexia nervosa: response clomiphene, citrate. *Psychological Medicine* 3:495–501.

Beumont, P. J. V.; George, G. C. W.; Pimstone, B. L.; and Vinik, A. I. 1976. Body weight and the pituitary response to hypothalamic-releasing hormones in patients with anorexia nervosa. *Journal of Clinical Endocrinology and Metabolism* 43:487–496.

Brown, G. M.; Garfinkel, P. E.; Jeuniewic, N.; Moldofsky, H.; and Stancer, H. C. 1977. Endocrine profiles in anorexia nervosa. In R. Vigersky, ed. *Anorexia Nervosa.* New York: Raven.

Casper, R. C.; Davis, J. M.; and Pandey, C. H. 1977. The effect of the nutritional status and weight changes on hypothalamic function tests in anorexia nervosa. In R. Vigersky, ed. *Anorexia Nervosa.* New York: Raven.

Diagnostic and Statistical Manual of Mental Disorders, 3 ed. (*DSM-III*). 1980. Washington, D.C.: American Psychiatric Association.

Friedman, E. J.; Gerner, R.; Stolar, M.; and Kramer, M. 1984. Psychological and endocrine evaluation of bulimia. Paper presented at American Psychiatric Association Annual Meeting, Los Angeles, May.

Frisch, R. E., and McArthur, J. W. 1974. Menstrual cycles: fatness as a determinant of minimum weight for height necessary for their maintenance or onset. *Science* 1985:949–951.

Garfinkel, P. E.; Brown, G. M.; Stancer, H. C.; and Moldofsky, H. 1975. Hypothalamic pituitary function in anorexia nervosa. *Archives of General Psychiatry* 32:739–744.

Gwirtsman, H. E.; Byrne, P.; Yager, J.; and Gerner, R. 1983. Neuroendocrine abnormalities in bulimia. *American Journal of Psychiatry* 140:559–563.

Hudson, J. I.; Pope, H. G.; Jonas, J. M.; Laffler, P. S.; Hudson, M. S.; and Melby, J. C. 1983. Hypothalamic-pituitary-adrenal-axis-hyperactivity in bulimia. *Psychiatric Research* 8:111–117.

Hurd, H. P.; Palumbo, P. J.; and Gharib, H. 1977. Hypothalamic-endocrine dysfunction in anorexia nervosa. *Mayo Clinic Proceedings* 52:711–716.

Kaye, W., and Gwirtsman, H. 1984. Paper presented at the First International Conference on Eating Disorders, New York.

Lundbert, P. O.; Walinder, J.; Werner, I.; and Wide, L. 1972. Effects of thyrotropin releasing hormone on plasma levels of TSH, FSH, LH, and GH in anorexia nervosa. *European Journal of Clinical Investigation* 2:150–153.

Vigersky, R. A., and Loriaux, D. L. 1977. Anorexia nervosa as a model of hypothalamic dysfunction. In R. Vigersky, ed. *Anorexia Nervosa*. New York: Raven.

23 IS BULIMIA AN AFFECTIVE DISORDER?

DAVID B. HERZOG

The relationship between eating disorders and affective disorders has generated considerable interest in the past decade. The early studies investigated anorectic subjects and families. Literature addressing normal-weight bulimia and its relationship to affective illness only first appeared in 1982. Since bulimia was first described as a syndrome distinct from anorexia nervosa (*DSM-III* 1980), affective changes have been acknowledged as an integral part of this disorder. The Axis I description of bulimia includes "depressed mood after a binge" as one of the five criteria for its diagnosis. Numerous studies support the coexistence of bulimia and depression, although the exact nature of this association is not yet understood.

One source of evidence relating bulimia and depression derives from the study of bulimia as a symptom in anorexia nervosa. Research has demonstrated that anorectics with bulimia are twice as likely to be depressed as those who restrict their intake (Casper, Eckert, Halmi, Goldberg, and Davis 1980; Garfinkel, Moldofsky, and Garner 1980; Strober 1982). Recent data also suggest that anorectics with bulimic symptomatology are more similar to normal-weight bulimics than to restrictive anorectics (Garner, Garfinkel, and O'Shaugnessy 1983). Although this chapter is based on research with bulimics of normal weight, the presence or absence of bulimia may provide for a more accurate characterization of eating-disordered patients than does weight loss.

The nature of the depression observed in bulimics is not clear; it may be a mood, a symptom, or a syndrome. Johnson and Larson (1982) employed an innovative sampling technique to study the moods and behaviors of bulimic women. For one week, the patients and normal controls were asked to fill out self-report diaries in response to the signals of an electronic pager. These signals occurred at random times throughout the day. The investigators found that the bulimics reported significantly more negative states than did the normal controls on six of eight mood items. Specifically, these women reported themselves as being sadder, lonelier, and weaker as well as being more irritable, passive, and constrained than did the control group. Additionally, the patients with bulimia reported significantly more variability in mood on all six items. Johnson and Larson suggest that the women who experience such dysphoric and fluctuating moods may be at risk for addictive behaviors. They propose that the uncontrolled eating emerges as an attempt to modulate these mood swings. The discovery of purging thus allows the women to incorporate binging as a mechanism of tension reduction without incurring the undesirable weight gain. According to this model, the bulimic symptoms may eventually take on a life of their own.

This sequence of events is but one possible explanation for the association between bulimia and depression. The four hypotheses that follow provide a framework for the exploration of this link: (1) depression leads to the eating-disordered state; (2) depression is a reaction to the bulimic behaviors; (3) bulimia and depression are separate, but often coexisting, conditions; and (4) bulimia and depressive illness reflect similar dispositions—biochemical, genetic, etc.—that increase the likelihood of their occurring together.

This chapter presents the five major sources of evidence relating bulimia to affective illness. The categories of evidence are as follows: (1) current and previous depressive symptomatology; (2) current and previous depressive syndrome; (3) familial aggregation and genetic predisposition; (4) biologic abnormalities; and (5) response to antidepressant treatment.

Current and Previous Symptomatology

Clinicians frequently describe bulimic patients as being sad, lonely, and constricted. The bulimics perceive themselves as being inadequate and socially maladjusted (Norman and Herzog 1984). Using self-report questionnaires, several investigations have documented the presence of depressive symptoms in bulimic patients. In a survey of 316 bulimic women, Johnson, Stuckey, Lewis, and Schwartz (1982) found that 62 percent described themselves as being either "often" or "always" depressed. These women also scored significantly higher on the depression scale of the Symptom Checklist-90 (SCL-90) than did normal controls. Similarly, Weiss and Ebert (1983) found that the bulimic patients rated themselves as being significantly more depressed on both the SCL-90 and the Piers-Harris Self Esteem Scale in comparison with normal-weight controls.

In an assessment of the first thirty bulimics presenting to the Eating Disorders Unit at Massachusetts General Hospital, 75 percent reported at least three symptoms of major depressive disorder (Herzog 1982). Fifty-five consecutive bulimic patients presenting for evaluation at the same clinic placed in the mildly depressed range on two subscales of the Schedule for Affective Disorders and Schizophrenia—Change Version (SADS-C): the Depressive Syndrome Subscale and the Extracted Hamilton Depression Rating Scale (Herzog 1984). Several investigators have also found that bulimics receive high scores on the depression subscale of the Minnesota Multiphasic Personality Inventory (MMPI) (Norman and Herzog 1983; Pyle, Mitchell, and Eckert 1981).

Current and Previous Depressive Syndrome

Two studies have assessed depression in bulimia. Hudson, Pope, Jonas, and Yurgelun-Todd (1983b) administered the National Institute of Mental Health Diagnostic Interview Schedule to forty-nine bulimic patients. They found that thirty-six (73 percent) of the bulimics displayed a lifetime diagnosis of major affective disorder. Seven (14 percent) of the patients displayed a DSM-III diagnosis of bipolar disorder, and twenty-nine (59 percent) a DSM-III diagnosis of major depression. These results were then compared with the DSM-III diagnoses of two study groups: forty-one first-degree relatives of fifteen probands with DSM-III schizophrenia, and fifty first-degree relatives of fifteen probands with DSM-III bipolar disorder. The lifetime rates of major affective disorder found in the relatives of schizophrenic and bipolar probands were 12 and 32 percent, respectively. The bulimics displayed a lifetime rate of major affective disorder significantly greater than that found in both comparison populations. No data are reported on the relatives of probands with unipolar depression.

In a recent study of the prevalence of depressive syndrome in bulimic patients presenting to the Eating Disorders Unit at Massachusetts General Hospital, thirteen (23.6 percent) of fifty-five met DSM-III criteria for major depressive disorder on the basis of a semistructured interview, the SADS-C (Herzog 1984). Twenty-seven (49.1 percent) of the fifty-five patients met DSM-III criteria for major depressive episode (MDE) on the basis of an unstructured psychiatric interview. The results demonstrate poor intertest reliability between the unstructured interview and the SADS-C measures. The more frequent diagnosis of MDE may reflect the added information of nonverbal cues present in an unstructured interview. The patient may also have had more difficulty hiding or denying her depression in the unstructured setting.

Familial Aggregation and Genetic Disposition

Two family-history studies of bulimic patients have been reported (Hudson, Pope, Jonas, and Yurgelun-Todd 1983a; Stern, Dixon, Nemzer, Lake, Sansone, Smeltzer, Lantz, and Schrier 1984). Using the family-history method, Hudson and colleagues studied twenty-five first-degree relatives of fifty-five patients with bulimia. Forty-one cases of major affective disorder were diagnosed, thirty-eight of forty-one exhibiting a major depression. The investigators, using the Weinberg shorter methods (Slater and Cowie 1971), calculated a 26 percent morbid risk for major affective disorder in the first-degree relatives of the bulimic patients. The relatives of the bulimics were then compared with the first-degree relatives of patients meeting DSM-III criteria for bipolar disorder, schizophrenia, and borderline personality disorder. They found a significantly greater percentage of familial affective disorder in patients with bulimia than in patients with schizophrenia or borderline personality disorder. When compared with the families of bipolar patients, no significant difference was observed. These findings were confirmed by the measure of morbid risk as well. The investigators did not compare the families of bulimics to those of unipolar depressed patients.

A second family-history study of bulimic patients presented contrasting results. Stern et al. (1984) found a nonsignificant difference in the lifetime prevalence of affective disorder in first- and second-degree relatives of bulimic women and controls. However, as Stern et al. note, these results do not preclude the possibility of a genetic link between bulimia and affective illness. Our understanding of the genetic role is severely limited by the absence of data reporting the incidence of bulimia in the first-degree relatives of depressed patients.

Biologic Abnormalities

The only biologic source of evidence suggesting an association between bulimia and affective disorders derives from two neuroendocrine abnormalities. Nonsuppression of plasma cortisol after dexamethasone administration has been reported in about 50 percent of patients with major depression (Brown and Shuey 1980). According to one study, twelve (67 percent) of eighteen bulimics had clearly abnormal dexamethasone suppression tests (Gwirtsman, Roy-Byrne, Yager, and Gerner 1983). Another study reports that twenty-two (47 percent) of forty-seven bulimic subjects were nonsuppressors of plasma cortisol in comparison with two (9 percent) of the control group (Hudson, Pope, Jonas, Laffer, Hudson, and Melby 1983). In a third study, fourteen (50 percent) of twenty-eight bulimic subjects failed to suppress plasma cortisol; however, nonsuppression did not correlate with severity of depression, body weight, duration of bulimia, or presence of abnormal eating behaviors (Mitchell, Pyle, Hatsukami, and Boutacoff 1984).

A second neuroendocrine abnormality has been demonstrated using the thyrotropin releasing–hormone (TRH) test. Research has shown that the thyrotropin response to TRH is abnormally blunted in patients with major depressive disorder (Gold, Pottash, Extein, Martin, Howard, Mueller, and Sweeney 1981). In a recent study of ten bulimics, 80 percent (eight) had blunted TRH tests (Gwirtsman et al. 1983). Although the results of these endocrine tests are supportive of a relationship between major depression and bulimia, other factors may account for these findings as well. The neuroendocrine abnormalities may, for example, reflect weight loss, dietary changes, stress, or noncompliance. Alternatively, the two disorders may share one or more common nonspecific neuroendocrine abnormalities. No data are available to distinguish between these hypotheses.

Response to Antidepressant Treatment

Reports on the clinical efficacy of antidepressants in the treatment of bulimia vary substantially. Two studies report improvement in both depressive symptoms and bulimic behaviors in response to treatment with antidepressants (Pope, Hudson, Jonas, and Yurgelun-Todd 1983; Walsh, Stewart, Roose, Gladis, and Glassman 1984). Others suggest that the drugs are effective only in the alleviation of depression (Mitchell and

Groat 1984). In one trial using mianserin, the drug-treated group reported no more improvement in either eating behavior or depression than did the placebo group (Sabine, Yonace, Farrington, Barratt, and Wakeling 1983).

The reported outcome of each study depends on a number of factors, some of which are extraneous to the drug itself. For example, Pope et al. (1983) report that 90 percent (eighteen of twenty) of their patients responded positively to imipramine. The subjects who participated in this study were all recruited for a drug study and may, therefore, have been unusually motivated to improve their condition. Another study limited its sample to bulimics with atypical depression and anxiety (Walsh et al. 1984).

A second important issue concerns the definition of outcome. Most investigators have defined response to antidepressants as a 50 percent reduction in binge-eating. In a recent follow-up study at the Massachusetts General Hospital Eating Disorders Unit, we found that only five (23 percent) of twenty-two of our patients maintained both a remission of depression and a decrease in binge-eating over three months. Our results might have been as positive as those mentioned above had we not expanded on the criteria defining response. We defined a true response as a 50 percent reduction in binging and no relapse or increase in depression or suicidality over a three-month period. Our less than promising results may also reflect the less than optimal dosages we administered to some patients, given the possibility of adverse side effects.

One final issue pertains to the differential effects of antidepressants. In the same study of twenty-two patients, we found that the patients whose binge-eating improved often showed no decrease in depressive symptomatology. Likewise, successful drug treatment of depression often did not eliminate the bulimic behavior. Mitchell and Groat (1984) found that the bulimics who were depressed had less of an antibinge response to drugs than those who were not. These findings suggest that antidepressants may have separate and possibly unrelated antibinge and antidepressant effects in the treatment of bulimia.

Conclusions

The available data do not allow for any definitive conclusion on the relationship between bulimia and affective disorders. We cannot verify or exclude any of the four associations mentioned earlier. Prospective, longitudinal studies that follow changes in depressive symptom profiles and depressive syndrome are needed. It is possible that the relationship between bulimia and affective illness may be better understood as the heterogeneity of bulimia is taken into account. For example, bulimics who are chemically dependent may be more closely linked to affective illness. Further studies are also necessary to clarify the biological and genetic relationship between affective disorders and bulimia. Such information will allow for a more specific and successful treatment of this syndrome.

NOTE

The author gratefully acknowledges the editorial assistance of Ms. Ingrid Ott.

REFERENCES

Brown, W., and Shuey, I. 1980. Response to dexamethasone and subtype of depression. *Archives of General Psychiatry* 37:747–751.

Casper, R. C.; Eckert, E. D.; Halmi, K. A.; Goldberg, S. C.; and Davis, J. M. 1980. Bulimia: its incidence and clinical importance in patients with anorexia nervosa. *Archives of General Psychiatry* 37:1030–1035.

Diagnostic and Statistical Manual of Mental Disorders, 3d ed. (*DSM-III*). 1980. Washington, D.C.: American Psychiatric Association.

Garfinkel, P. E.; Moldofsky, H.; and Garner, D. M. 1980. The heterogeneity of anorexia nervosa. *Archives of General Psychiatry* 37:1036–1040.

Garner, D. M.; Garfinkel, P. E.; and O'Shaughnessy, M. 1983. Understanding anorexia nervosa and bulimia: clinical and psychometric comparison between bulimia in anorexia nervosa and bulimia in normal weight women. Report of the Fourth Ross Conference on Medical Research. Columbus, Ohio: Ross Laboratories.

Gold, M. S.; Pottash, A. L.; Extein, I.; Martin, D. M.; Howard, E.; Mueller, E. A.; and Sweeney, D. R. 1981. The TRH test in the diagnosis of major and minor depression. *Psychoneuroendocrinology* 6:157–169.

Gwirtsman, H. E.; Roy-Byrne, P.; Yager, J.; and Gerner, R. H. 1983. Neuroendocrine abnormalities in bulimia. *American Journal of Psychiatry* 140:559–563

Herzog, D. B. 1982. Bulimia: the secretive syndrome. *Psychosomatics* 23:481–487.

Herzog, D. B. 1984. Are anorectics and bulimics depressed? *American Journal of Psychiatry* 141:1594–1597.

Hudson, J. I.; Pope, H. G.; Jonas, J. M.; Laffer, P. S.; Hudson, M. S.; and Melby, J. C. 1983. Hypothalamic-pituitary-adrenal-axis hyperactivity in bulimia. *Psychiatry Research* 8:111–117.

Hudson, J. I.; Pope, H. G.; Jonas, J. M.; and Yurgelun-Todd, D. 1983a. Family history study of anorexia nervosa and bulimia. *British Journal of Psychiatry* 142:133–138.

Hudson, J. I.; Pope, H. G.; Jonas, J. M.; and Yurgelun-Todd, D. 1983b. Phenomenologic relationship of eating disorders to major affective disorder. *Psychiatry Research* 9:345–354.

Johnson, C. L., and Larson, R. 1982. Bulimia: an analysis of moods and behavior. *Psychosomatic Medicine* 44:341–351.

Johnson, C. L.; Stuckey, M. D.; Lewis, L. D.; and Schwartz, D. M. 1982. Bulimia: a descriptive survey of 316 cases. *International Journal of Eating Disorders* 2:3–16.

Mitchell, J. E., and Groat, R. 1984. A placebo-controlled, double-blind trial of amitriptyline in bulimia. *Journal of Clinical Psychopharmacology* 140:559–563.

Mitchell, J. E.; Pyle, R. L.; Hatsukami, D.; and Boutacoff, L. I. 1984. The dexamethasone suppression test in patients with bulimia. *Journal of Clinical Psychiatry* 45:508–511.

Norman, D. K., and Herzog, D. B. 1983. Bulimia, anorexia nervosa and anorexia nervosa with bulimia: a comparative analysis of MMPI profiles. *International Journal of Eating Disorders* 2:43–52.

Pope, H. G.; Hudson, J. I.; Jonas, J. M.; and Yurgelun-Todd, D. 1983. Bulimia treated with imipramine: a placebo-controlled, double-blind study. *American Journal of Psychiatry* 140:554–558.

Pyle, R. L.; Mitchell, J. E.; and Eckert, E. D. 1981. Bulimia: a report of 34 cases. *Journal of Clinical Psychiatry* 42:60–64.

Sabine, E. J.; Yonace, A.; Farrington, A. J.; Barratt, K. H.; and Wakeling, A. 1983. Bulimia nervosa: a placebo-controlled, double-blind therapeutic trial of mianserin. *British Journal of Clinical Pharmacology* 15:195S–202S.

Slater, E., and Cowie, U. 1971. *The Genetics of Mental Disorder*. London: Oxford University Press.

Stern, S. L.; Dixon, K. N.; Nemzer, E.; Lake, M. D.; Sansone, R. A.;

Smeltzer, D. J.; Lantz, S.; and Schrier, S. S. 1984. Affective disorder in the families of women with normal weight bulimia. *American Journal of Psychiatry* 141:1224–1227.

Strober, M. 1982. Validity of the bulimia-restrictor distinction in anorexia nervosa: parental personality characteristics and family psychiatric morbidity. *Journal of Nervous and Mental Disease* 179:345–351.

Walsh, B. T.; Stewart, J. W.; Roose, S. P.; Gladis, M.; and Glassman, A. H. 1984. Treatment of bulimia with phenelzine. *Archives of General Psychiatry* 41:1105–1109.

Weiss, S. R., and Ebert, M. 1983. Psychological and behavioral characteristics of normal-weight bulimics and normal-weight controls. *Psychosomatic Medicine* 49:293–303.

24 MEDICATION IN THE TREATMENT OF BULIMIA

B. TIMOTHY WALSH

A variety of approaches to the treatment of bulimia has been explored in the last ten years, including the use of medication. The use of drugs in this syndrome has been based primarily on one of two conceptual models. In the mid 1970s, a group of investigators proposed that bulimia was a form of seizure disorder and suggested that anticonvulsant medication was of significant benefit. In recent years, several groups have noted links between bulimia and affective illness and have begun to explore the usefulness of antidepressant agents.

Anticonvulsants

Green and Rau described compulsive eating in patients of below-normal, normal, and above-normal body weights (Green and Rau 1974, 1977; Rau and Green 1975; Rau, Struve, and Green 1979). These authors were struck by patients' descriptions of the binges as being unpredictable, uncontrollable, and at times preceded by a strange state that could be likened to an aura. They obtained EEGs for patients with "compulsive eating" (who would now almost certainly be called bulimic) and found a high frequency of mildly abnormal results. They therefore proposed that "compulsive eaters have a primary neurologic disorder similar to epilepsy" and treated patients with these characteristics with the anticonvulsant phenytoin. In forty-seven patients treated openly with this drug, the authors noted impressive improvement in 57 percent.

Only two studies have used placebo-controlled methods in their attempts to test the utility of anticonvulsant agents in the treatment of bulimia. Wermuth, Davis, Hollister, and Stunkard (1977) published the results of a double-blind, placebo-controlled crossover trial of phenytoin in twenty patients suffering from binge-eating. All patients were female and ranged in weight from forty to 112 killograms at the time the study was initiated. Patients were randomly assigned to receive either six weeks of phenytoin (300 milligrams daily) followed by six weeks of placebo or the opposite sequence. In the ten patients who received phenytoin first, there was a significant decline in binge frequency when the drug was initiated. However, contrary to the investigators' expectations, this symptomatic improvement persisted through the placebo period. Thus, in this group, there was no difference between the results for phenytoin and placebo. In the group that received placebo first, there was no change in binge frequency during the first six weeks, but the patients did improve when they were switched to phenytoin. Overall, six of the nineteen patients who completed the trial were felt to have improved markedly on phenytoin, but only one patient ceased binging entirely. Four of these six markedly improved patients continued phenytoin beyond the study period, and, though they remained on phenytoin, two of the four relapsed. The investigators obtained EEGs for all twenty patients, and definite EEG abnormalities were found in only three. The patients' improvement while they were being treated with phenytoin was not clearly associated with either the presence of pretreatment abnormality in the EEG or the plasma level of the drug.

Greenway, Dahms, and Bray (1977) reported a trial of similar design in obese women. Interpretation of this study is hampered by the lack of clear diagnostic criteria and by a small sample size. Nonetheless, while the seven women probably had bulimia, none had significant pretreatment EEG abnormalities, and, in a double-blind crossover study of phenytoin versus placebo, there was no indication of benefit from treatment with phenytoin.

The studies of Wermuth et al. (1977) and Greenway et al. (1977) are the only controlled trials of phenytoin in the treatment of bulimia. Additional well-designed trials are needed to assess more completely the value of phenytoin in the treatment of this syndrome. While the implications of the available studies are limited by the selection criteria, crossover design, and small sample size, the data do indicate that the initial reports of Green and Rau (1974, 1977) were overly optimistic. Whatever therapeutic effects phenytoin has in binge-eating are not easily attributable to its conventional anticonvulsant activity. Unlike its effects on seizures, phenytoin's effects on bulimia are related neither to the patient's EEG abnormalities nor to the plasma level of the drug. Furthermore, the degree of improvement resulting from treatment with phenytoin seems to be less than that reported resulting from treatment with antidepressants—and more difficult to sustain.

A recent report describes preliminary results from a double-blind, placebo-controlled trial of the anticonvulsant carbamazepine (Kaplan, Garfinkel, Darby, and Garner 1983). Five of six normal-weight patients had either no response or an equivocal response to this drug. However, one patient who may have also had a mild bipolar mood disturbance responded dramatically to carbamazepine and relapsed when she was switched to placebo. Carbamazepine is widely used in the treatment of seizure disorders. It has a chemical structure similar to that of the tricyclic antidepressants and has been shown to be effective in the treatment of bipolar affective illness. Therefore, if further investigation suggests that some patients with bulimia do benefit from treatment with this medication, it will be difficult to attribute its effects purely to its anticonvulsant activity.

Antidepressants

There has been increasing interest in whether medications usually used to treat depression might have value in the treatment of bulimia. As clinicians began to see an increasing number of patients with bulimia, they became more aware that mood disturbances, particularly major depressive episodes or dysthymia, were frequently present in bulimic patients. Despite the evidence that antidepressant drugs have some therapeutic efficacy in the treatment of bulimia, this observation alone does not prove that bulimic patients are depressed. The medications used to treat depression affect more than just mood, and it appears that some nondepressed bulimic patients derive benefit from treatment with antidepressants. While there is growing evidence of links between affective illness and eating disorders, the relationship between bulimia and depression is not entirely clear, and our understanding of how treatment with antidepressants may be of benefit is far from complete.

There have been isolated case reports of successful treatment of bulimia with antidepressant medication since 1978 (Rich 1978). The first series of patients treated with antidepressants were described by Pope and Hudson (1982), who used tricyclic antidepressants, and by Walsh,

Stewart, Wright, Harrison, Roose, and Glassman (1982), who used monoamine oxidase inhibitors. These reports of open experience have been followed by several double-blind, placebo-controlled trials. Pope, Hudson, Jonas, and Yurgelun-Todd (1983) reported a trial of imipramine (200 milligrams daily) in twenty-two normal-weight patients with bulimia. In the nine patients who were assigned to receive imipramine and completed the trial, there was a 70 percent reduction in binges per week, compared to essentially no change in the patients assigned to placebo. Of the twenty patients who received imipramine either during the study or later on an open-trial basis, seven (35 percent) ceased binging entirely and eighteen (90 percent) showed at least a 50 percent reduction in binge frequency.

Hughes, Wells, and Cunningham (1984) reported similar results in a double-blind trial of desipramine versus placebo in the treatment of twenty-two outpatients with bulimia. Results of treatment with desipramine (200 milligrams daily) were strikingly superior to results of placebo treatment, and fifteen (68 percent) of the twenty-two patients treated with desipramine either during the study or on follow-up achieved total symptomatic remission.

Walsh, Stewart, Roose, Gladis, and Glassman (1984) reported the results of a double-blind, placebo-controlled trial of phenelzine (sixty to ninety milligrams per day) in the treatment of normal-weight women with bulimia. Of twenty patients who completed the ten-week protocol, nine were treated with phenelzine and eleven with placebo. Although the groups were comparable at the time of randomization, at completion of the drug treatment the phenelzine-treated group reported significantly fewer binges per week compared to the placebo-treated group (2.6 vs. 10.5). Five of the nine phenelzine-treated patients ceased binging entirely, and the other four reduced their binge frequency by at least 50 percent; none of the eleven placebo-treated patients stopped binging, and only two reduced their binge frequency by 50 percent or more.

Thus, three double-blind, placebo-controlled trials of normal-weight patients with bulimia have found evidence of a significant benefit from treatment with antidepressant medication. On the other hand, two double-blind, placebo-controlled trials have failed to find an advantage for drug treatment over placebo treatment. Sabine, Yonace, Farrington, Barratt, and Wakeling (1983) used the new antidepressant mianserin and found that both placebo- and drug-treated groups improved significantly and that the active drug provided no additional benefits. This study used only a modest dose (sixty milligrams per day) of mianserin and appears to have treated a less severely ill group of patients than did the other placebo-controlled trials of antidepressants.

Mitchell and Groat (1984) reported a double-blind, placebo-controlled trial of amitriptyline in the treatment of thirty-two women with bulimia. While the drug-treated group was significantly less depressed at study termination than the placebo-treated group, both groups improved equally in terms of eating behavior. Plasma-level measurements indicate that, at the dose used in this study (150 milligrams daily), a significant number of patients may not have received adequate drug treatment.

There are now five reported double-blind, placebo-controlled trials of antidepressant agents in the treatment of normal-weight patients with bulimia. All five trials have found substantial improvement in drug-treated patients, but in two studies there was substantial improvement in placebo-treated patients as well. Because of statistical variability, one would not expect every placebo-controlled trial of an antidepressant to demonstrate superiority even if there is a valid difference between the two treatments. Furthermore, the two trials that failed to find drug-placebo difference were those that used the lowest drug doses, that is, compared to the doses usually used in the treatment of depression. Thus, there is now reasonably strong evidence that tricyclic antidepressants and monoamine oxidase inhibitors, in doses typically used to treat major depression, have some therapeutic effect in the short-term treatment of normal-weight patients with chronic and moderately severe bulimia.

A number of questions about the role of antidepressant medication in the treatment of bulimia remain unanswered. The placebo-controlled trials that have found a significant advantage for the drug treatment have treated patients with moderate-to-severe and chronic bulimia for relatively short periods of time. Whether antidepressants are more effective than placebo in the treatment of milder and less chronic forms of this syndrome is unknown. Virtually all patients treated with medication have been adults; whether medications are as useful in adolescents has not been evaluated. It is also unknown how long patients who respond to antidepressant medication need to remain on the medication and how they fare after the drug is discontinued.

Recommendations and Guidelines

Despite these uncertainties, several guidelines can be offered concerning the use of medication in the treatment of bulimia. Any form of treatment should be a collaborative venture between therapist and patient. Because of side effects, the hazards of overdose, and the necessity of compliance to ensure an adequate trial, collaboration is critical when medications are being used. It should be emphasized that the antidepressant medications that appear to be useful in the treatment of bulimia are lethal in overdose and that because of the propensity of patients with bulimia to be depressed and to be impulsive, the risk of suicide must be carefully evaluated, especially in an adolescent. Another problem in treating bulimic patients with medication is ensuring that the drug is not only ingested but also absorbed. Patients must take the medication when they can be relatively sure they will not engage in purging behavior for several hours; some find that taking the medication at bedtime or immediately on arising is most convenient, but these considerations must be specifically reviewed by the psychiatrist. Plasma-level measurements, discussed below, can be useful in ascertaining if the drug is in fact getting into the bloodstream in adequate amounts.

Some clinicians working in this area have the impression that monoamine oxidase inhibitors may be the single most effective type of antidepressant in the treatment of bulimia. However, monoamine oxidase inhibitors are substantially more difficult to use, both because of a high frequency of side effects and because of the necessity for the patient to remain on a strict tyramine-free diet. Therefore, treatment is probably best initiated with a tricyclic antidepressant drug. It may be particularly advantageous to use imipramine, desipramine, or nortriptyline, because the plasma levels required for antidepressant efficacy of these drugs are reasonably well established. Although it is not known whether the plasma levels needed to treat bulimia are the same as those needed to treat depression, the psychiatrist can use the latter as a guide to adjusting dosage and as a means of assessing a patient's compliance. A full discussion of the use of plasma levels is beyond the scope of this review, but, in brief, plasma levels of the tricyclic antidepressants named above should be obtained (1) after the patient has been on a stable daily dosage for five to seven days and (2) approximately twelve hours after the last dose. For optimal antidepressant efficacy, in patients taking imipramine the plasma levels of imipramine plus its major metabolite, desipramine, should be greater than 200 nanograms per milliliter; in patients taking nortriptyline, the plasma level of nortriptyline should be between fifty and 150 nanograms per milliliter; and, in patients taking desipramine, the plasma level of desipramine should be greater than 125 nanograms per milliliter

(Glassman, Schildkraut, Orsulak, Cooper, Kupfer, Shader, Davis, Carroll, Perel, Klerman, and Greenblatt 1985). Typical daily dosages required to achieve these levels are 200 milligrams of imipramine, seventy-five milligrams of nortriptyline, and 200 milligrams of desipramine, respectively. However, rates of metabolism vary enormously between patients, making determination of plasma levels very useful in ensuring that adequate dosages of drug are being used.

If results of treatment with a tricyclic antidepressant are unsatisfactory, a trial of a monoamine oxidase inhibitor such as phenelzine can be considered for treatment of patients who are sufficiently reliable to adhere carefully to the tyramine-free diet. Phenelzine in a daily dosage of one milligram per kilogram body weight generally provides 80 percent or greater inhibition of platelet monoamine oxidase activity, a level believed necessary for optimal antidepressant effect. Treatment with phenytoin, as already discussed, and with the recently introduced antidepressant trazodone may also be of some merit. In the use of any of these medications, it is crucial that the drug be used in an adequate amount, as already outlined, and for an adequate duration—that is, at least three weeks at full dosage—before coming to a conclusion about the drug's effect.

Conclusions

Recent double-blind, placebo-controlled studies suggest that psychotropic medication, especially antidepressants, may be of use in the treatment of normal-weight patients with bulimia. Further studies are needed to clarify which bulimic patients respond to medication, to define the long-term outcome of drug treatment, and to investigate whether it is advantageous to combine medication with other forms of treatment.

NOTE

The author would like to acknowledge the support of NIH grants MH-38355 and MH-00383, which assisted some of the work reviewed.

REFERENCES

Glassman, A. H.; Schildkraut, J. J.; Orsulak, P. J.; Cooper, T. B.; Kupfer, D. J.; Shader, R. I.; Davis, J. M.; Carroll, B.; Perel, J. M.;

Klerman, G. L.; and Greenblatt, D. J. 1985. Tricyclic antidepressants—blood level measurements and clinical outcome: an APA Task Force Report. *American Journal of Psychiatry* 142:155–162.

Green, R. S., and Rau, J. H. 1974. Treatment of compulsive eating disturbances with anticonvulsant medication. *American Journal of Psychiatry* 131:428–432.

Green, R. S., and Rau, J. H. 1977. The use of diphenylhydantoin in compulsive eating disorders: further studies. In R. A. Vigersky, ed. *Anorexia Nervosa*. New York: Raven.

Greenway, F. L.; Dahms, W. T.; and Bray, G. A. 1977. Phenytoin as a treatment of obesity associated with compulsive eating. *Current Therapeutic Research* 21:338–342.

Hughes, P. L.; Wells, L. A.; and Cunningham, J. C. 1984. A controlled trial using desipramine for bulimia. Paper presented at the 137th Annual Meeting of the American Psychiatric Association, May.

Kaplan, A. S.; Garfinkel, P. E.; Darby, P. L.; and Garner, D. M. 1983. Carbamazepine in the treatment of bulimia. *American Journal of Psychiatry* 140:1225–1226.

Mitchell, J. E., and Groat, R. 1984. A placebo-controlled, double-blind trial of amitriptyline in bulimia. *Journal of Clinical Psychopharmacology* 4:186–193.

Pope, H. G., and Hudson, J. I. 1982. Treatment of bulimia with antidepressants. *Psychopharmacology* 78:176–179.

Pope, H. G.; Hudson, J. I.; Jonas, J. M.; and Yurgelun-Todd, D. 1983. Bulimia treated with imipramine: a placebo-controlled, double-blind study. *American Journal of Psychiatry* 140:554–558.

Rau, J. H., and Green, R. S. 1975. Compulsive eating: a neuropsychologic approach to certain eating disorders. *Comprehensive Psychiatry* 16:223–231.

Rau, J. H.; Struve, F. A.; and Green, R. S. 1979. Electroencephalographic correlates of compulsive eating. *Clinical Electroencephalography* 10:180–189.

Rich, C. L. 1978. Self-induced vomiting: psychiatric considerations. *Journal of the American Medical Association* 239:2688–2689.

Sabine, E. J.; Yonace, A.; Farrington, A. J.; Barratt, K. H.; and Wakeling, A. 1983. Bulimia nervosa: a placebo-controlled double-blind therapeutic trial of mianserin. *British Journal of Clinical Pharmacology* 15:195S–202S.

Walsh, B. T.; Stewart, J. W.; Roose, S. P.; Gladis, M.; and Glassman,

A. H. 1984. Treatment of bulimia with phenelzine: a double-blind, placebo-controlled study. *Archives of General Psychiatry* 41:1105–1109.

Walsh, B. T.; Stewart, J. W.; Wright, L.; Harrison, W.; Roose, S. P.; and Glassman, A. H. 1982. Treatment of bulimia with monoamine oxidase inhibitors. *American Journal of Psychiatry* 139:1629–1630.

Wermuth, B. M.; Davis, K. L.; Hollister, L. E.; and Stunkard, A. J. 1977. Phenytoin treatment of the binge-eating syndrome. *American Journal of Psychiatry* 134:1249–1253.

PART IV

TODAY'S ADOLESCENT PSYCHIATRY: WHICH ADOLESCENTS TO TREAT AND HOW?

INTRODUCTION:
TODAY'S ADOLESCENT PSYCHIATRY:
WHICH ADOLESCENTS TO TREAT
AND HOW?

FRANÇOIS LADAME

In March, 1984, an international conference brought together in Geneva Evelyne Kestemberg (France), James Masterson (U.S.A.), Moses Laufer (England), Brian Muir (England), and Luc Kaufmann (Switzerland).[1] This meeting marked the tenth anniversary of the Geneva Adolescent Psychiatric Unit (Unité de Psychiatrie de l'Adolescence). Since 1973, Geneva has had an adolescent outpatient center for treatment and consultation of adolescents, distinct from available services provided for children and adults. During the last decade, adolescent psychiatry as such has become recognized, and understandably so, as a direct reflection of a specific developmental phase. We now also realize the multiplicity of psychological problems with which we are faced and the need to do everything possible in order to prevent eventual chronic mental illness in adulthood.

Experience has shown that transitory or situational disturbances rarely require a specialist's help as long as they correspond to a specific definition that is based on careful assessment of the entire personality organization. In this case, we are faced with mere stumbling blocks in the developmental process, linked to outside circumstances particularly unfavorable but transitory, as well as excessive internal pressures inherently part of the psychic process, or, more generally speaking, the association of both.

Section IV published with permission of Presses Universitaires de France.

A crisis is resolved through change, and development continues normally. Adolescents going through critical periods are not subjected to the repetition compulsion and can usually find support from outside sources—containment or stimulation—in order to face temporary interruptions in the growth process.

It appears to me that the field of adolescent psychiatry is circumscribed through its specificity around what Laufer has called deadlock in development. For those adolescents who find themselves in a cul-de-sac situation, progression as well as regression become impossible. Anxiety-provoking adjustments lead to symptom formation the structure of which is a paradoxical expression of both levels, being incompatible albeit concomitant. Adolescent psychiatric or psychotherapeutic assessment consists of establishing whether we are dealing with a transitory difficulty or a breakdown. The contrasting pair, binding and unbinding, represents a central coordinate insofar as a break in the different psychic ties signifies developmental arrest. Binding and unbinding concern both body and psyche, object and narcissistic cathexis, pleasure and displeasure, excitement and tranquillity, and delay in satisfaction and immediate abandonment of drive, which in the final analysis refers to primary masochism as representing the initial tie.

In our service in Geneva, with each new case, we first try to establish whether we are dealing with developmental deadlock and, if so, how it fits in with borderline pathology, predominant narcissistic disturbances, or psychotic functioning. These differences are more important than may meet the eye. They have the important advantage of facilitating exchanges with colleagues treating patients of other ages and, furthermore, have direct repercussions on therapeutic possibilities and preparation, the treatment framework, and the risks of failure. Failure is most likely to occur when the narcissistic pathology is in the foreground, as these adolescents have to fight their dependency needs and their massive defenses associated with self-sufficient omnipotence. On the other hand, patients with more typical borderline pathologies have greater and more urgent needs for dependency. Finally, adolescents with clearly established psychotic functioning (as opposed to those with psychotic episodes as, e.g., in a suicide attempt) are often submissive to external figures who represent more or less virtuous or powerful maternal images, which reduces the risk of therapeutic failure.

In the course of many years, our work in Geneva has enabled us to acquire a great deal of experience with long, intensive psychotherapies (three weekly sessions for as long as necessary, and generally with the patient facing the therapist, at least in the beginning) or psychoanalyses (four weekly sessions with the patient lying down) with borderline, narcissistic, or psychotic adolescents. These treatments are based on a very important concept: transference psychosis. I cannot imagine long psychoanalytic treatment of such patients without transference psychosis, which refers to the state in which within/without, past/present, and internal/external reality are confused or even excessively condensed. It is only through transference psychosis within the here and now of the analytic framework that the patient can relive his breakdown and progressively understand its meaning.

The most important aspect of developmental breakdown is to maintain the idealization of the ideal body image that is pregenital and implies sexuality in a broad sense but without the need to join with a complementary object. This break in body representation is accompanied by overwhelming nonintegratable drives and/or the risk of disappearance of the object. These two states are qualitatively different from the growth of the sexual and aggressive drives that accompany normal adolescence as well as from the usual changes in identificatory patterns. Here we are dealing with a type of "raw" force, undifferentiated or poorly differentiated, and a danger of a breakdown in the identificatory process with consequent panic.

When this particular constellation occurs, some therapists advocate caution and prefer to function as a stimulus barrier rather than engage in a too intensive therapeutic situation with the potential danger of a *folie à deux*. When the therapist adopts a more cautious attitude with the patients we refer to here, and, even if it permits the slowing down of the counterdevelopmental process, there is the disadvantage of not getting to the heart of the illness and breakdown. This is the reason why we prefer, each time that it is possible, treatment that aims at undoing the pathological process, even though this obliges us to deal with transference psychosis, its repercussions, and the commitment it implies, as emphasized by Laufer.

It is not possible for a therapist to function efficiently without models: a model of adolescent psychic development followed by a model for therapeutic care. In private practice, the therapist may prefer only one technique that he will constantly try to perfect and will pass on to colleagues those adolescents whom he does not think he can help or who think that the proposed treatment cannot help them. In our public mental health service, which is *a fortiori* the only one of its kind in Geneva, the situation is more complex. The Geneva adolescent psychiatric unit covers a multiple population (with the exception, however, of mentally retarded patients, exclusively forensic situations, and chronic drug addicts). There are few alternative consultation possibilities because of the limited number of private therapists and the consequent costs involved.

Our theoretical reference is the psychoanalytic model. Our views of adolescence as a specific contributing factor to later psychic organization, as well as the characteristics of psychopathology and the aims of treatment in case of developmental breakdown, are all based on psychoanalytic theory in a developmental perspective. Even though these options are recognized and accepted, clinical reality obliges us sometimes to look for solutions that may not be optimal (in which case they should be the least harmful and guarantee an opening for the future). Clinical reality may oblige us to deal with family confusion when parents have lost their containment capacities and are helpless witnesses to the deteriorating psychic state of their adolescent child—whom we may never get to see at all or see only for a short time. We have to accept the fact that our status is that of a public service agency, and, as such, we must keep our doors open to all. This does not mean that we compromise our basic theoretical position but, rather, that we attempt to recognize mutual points of view.

The symposium's syllabus (that I established with Philippe Jeammet) is a reflection of this position. The choice of lecturers was based on the clarity of their ideas, their professionalism, and their authority in their respective fields. The first half was intended to allow a confrontation among E. Kestemberg, J. F. Masterson, and M. Laufer. Even though these three speakers all adhere to the psychoanalytic model, they nevertheless differ in some of their theoretical conceptions and the way they put their views into practice. It is true that the differences concern form more than content. As far as we know, Kestemberg, Masterson, and Laufer have never had the opportunity of presenting and confronting their clinical methods as well as their respective theoretical positions.

The second half of the symposium concerned two complementary aspects of outpatient individual psychotherapy or psychoanalysis: the family therapy approach, L. Kaufmann, and residential treatment, B. Muir. Personally, I am convinced that family intervention or even family psychotherapy *stricto sensu* cannot undo the psychopathology of an adolescent who has suffered a developmental breakdown. However, this approach may represent the best possible solution at a given time. The family approach may help reestablish hierarchical family organization or eliminate a symptom that may otherwise become autonomous and consequently destructive for the psychic economy. It may also help prepare the groundwork for future individual treatment. However, in situations where we deal with transitory difficulties but where the danger of developing more chronic disturbances cannot be excluded rapidly with any amount of certainty, I believe in the therapeutic effectiveness of family psychotherapy. Theoretically, we can associate these problems to assessment. Unfortunately, in practice, more often than not we are faced with a clinical reality that does not allow us adequate freedom of choice. It is also true, as Kaufmann reminds us, that a general theory of psychotherapy should include pertinent criteria to evaluate the predominance of either intra- or intersubjective disturbances. However, such criteria are still lacking and, in this respect, the Geneva meeting has not made any progress. This would be the only way to extricate ourselves from the perfectly sterile "holy wars," of which some systemic thinkers are unconditional supporters, in order to study complementary perspectives.

Adult psychiatric care over the last few years has been able to measurably reduce both the number and length of psychiatric hospitalizations with increased use of outpatient facilities and with the help of more flexible structures in times of crisis. Unfortunately, we tend to forget that an adult patient's psychic reality is not the same as an adolescent's, whether it be the psychic phase of development or, more generally speaking, the psychosocial condition. Both my colleagues and I are convinced that a certain number of adolescents imprisoned in developmental deadlock require long-term residential treatment if we hope to achieve a long-lasting cure of psychopathology and spare these patients future mental illness. We refer to those patients who act out in order to defend themselves against paranoid anxieties and attraction for dependency (i.e., make greater use of simple projection than projective identificatory mechanisms). In Geneva, we do not have this kind of institution or even short-term facilities for adolescents. It seemed important to include, in these chapters on adolescent psychiatry, a space for a discussion of long-term hospitalizations. Psychoanalytic hospitals are particularly rare; in Richmond, close to London, we have the Cassel Hospital with an adolescent unit. The association of individual psychotherapy with nursing care has been highly perfected, as is illustrated by Muir. This collaborative effort constitutes an opportunity for internal change as well as community life experience leading to, in the latter stage, successful outpatient treatment.

The articles that follow do not constitute a treatise on adolescent psychiatry, but they give a clear picture of how one can conceptualize the problems with which we are confronted on the basis of specific models of psychic functioning and development. They enable us to view the treatment of adolescents in a perspective that aims at curing the psychopathology rather than resorting to makeshift patchwork that only defers the problem to later.

NOTE

Translated from French by I. Frank, C. Kaelin, and J. Preiswerk.

25 ADOLESCENT PATHOLOGY: COMMENCEMENT, PASSAGE, OR CATASTROPHE

EVELYNE KESTEMBERG

First of all, I want to focus on the uniqueness of adolescence. For the psychoanalyst—and it is as such that I speak—the adolescent stage is a true challenge, because it is a difficult time for the individual to undergo analysis. We seem to know less about adolescence than other periods of life because we rarely undertake analysis with adolescent patients. We do, however, have much experience with adolescents because we can and do engage in long face-to-face psychotherapies.

I think that adolescence is a period that fascinates us all. It remains in our memory—a bit estranged, a bit nostalgic, a bit withheld. However, adolescence is neither merely Hamlet wondering whether "to be or not to be" nor always Rimbaud—because few have such genius—but is it often Cherubin. It is a springing forth. It is the ability to go from one state to another that is entirely different and to land on one's feet.

There is no lack of paradox. Although it is a wholly unique period, adolescence borrows symptoms and character traits from other stages in life. Very dramatic events and ways of self-expression are used (e.g., suicide). These themselves are not significant of adolescence, but it is the place that they occupy in this very specific organization that is indeed the real paradox.

When I say that adolescence is something entirely apart, I have to set forth a series of remarks for which I implore your indulgence. Adolescence is a unique period in human development in that it opens at a very precise moment and closes with a metamorphosis, all within a relatively short span of time in the course of an individual human existence. The past—that is to say, childhood—takes on its full importance, and although things are prepared for in childhood, they take their final shape in adolescence.

It is during adolescence—in the course of this period of crisis, commencement, and passage—that a catastrophe may take place. When I say catastrophe I mean in the sense explicated by Thom, the mathematician, for whom a catastrophe is that which, in a complex organization of elements, disturbs the previously established links that permitted those elements to remain in equilibrium. During adolescence a catastrophe may occur during which the elements, formerly set in place and in equilibrium, are cut off from one another and give way to a new—or apparently new—organization that reaches back into the past. I am, of course, speaking of elements within the psychic apparatus. On the one hand we are confronted with the organization of an adult psychosis that takes shape during adolescence. On the other hand, dramatic events may take place (drugs, serious intellectual inhibition, attempted suicide, morosity, bizzare behavior) without a catastrophe ensuing. This may just be a passage during which there is not a rupture among the different constituents of the psychic apparatus. Growth may take a more favorable course once the storm has blown over.

So it is that this period, during which the future of the adult takes shape, occurs at the precise moment that the body becomes permanently sexual. This is something that must be taken into account, because it means a fundamental reorganization of the entire psychic system. All the components of infantile sexuality are reorganized in anticipation of this new, awaited, and hoped for body. But, as you know, in many cases this new body is immediately rejected, because it is the seat of new sensorial, affective, and representational stimulation. There follow new ways of behavior and new cathexis. I am not only thinking of masturbation, for example, but of the ways of looking at oneself and one's peers, as well as the way one refuses to look or the way one feels that he is being looked at by others. This implies a major importance of autoerotism in counterpoint to object cathexis, because this body makes it necessary for a stimulus barrier to be put into place.

Second, this body excitation, a term that I use in its broadest sense, along with all the psychic apparatus that accompanies it, brings about a resexualization of the sublimated desexualization or a socialization of the latency period. This is perhaps one of the most important events, because this resexualization may become the entire task of the psyche—that is to say, it may encompass intellectual functioning that then becomes subordinated. Should this be the case, we are faced with many serious difficulties. Relationships with the peer group are also to a large extent resexualized—but in a simpler fashion, because this movement is intended, at the same time, to ward off the sexual differences of these same peers. In other words, to stamp out sexuality under the pretext of showing it off or making use of it is, in any event, to stamp out its specific nature.

This new body, these new excitations, this new way of looking and behaving with regard to this body, give rise to a whole series of reaction formations and countercathexes. These are expressed by bizarre behavior, slovenliness, obnoxious attitudes, withdrawal, and other traits that do not necessarily correspond to an "installed" character but that are more or less behavioral paraphrasing—by reaction formations—that finally results in intellectual inhibition that in itself is very complex.

In the best of situations, things will not go beyond this plethora of countercathexes and reaction formations that are destined to establish a distance between the subject and his body, in spite of the fact that sexual pragmatism, for example, may take on a completely disproportionate importance in what seems to be an object cathexis. In more serious cases, there will be a cleavage with this body such that it will not only be rejected and isolated through the use of defense mechanisms but actually separated in a completely desperate attempt to be rid of it altogether. One of the most striking examples of this response is anorexia nervosa.

With respect to the body during adolescence, then, while one aspect of castration is abolished—that which says, "I am little in comparison to adults who are big"—another aspect prevails. The adolescent must choose once and for all to be a man or a woman. He has to renounce having both sexes, renounce ambiguous ambisexual, archaic imagos that carry with them—or upon which are placed—the ego ideals. This also implies that one must inevitably readjust the relationship with parental representations and with one's actual parents from day to day—but most especially with the idea one has of one's parents, owing to the fact that the relationship with them is more sexualized than it has ever been before. There is also the necessity of integrating infantile sexuality—or, on the contrary, evacuating it. The adolescent is confronted with sexual differences and with the sexual relations of his parents, as well as the fact that now he himself can have the very same sort of sexual relations that his

457

parents have together. The fact that he now has this potentiality and feels it within his body—the fact that his body is identical to that of an adult—means that he may refuse to assume the identity of his parents. This is true to a large extent, but in the most favorable cases, it is only temporary. Troubles with identity and with identification will take place and perhaps take root.

This may lead to one of the most serious consequences of the adolescent crisis—depression, owing to the loss of infantile representations and one's infantile self, which means the loss of a part of oneself. The extent of this depression is something that must be carefully weighed when assessing an adolescent. This depression is accompanied by an inflated ego ideal and identification processes. This is not unusual but typical, and it could be useful, for example, in promoting certain moments of asceticism. It could, however, aggravate the depression, since it widens the gap between what the adolescent wishes to be in his fantasies—both conscious and unconscious—and what he actually sees himself as being or what he accepts as being the reality of his existence.

In very drastic cases, we have the following situation: rejection of the body and an attempt at ridding oneself of one's own body, depression, and idealization. In less drastic cases, even though we may see this response take shape through different behavior patterns, it is not necessarily the definitive way that things may or must turn out. This is where adolescent symptoms are deceitful. We may be confronted with apparently dramatic symptoms that express those three elements of repudiation of the body, depression, and idealization. Yet these symptoms may give way with remarkable ease on the occasion of a meeting either with a therapist or someone who is not a therapist. It is then that the adolescent can choose either to identify with the person he has seen or to accept the recognition of this person who lets him remain what he was.

Perhaps one of the most spectacular examples that I have seen in this respect is the evolution that took place in an adolescent who came in, settled himself down, said, "Things are going badly," and then did not say another word. I let him remain silent. A quarter of an hour later I asked him, "Is that all right now?" He answered, "Yes, I want to come again." I said, "Okay." And so he came back a dozen times, always just as silent, looking but apparently not seeing. Then I learned—not from him but, as is often the case with adolescents, from his parents—that he had given up his studies and that the situation seemed totally catastrophic. On one of the last times I saw him, he said, "You know, I have to tell you, I've gone back to my studies." I said, "Oh, because you had left them?" He asked me, "You mean you didn't know?" I said, "I knew, but not through you." And to this he responded, "Well that's only natural." This sort of extraordinary attitude, defiant and yet confident, permitted us to get along well together on this basis. He was able to emerge from the universe to which he had withdrawn without too much effort, even though it took him several months. To be truthful, I never understood what took place, but I think he appreciated the fact that I respected his way of consulting me, which in his case meant not speaking to me and my letting him come when he wanted at intervals that he more or less chose himself. However, when he had planned on coming and did not show up or when he came late, I told him that he could not do that. So there was a minimum of framework. Some months after he had gone back to his studies, he wrote a long letter explaining all his difficulties and telling me how much his having met with me had saved him from becoming "psychiatric."

I mention this case because these are the actual words used by today's adolescents; they are afraid of becoming "psychiatric." This use of the word psychiatry should give us food for thought. The adolescents of today fear, as do we all, madness. Only they no longer call it madness; they call it psychiatry! I find this very interesting, because it is quite important for us to realize the extent of the impact that our spoken words may have—as well as the impact of the very fact that we try to understand them or put them in a framework. This fear of becoming "psychiatric" is not specific to adolescence; perhaps not children, but certain adults I know express themselves in this way, too.

Coming back to my line of thought, I must note that in adolescence we are confronted with a period of life in which the oedipal constellation—reactivated by the inevitability of a sexualized body and the excitations it provides and by the resulting difficulties that appear in the patient's psyche—is upset in its balance. This development causes the patient to question all the components of infantile sexuality, all former internal adjustments and organization, such as socialization, certain sublimations, and many of the defense mechanisms that were destined to structure the decline of the oedipal period. The questioning of former identifications brings about an identity crisis, which will either be overcome or not.

This is the framework within which my thoughts have developed. Let me add that when I have to assess what is taking place concerning an

459

adolescent, these are the criteria I use. On the ordinate I place the different disorders that the adolescent presents—above all, the extent of depression, the importance of the ego ideal, the identity crisis, the pitfalls of identification, and the rejection of physical excitations and infantile sexuality. This is to say that I take into account either new reaction formations, if these exist, or, on the contrary, the disappearance of what former symptoms may have been present. On the abscissa I place the new economy of autoerotic cathexis, that is to say, narcissistic cathexis, object cathexis, and the evaluation of object implication in narcissistic cathexis. Inversely, I also consider the autoerotic aspects of object cathexis, such as certain peer relationships. I place much value on intellectual functioning, because inhibition on this level may have a dramatic effect on the scope of the depression itself and because poor intellectual functioning deprives the adolescent of the pleasure of activity that is autonomous with respect to his parents. I also weigh the importance, the economy, and the scope of reaction formations, because they may be of such a nature as to weaken the ego so greatly that identifications cannot be restored. This may lead to a catastrophe. Faced with excitations of a violent nature that indicate the extent of countercathexis and reaction formation, I try to discover what inner resources are still available in order to render former internal organization more supple, avoid a rupture, and reintegrate those organizations that had previously been established.

Case Example

In order to illustrate this outline, I would like to relate a clinical case. I have not chosen a simple case that could be easily labeled right from the start. I will submit the treatment and the assessment of a young patient, a young man whose treatment ended ten years ago, for your wise consideration. I had decided on an outpatient treatment, with no recourse other than psychotherapy. I now have a ten-year perspective, and I also know what has become of this young man since.

This adolescent was fifteen years old when I met him. As is often the case, I met not him but his parents first. I say this is often the case because generally I do not meet with the parents alone; I prefer to meet parents when they bring the adolescent and to see them alone after explaining to the patient that it is now the parents' turn to speak. I prefer this method because I like the adolescent to hear what his parents think about him and how they see him, since he himself so often expresses what he thinks of them. This first confrontation of different viewpoints is generally useful. In this particular case, the parents had come to see me, saying that they were extremely worried about their son, the eldest of their two sons and two daughters, in whom they had evidently put all their hopes. They were most upset because this child, who had up until now fulfilled their expectations, had refused to continue his scholarly efforts, was frighteningly filthy, and bought all sorts of abominable animals into their house. He refused to speak and was totally uncouth. His parents, truly nice people, were sufficiently masochistic to accept his animals and even his filth, but, as is often the case, they could not accept his intellectual failure and the fact that he rejected his former brilliant school career.

This is about the way things were presented. As for his early childhood, he had been desired and had given no problems to his parents. He had walked, talked, and been toilet trained at an early age. He had gone to school without any mishap; in short, there had apparently been no major problems. He accepted his brother and sisters fairly well and had just the right amount of ill temper.

What the parents did not tell me—and what I only learned later—was that as a child (and I have often noticed this in difficult developments) he had organized, at a very early stage, something that suggested the existence of obsessional neurosis, a haunting doubt. He collected lots of things, but this had not seemed to be a source of much worry. On the other hand, what he told me much later was that since the age of five years, as soon as he did anything, he immediately felt he had to undo it; he became seized with doubt and uncontrollable fear. For example, he would decide to play such-and-such a game and then would be overcome by a state of panic, wondering if he was or was not going to play what he had decided. My long experience as a child analyst has taught me that children who are subject to this sort of doubting, which is directly related to concern about death, usually have a difficult adolescent period. Children with this profile are more likely heading toward a catastrophe than toward a commencement or a passage!

Let us go back to our young man. I asked the parents, "Is your son himself willing to come?" And what they answered was so evident that it made me realize that although we may often ask silly questions, we do not always get silly answers: "How do you expect us to know, because whenever we say anything he always says 'no'?" Of course, I should have foreseen this. Nevertheless, I did want to know whether or not the boy was willing, and so I told the parents to bring him along and that I would then see. They came back with their son, who, in their presence, stared at me with a completely facetious expression. He was remarkably dirty. The contrast between his appearance and that of his refined, elegant parents was unbearably provocative.

Then I saw the boy alone. I said, "Okay, listen, let's talk seriously. Do you want to come or not? If you don't want to come, there's nothing I can do, so we can just leave things the way they are and not bother." After a moment's silence, he answered that he did want to come and that in actual fact he was not feeling well. He said he was not well because nothing interested him, and shortly he began to let me know about his depressive experience. He did not say, "I'm sad," "I'm worried," or "I'm unhappy"; he said, "Nothing interests me." This was the beginning. First he came twice a week, and then we agreed together on three sessions per week. It was a long treatment. I am not going to tell you about all of it in detail; I will just present you with the outstanding moments. First, I will describe his behavior and the effect it had on me. I feel this to be a useful approach because what we ourselves feel seems to me to be of vital importance for the treatment and the assessment of adolescents. This boy had a very particular way of behaving. We would sit facing each other. He would sit on just one quarter of his buttocks, twisting himself three-quarters around in a complicated way so as not to look at me and yet to be able to see me. He did not hide his face with his hands and peek out through his fingers the way little children do. He would turn his head from one side to the other continuously, like a metronome, in order to have a glimpse of me en passant. He would make a face each time he thought that I could tell he was looking at me. This would go on for three-quarters of an hour. I must admit that it was rather tiring, but at the same time it gave me the feeling that something was being conveyed from him to me. I was thus able to imagine that his arrogant attitude, his increasing un-cleanliness, his silence, and even the insults that were to follow were not only defense mechanisms but the sign of an overwhelming cathexis that he found intolerable. This perception of "overwhelmingness" brought to my mind at that moment the image of a psychotic type of organization, even though the boy was only fifteen years old.

When he began to talk (between two peeks, so to speak), he declared that if he had stopped going to school it was because it was absurd to go; what one did in school was completely ridiculous. Of course he had been mentioned for the "*concours général* (an especially difficult competition held for the best students in all French high schools), but what could be more idiotic than that?" Of course it would please his parents, but his parents "could go . . . they were . . . ." I will leave his words to your imagination. He had greater ambitions; he had decided to serve God. I wondered at the time whether he was going through a mystical crisis, which I would have considered a favorable sign, or was considering joining a sect, which would have been less encouraging, or had hallucinations about being God's servant.

In fact it was neither a hallucination nor a mystical crisis. It was his ideal. He had contemplated how to serve God and thought that one way was, as Corneille's Polyeucte would have said, to embrace "the delicious springs of fertile misery." He gave up everything that was pleasurable, enjoyable, and good in favor of an ascetism carried to its utmost, with of course all that this meant to his parents. I brought this to his attention. I said that it was all very well to serve God but that God had also professed the love of one's fellow man and that with regard to his parents this love did not seem to be in evidence! He answered me with a confused passage from the Gospels. This was as far as we had come, but, in passing, I was able to pinpoint his aggressiveness and reassure myself as to his psychosis.

At this point, a behavior pattern started that lasted two and a half years and probably should have alarmed me more than it did. He began to insult me in an absolutely crude manner and to send me injurious letters twice a day. It was completely crazy. There were vile insults on the envelope and on every visible piece of paper. The letters were not sealed, or if they were it was in envelopes covered with obscene filth, drawings such as can be seen in public washrooms. He sent postcards of the same nature, which displayed a mixture of phallic exhibitionism and excremental language that was entirely overt and astonishing. Incessantly I received the same letters. The postman thought it was funny; I did not. Furthermore, I was extremely worried to see him carried away by an excitation over which he had no control. He was even more out of control when it became time for us to take leave of each other for the holidays. This led to bizarre acting out: on one occasion he tried to strangle me a bit; on another, he stalked around my house, and one evening when I had some colleagues over for supervision, he thought of nothing better to do than to put a padlock on the garden gate and lock us in. I found myself in a very difficult situation, not because we were locked in—a locksmith came to let us out—but because I knew this to be his work yet could not come out and say so because I had not seen him do it. I was certain he was the one, and I wanted to see how long he could hold out without mentioning it to me. I spoke to him about his letters, asking him what effect he thought they had on me. He answered (and this reassured me), "I don't give a damn; I just feel like sending them." I told myself that this burst of filth, while it did not denote an extraordinary self-control, was at least in some way connected with him. He was not completely alienated from his action, and I could use this as material for his analysis. On the other hand, the incident of the garden gate was very difficult to handle because I could not speak of it. He did not speak of it either. We took leave of each other for the holidays. He continued to send me insulting letters, and, after holiday time, he did not show up for his sessions. However, he continued prowling about my house. He had not been in my house for some time, but I could see him lurking about. I wondered what to do—should I show him that I knew, do nothing at all, or wait. In the end I decided to wait. When he came back he spent a number of sessions without saying anything, and then he blurted forth, "I saw you with your husband, and don't try to deny it!" This was all in his head, and he had "seen" it. Thereupon ensued a kind of unleashing (I cannot think of a better word) of the picture he had of his parents, whom he had perhaps seen, and all this meant that his parents were the way they were and that one is never alone. This was a lapsus, and that is why I mention it. I suggested that in these circumstances perhaps he always felt very much alone, and he came to the conclusion that even with God he felt alone and said that he had given up serving God.

At this point I was very concerned and wondered how all of this was going to terminate. He decided that he would continue coming. He became cleaner. He did not talk much, but I was especially worried by his outbursts and unleashing of enactments, of his completely "crazy" way of behaving. Then one day he finally said, "I think I'm going to tell you my dream." What a relief I felt! He told me of a very simple dream: he came into my house, it was closed, nobody was home; he went in; he stood there; he was feeling very well; he was in my office; he sat in my armchair. Indeed, he would "sit in my armchair" and would spend a lot of time analyzing me, that is to say, he would interpret every one of my moves, all that I did or did not do. Once, things were relaxed enough so that I was able to say that, in any case, one thing that I did do was continue my studies. To this he answered: "Yes, that's true, but I intend to go back to mine." And so it was that he decided to take up his studies three months later. He was almost seventeen and had lost two years.

At this point I want to bring your attention to the coexistence of two factors: not only did he tell me of his childhood memories but also of his transvestite behavior when he was a child. He would put on his mother's clothes, expecially her bra, and look at himself in the mirror. Then he would wonder if someone had seen him or not. This goes back to his doubts, which I mentioned earlier but about which he had never spoken. Then, through association and after a long process of elaboration, he spoke to me of his childhood homosexual experiences and of how this had disgusted him. He also spoke of his recent liaison with a friend. Had I been his mother, I would have considered this friend "a bad influence." As a matter of fact, his friend drank and took drugs, as did my patient later on. He later broke off with this friend, but he was able to relate to himself through this peer (even though he was not perfect and had problems, he did have many things to offer, despite the fact that he used drugs) and to recognize his own depression through the depression of another. This awareness of another, this ability to identify himself with someone other than me, seemed to be a favorable omen.

I left things as they were. We kept on with our three sessions. I had considered having him hospitalized, but in the end I had decided not to do so. From a more and more confirmed homosexuality—not necessarily in his actions but in the fact that he himself accepted and recognized it—he passed to admiration of his father, which he entirely regained. He began to feel that I was really just a pitiful woman, and he did not know if he would keep coming much longer.

Conclusions

At just about the time when he stopped considering me to be a pitiful woman who desperately needed him in order to survive, he resumed his studies, found other friends, rediscovered his father—for whom he had a certain respect—and once again was able to work and to dream. The business of the letters was over; the incident concerning the lock on the garden gate was brought out into the open. Then he said that he wanted to end his treatment at this point. This was the first time that he had actually used the term treatment. I said that I was willing and that he should decide when. However, I told him of my feeling that he should undergo analysis later on, because he was interested in what went on within himself. He listened to me with pleasure. We stopped the sessions two weeks after his decision. I learned that he started an analysis three years ago. You will not be surprised to learn that he also began to study psychiatry.

I will stop here. I think that this very complex case raises many questions. In treating this patient I chose not to deviate from a psychotherapeutical approach, not to give too much credit to the idea of a psychosis, and to believe that the dice had not been irrevocably tossed in order to be able to keep on believing that this was a passage and not entirely a catastrophe.

NOTE

This article was translated from French by S. Clot.

JAMES F. MASTERSON

A key consideration in psychotherapeutic work with the borderline patient (adolescent or adult) is the identification, tracking, and bringing to
the patient's awareness the clinical vicissitudes of the operation of the
borderline triad: separation-individuation or self-activation leads to
anxiety and depression, which leads to defense. Confrontation of the
defense leads to awareness of the underlying abandonment depression,
which can then be worked through.

The borderline triad, similar to drive derivative defense constellations
in neurotic patients, does not necessarily announce its presence dramatically and clearly, although sometimes it may. More commonly, the clarity
is masked, and the therapist's attention must be given evenly and objectively to all levels of his or her patient's reporting to avoid imposing the
theme on the patient. Rather, as he listens, the clinical details of the
sequence become so evident, so stereotypical, and so repetitive that,
through observation, hypothesis testing, and confirmative patient response, the therapist can establish its validity. The therapist must then
carefully and gradually bring this knowledge to the patient's awareness
through confrontation as the patient becomes emotionally "ready" to
deal with the affective consequences.

The following case example illustrates this process:

Jean, Age Seventeen

Chief complaint.—Jean complained of difficulty managing her weight,
either "pigging out" and gaining thirty to forty pounds or drastically
dieting for the past four years. These complaints had increased in severity

in the past two years, following her sister's marriage. She avoided going to school when overweight because she felt she was so "disgusting," and in the last year she had missed fifty days. She reported being depressed but not suicidal and of being more in conflict with the father than the mother. Jean had had two years of prior treatment twice a week, without any change.

The mother's complaints were: Jean was unmotivated, irresponsible, did not take care of herself, her clothes, or her room, and she slept all day, demanded the mother's time, and was disrespectful and wanted to be waited on.

The father's complaints were: she was selfish, lazy, demanding, and spoiled, did nothing for anyone else, she expected to be waited on, and she tried to get everything she could out of him.

Past history.—Jean was born to an upper-middle-class family, the second of three children, with a sister six years older who had adapted quite well and a brother two years younger who in the family was viewed as the "ideal" son. Jean was described as essentially a "contented and happy baby." At her brother's birth she had temporary loss of bowel control and a retreat to the bottle. She used a pacifier until age three. Early development was otherwise normal. She evidently had no difficulty starting school, where she did well and had no problems socially or any later evidence of childhood symptomatology. There was much rivalry between her and her younger brother. There were four changes of residence between ages seven and fifteen.

Menarche occurred at age fourteen without menstrual problems. She had had dating relationships with boys but little sexual activity, feeling that boys were "out to get what they could from her." She had just graduated from high school and was planning to go away to college. Her principal outside interest was singing.

A brief evaluation of the parents showed the father to be narcissistic, angry, and demanding. He had been sent to a boarding school by his father because of stealing and discipline problems. He was very successful in business. The mother's father died when she was a child, and her mother remarried when she was an adolescent. The mother graduated from high school and then married the father at age twenty; she had had two abortions and three children by age twenty-seven. Although she was an attractive, compliant woman on the surface, Jean described mother as idealizing father but unable to be physically affectionate and extremely resentful of the burden of being a mother, particularly for the patient.

Psychiatric examination.—Jean's physical appearance was striking: that of a very attractive teenager trying to look like a chorus girl in her mid-twenties—dyed blond hair, excessive lipstick and makeup, and wearing a revealing dress and spike heels. She was depressed, angry, and detached. There was no thinking disorder, and there was adequate and appropriate affect.

She described her prior treatment as follows: "The therapist said at first that my problems were 'normal and not to worry,' so I let go and got worse. Then she told me that I was in conflict with my mother. How could that be when I love my mother?" Jean would report other people's—that is, mother's, father's, therapist's—opinions about her, but had great trouble describing her own feelings and thoughts. She had no delusion of body image but was able to see herself as both thin and fat.

FIRST COURSE OF PSYCHOTHERAPY (THREE MONTHS)

Jean was seen three times a week throughout the summer. The therapist confronted the patient with the self-destructive and maladaptive aspects of her regressive and avoidant behavior and tried to help her get in touch with her feeling states. Despite the efforts of a very competent therapist, the patient resisted therapy, and there was no progress. At the end of the summer, against our emphatic advice that she should continue treatment, she left to follow through on the original plan to go away to college. She managed to get through the first semester, having great trouble with depression, dieting, and binge-eating. Finally, in the middle of the second semester, she was no longer able to manage because she was again missing classes. She dropped out and returned to see me for consultation.

The prior work had convinced me that Jean's diagnosis was a false-self type of borderline personality disorder: that her pathological defenses had become identified as her self-image, and that she would be a difficult treatment case, especially in the light of the two failed attempts. I decided to undertake the treatment, and as a condition recommended that she should not live at home and should have a job. These environmental arrangements were suggested to deal with two aspects of her psychopathology: to physically remove her from constant contact with negative parental projections and to place her in an environment where she was required to take responsibility for herself, thus providing an obstacle to her regressive, dependent behavior whose defensive function was to

469

avoid the internal experience of anxiety and depression. I recognized that this recommendation ran the risk of resonating with her rewarding unit and reinforcing resistance that would have to be dealt with later in the treatment, but I felt the risk had to be taken since her regressive environment had played such an important role in defeating previous psychotherapy.

In the first few months of treatment, observations about her psychodynamics and intrapsychic structure and the clinical manifestations of her borderline triad made it possible to design a therapeutic plan. It appeared that the patient had been the repository or container of the negative projections of both the parents and that she was required to perform this function to process these feelings for the parents, in order that they not feel painful dependency and guilt. For example, the father, through the process of projective identification, projected his despised dependent self-image on the patient and saw her as no good, lazy, demanding, and doing nothing for herself. The patient, therefore, had to identify with this projection of the father and act in this manner in order to defend him against his awareness of his own dependency needs.

The mother projected a different set of negatives. An empty, dependent, passive, depressed, compliant borderline woman in great conflict with her narcissistic husband, she felt the deprivation of having to be a mother and take care of these children when she felt so needy, empty, and deprived of dependency satisfactions herself. On the one hand, the mother clung to the patient, rewarding the patient's regressive behavior and withdrawing from her individuative behavior to defend against her own depression, thereby preventing the patient from separating. In addition, the mother projected her guilt and depression onto the patient, who was required to contain and process these painful affects. Paradoxically, at the same time, Jean had to play the role of the mother's mother and listen to her problems and try to give her advice.

When Jean was born the parents, who had badly wanted a boy, were terribly disappointed. When the next child was a boy, they demonstrated in the most gross and obvious ways their preference for him. The patient, therefore, had to carry the father's negative feelings and the mother's depression and dependency needs. Jean did this by identifying with these projections and behaving in a compliant, helpless, dependent, little-girl fashion. The theme revolved around her own self-activation or assertion. If she did act in an autonomous or self-activated manner, both mother and father would attack her. In other words, as long as the patient was "bad," the parents could feel "good."

These themes were then internalized or introjected by the patient to form the patient's intrapsychic structure: a rewarding object relations part-unit (RORU) consisting of a maternal part-object, which the patient experienced as loving, caretaking, with a heavy emphasis on reward for regressive, dependent, helpless, clinging behavior. The self-representation was of being helpless and clinging; the affect that linked these two was very clearly one of feeling loved based on the mother's verbalizations, not on the reality of her behavior. The withdrawing object relations part-unit (WORU) consisted of a part-object representation of an attacking "witch" that was deeply defended against by splitting. The part-self representation was of being nothing, worthless, undeserving, useless. The affect that linked this part-object and part-self representation—abandonment depression—did not emerge until much later in the work and had as its major component a severe separation panic when she was alone or managed herself independently. The other ingredients of the abandonment depression were also present: depression, guilt, helplessness and hopelessness, a massive rage, that was also heavily defended against, and an absence of any feeling of self-entitlement.

THE BORDERLINE TRIAD

The borderline triad—individuation leads to depression which leads to defense—operated in the following manner: Jean's behavior was regressed in the sense that she avoided self-activation or individuation at all costs through compliant behavior with others—not operating in an autonomous or independent fashion. The abandonment depression and the separation panic with underlying rage were stimulated whenever: (1) an external situation like going away to college involved separation and required more individuation; or (2) she happened to make a more individuated move in her psyche; or (3) she was exposed to a neglectful or seductive experience at the hands of either parent. These separation and individuation stresses would trigger the depression (WORU) that would then trigger a bulimic episode in order to relieve it (RORU). Beyond this, and far more significant clinically, was a defensive detachment of affect. The patient would describe herself as feeling nothing at all and

471

being preoccupied mainly with what I would call rewarding part-unit daydreams. Teachers in grammar school complained of her "day-dreaming."

Through the operation of the splitting defense, she maintained that she had more problems with her father than with her mother despite many episodes of the mother offering material and physical rewards of regressive and clinging behavior. The patient accepted these only to later binge-eat in order to deal with the rage and depression that these seductions impelled.

PLAN OF TREATMENT

The treatment plan was to confront the maladaptive or self-destructive aspects of her regressive, clinging, and avoiding defenses and at the same time to try to help her overcome the detachment and get in touch with her affective states and how they related to her defensive behavior. She initially described overeating "only when alone . . . feeling desperate"; afterward feeling furious and hopeless and giving up, feeling her parents had given her everything, how could she "be this way"? She would then detach all feeling to enter the daydreaming state. She felt guilty, hopeless, and like a leech who had ruined father's life.

PSYCHOTHERAPY: FIRST YEAR
(THREE TIMES A WEEK)

My confrontations were as follows: Why did she not take better care of herself, her appearance, her apartment, her job? Why did she let other people dump on her? Why did she not activate herself and support herself? This issue became clarified in the first six months of treatment around discussions about two boyfriends whom she was then dating. One seemed healthier and more genuinely interested in her, but he made her so anxious that after dates with him she would have to binge-eat. Then she would avoid him. The other boy, narcissistic, clearly tried to exploit her solely for sexual purposes. She reported liking him and daydreaming about his caring for her. Her fantasy about the narcissistic boy was as follows: "He wants me. The rest of the world doesn't exist; it's just me and him—perfect. He's there—the first time anyone put me first."

Confrontation of the maladaptive vicissitudes of these two relationships made her aware that when she acted in a mature, independent fashion with the boy who really liked her, she became very anxious, "pigged out," and then wanted to avoid him. On the other hand, the one who was exploiting her relieved her anxiety about being independent, and she therefore felt better with him, although she was allowing herself to be abused, which inevitably ended up in reinforcing her bad feelings about herself. She integrated this confrontation, stopped seeing the narcissistic boy, and tried to maintain a relationship with the healthier one, but without much success. She was not yet ready to manage herself in an autonomous and independent fashion.

At one point, after a particularly neglectful act on the part of the mother, the patient had an outburst of rage and binge-eating, recognizing for the first time that she was expressing her anger and disappointment at her mother by the overeating, but it was quite superficial and did not last. She began to suspect that maybe she felt that her parents expected her to "screw up."

In the second six months she gained somewhat better control of her regressive defenses, affect began to emerge, and her ability to stay in touch with it improved. Work on her feelings and perceptions about herself and her relationship with her parents moved to center stage. She felt cheated, that she had been given nothing: "I'm stuck, and I don't feel I deserve it. I'm a bitter sufferer. My self is not important; I'm wasting my life away, lonely and depressed, so sick of no place to belong. I feel deserted. It's degrading to feel like nothing. I can't enjoy anything because of self-hatred. I'd just like to curl up and die. I feel dead, hopeless, and might as well daydream."

This session activated the patient's regressive defenses. She stayed in bed the next day—did not go to work or come to the next session. "I didn't care. I felt helpless, alone, nobody loves me. It's unfair. Everybody has their own life, but I'm stuck and I have no self. I want to feel needed, special, loved."

She now began to investigate the past a bit, saying: "As a child I always felt that way, but I also thought mother was so wonderful."

PSYCHOTHERAPY: SECOND YEAR

By the end of the first year, the patient's perceptions of parental scapegoating were deeper and more continuous. "My emotional instability is related to not being noticed or cared about. My failure is a reflection not of me but them. I felt like a 'thing.' All they seemed to care about is that they failed. How dare I think of failing and being depressed? It's like stabbing them in the back. My mother is so sweet on the surface. She makes me feel so guilty that I want to cry. They just want to be free from the burden of guilt. My father would sacrifice anything for his pride—his selfishness. How come my mother was never there for me? How dare she treat me as if I'm nothing? How dare Father tell me I should slave for him?" Here, for the first time, the patient is beginning to mobilize her aggression to support herself. The internalization of aggression defense is beginning to yield.

However, after the session she again became overwhelmed by guilt and depression. It then took several sessions of confrontation of the link between affect and defense to get back to the theme. For example, several weeks later she returned with: "Mother is a pitiful working machine; Father is a fraud, a fake, callous. I am a lost, helpless soul who belongs nowhere. My parents always have somebody else to blame, mainly me. They haunt me. They got me. I have no self. I'm at the bottom of the barrel. They wanted a boy, felt guilty about me, treated me as if I didn't exist. I had to bear their guilt."

This interview discharged some rage and depression. The patient's self-representation started to be restored. She said: "I felt good after that interview. When I'm not off in a detached state, I realize I'm smart enough to do anything, and I felt good about myself." Jean now was beginning to fight off the detachment defense after these sessions filled with rage and depression.

Several months later the emerging self-representation, the soundness of the therapeutic alliance, and the establishment of working through were further evidenced by a dramatic change in her appearance. She stopped dyeing her hair blond, removed the makeup and spike heels, and appeared as a natural eighteen-year-old brunette. She said proudly: "It's me." She also became more interested in singing and began to look for auditions with local bands. She was starting to express her newly restored self in reality. Still the enormous struggle with depression, detachment, and daydreaming continued.

A month later she was able to say: "I can see my own life coming together for the first time." About eighteen months into treatment, a dramatic incident occurred showing a further restoration of the self and self-supportive behavior. The mother again rewarded her regressive behavior, and the next morning she felt terribly depressed. "I didn't want to get out of bed, so I didn't. It's a constant battle. Then I felt over-whelmed, helpless, couldn't go on, couldn't handle it. Then I decided the hell with everything. I'm going to do something for me. Let them worry about it." In other words, she transferred affective investment from the object to the self-representation. She took off for two days by herself to think just about herself and let the feelings come. The parents called me in a panic, and all I could say was that I did not know where she was, but I thought that she would probably come to no harm. On return she said: "I decided I had me, and that's all I needed. I have to take care of me and not be so concerned about them. I have to break the pattern. I had to make a choice for myself and take the consequences, and now I have to follow through. I'm ready to do for me. I feel a solid grasp, a solid perspective." Nevertheless, she still continued to behave in the same compliant role with her parents, although she saw less of them.

Now the theme that had been played out in the environment began to emerge purely from her psyche: her attempts to activate herself precipi-tated all the symptoms that had formerly been precipitated by interac-tions with her parents. She would get depressed, binge, feel exhausted and detached: "When it's most important to support myself, it's most difficult. After the last interview, I felt positive about myself, but then I did it again. I gave up and cut off feeling and wanted to 'pig out.' I'm scared to death of that other person who gives up and wipes me out—the saboteur who pulls the wool over my eyes."

The progression-regression continued through the next several months. The persistence of regressions suggested that she might not be able to maintain the continuity of containment of affect necessary to create the conditions to work through the abandonment depression. I began to doubt her capacities. Did she not have the basic ego strength to work through? Was she part psychopathic, or had she been so rewarded for regression that she was unable to give it up? Or was she so masochistic that she could not give up the pleasure of the punishment?

I brought these concerns to her attention by saying that it seemed to me that she floated back and forth on issues about which she was quite clear. I was uncertain whether she did this because she was unable to control her behavior or because she chose not to. I noted that I did not observe the kind of struggle that would indicate that she was trying, but unable to control her behavior. I wondered why she seemed to give up on her self. This led to a renewal of her efforts to activate her self.

PSYCHOTHERAPHY: THIRD YEAR

Paradoxically, as Jean began the third year of treatment, for the first time she reported managing her separation panic about being alone without regressive acting out, detaching, or overeating. Several weeks later, in the setting of a separation stress resulting from my going away for a week, Jean again reported more mastery of her separation panic, "I left here scared. I went back to the apartment and realized that if I didn't instantly force myself into action, the infant would take over, and I would give up. I felt desperate, and I went jogging without even changing clothes. Afterward, I felt so relaxed and so good." The commitment to her self-representation overcame the regressive urge. I reinforced her efforts at mastery by pointing out how well she managed when she put her mind to it—the acknowledgment of her individuation she had never received. She continued, "But then, if I keep it up, I feel so lonely and angry at my fate, I have to blow it." These reports allayed for the moment my doubts as to her capacity.

Several weeks later the patient reported a dramatic dream outlining her WORU in the following context: "I was rereading my diary about my relationship with my parents, and I saw it was the same now as five years ago. I just wanted to give up. I couldn't sit there and feel bad, so I binged. I wanted something to knock me out and put me to sleep.

"I went to sleep and had the following dream: My mother was there telling me what to wear, but she didn't look like my mother. It was another woman, scary, with wicked eyes, a strange woman, a witch, an ugly monster who resented me and had it in for me. I was desperately trying to put the face of my mother back on the witch, trying to tell this woman with my eyes not to turn into the other woman, not to turn into a witch. I was holding my breath, and finally I was able to see my mother."

Her free associations: "I'm desperate to continue the fantasy of a loving mother. I can't bear to see anything different. As a child 'I used to feel uncomfortably bored.' That morning I had to drag myself out of bed to go to work. I wanted to quit. I was exhausted. I am brainwashed. It's too much to fight; I give up. My heart bleeds for myself and my innocence. Could it have been possible in the family that I was the good person?"

I interpreted that she seemed unable to handle the anger, disappointment, and depression at the perception of the mother's scapegoating (WORU). She would have to face these feelings about the witch in her head that were activated (WORU) every time she tried to individuate. She would have to master it in her head or it would continue to interfere with her emerging self-activation. She replied that when she sees the anger she panics and takes the anger out on herself by giving up and beating herself up.

The increasing capacity to contain and work through her abandonment depression rather than regress and act out to defend were illustrated in her reaction to my next vacation. She complained in the last interview of feeling empty, bored, and depressed and then reported the following dream: "I saw my little cat jump from a balcony, knew it was too high, screamed for help but no one heard. The cat jumped and was smashed on the floor. A helpless, innocent thing? Why did she leave me?" Her free associations: "People put me so low. There is nothing to my self! What difference could I make? I remember feeling this way when Mother had my brother. And then she ignored me even more."

For the first time I interpreted that she was reacting to my impending vacation as if it were a repetition of her mother's unavailability.

Discussion

ORIGIN OF BORDERLINE TRIAD

The parents verbalized love and affection despite their mutual neglect of Jean's individuative needs, and these verbalizations formed the basis for Jean's rewarding-unit fantasy. The father's negative feelings about dependency were projected onto the patient; the mother's negative feelings about independence as well as her depression were projected onto the patient.

CLINICAL PICTURE OF BORDERLINE TRIAD

Jean identified with these projections at the cost of her own individuation. Her self-representation of a good, obedient child linked with the affect of this unit—being taken care of—was allied with a pathological ego that required avoidance and denial of individuation, clinging, helpless, childlike behavior. The painful affects of separation panic, homicidal rage, and suicidal depression were managed by detachment of affect and binge-eating. She presented herself as a helpless, clinging, compliant, "beautiful" child who on the surface was loved for her childlike

477

behavior but who underneath was bad and wrong for her dependent needs.

THERAPEUTIC MANAGEMENT OF BORDERLINE TRIAD

This false-self, detached-affect facade had defeated the efforts of therapists to penetrate it for three years of psychotherapy and was the first clinical problem in treatment. In order to minimize regression and maximize the need for responsibility and self-activation, I required that she move out of the home and get a job in order to have to take care of herself. I began the task of dealing with the pathological ego through confrontation of the maladaptive and self-destructive aspects of her avoidance and clinging behavior as well as the detachment of affect involved in binge-eating. As a consequence of internalization of my confrontations, she began to take better care of herself, activate herself, and try to act in a more mature and independent fashion. She also attempted to get hold of and control the acting out through detachment and binge-eating. A pattern emerged of progressions that would lead to temporary control and movement ahead, followed by overwhelming need for regression. This process occupied the first year without the patient becoming aware of either the underlying affects that the regressions were to deal with or of what precipitated these affects.

In time, as she became better able to activate herself and to continuously control the defensive regression, she became more and more aware of two types of precipitating factors that produced painful affects that required regressive defense: (1) self-activation or individuative movement itself and (2) environmental separation experiences including parents' neglect or seduction.

There was also a relationship between the degree to which she was able to activate herself and the type of man she had a relationship with. During the first stage, when she could not activate herself, she had a very destructive boyfriend—a repetition of the relationship with the mother, whereby she had fantasies of loving and being loved by him, while in actuality he was narcissistically using her. As she moved into the second stage, her self began to emerge and she became better able to take care of herself and to activate herself. She dropped this boyfriend, and the next one at least verbalized and attempted to treat her more appropriately, but he, himself, was not able to be available because of his own problems.

After the second year of treatment, as her self-activation consolidated, she was now in her own apartment and managing both that and her job. A third male entered the scene who was the most appropriate so far in his feelings and behavior toward her. The regressions had become fewer and she had become more and more in touch with separation panic, homicidal rage, suicidal depression, and a profound lack of entitlement of self.

The progressive and regressive vacillations have often impelled me to seriously question whether Jean has the capacity to individuate and free herself from the bonds of the abandonment depression and separation panic. This issue, however, could not be put to the fundamental therapeutic test until the present phase of treatment, where it is seated securely in her psyche rather than in the environment, that is, where Jean perceives that any move toward self-activation or growth brings on a separation panic that she responds to by regressive defense. The issue has been joined, and progress is maintained, but its final resolution remains in doubt.

Conclusions

The case illustrates how the therapist uses the therapeutic technique of confrontation of the patient's pathological defenses to eventually bring the patient to the awareness of the operation of the borderline triad within her own psyche; individuation leads to depression, which leads to defense. It is the patient's awareness that this triad is deeply internalized and automatically triggered by separation and individuation precipitating stresses that secures the therapeutic alliance and binds the patient to treatment as the alternative of choice in dealing with her borderline problem.

27 ADOLESCENT PSYCHOPATHOLOGY AND AIMS OF TREATMENT

MOSES LAUFER

Those of us who work with the disturbed or ill adolescent are faced constantly with a range of views and techniques that may not only contradict one another but may also hold out a promise that one or another technique contains the correct approach to helping the adolescent with his or her psychopathology and to helping the therapist with his or her uncertainties. When an adolescent arouses in us feelings of helplessness, boredom, or anxiety, we ourselves may be prone to take hold of whatever it is that is there as an ally, whether or not that ally actually offers anything to the adolescent.

In these remarks, I have in mind the theme of the symposium. When we talk of which adolescents to treat, I would like to rephrase that for my presentation and ask instead, How do we imagine change to take place in the adolescent, and what part, if any, can we, as professional people, play in this process of change? And as regards the question of "How to treat?" I would be able to answer this if I could answer another question, which is, What is it that we are treating? Or what is going on in the mind of the adolescent that his present psychopathology is trying to express? Only after I have answered such questions would it be possible to address myself to aims of treatment.

I referred a moment ago to the range of views and techniques available to us; I have in mind my own experience when I began to work with the disturbed adolescent. I would like to tell you what these experiences were and also how I moved to the views I now hold about the nature of adolescent psychopathology and what our aims might be in treatment.

Perhaps I might start even further back. When I was a young adolescent in Canada, the brother of a close friend suddenly disappeared one night; or so I thought. A little while afterward my friend could tell me that his brother, aged eighteen, had gone crazy and had to be taken to a mental hospital by the police. Today this eighteen-year-old is just over sixty and he is still in a mental hospital. The secret has long passed, but the tragedy remains for him, for my friend, and for his family. That experience frightened me and has stayed with me, but it has also been a reminder of the suddenness, or so it seems, of the illnesses that transform the lives of so many adolescents. I tell you this story partly because I am convinced that this adolescent was not at all psychotic but that he had had an acute psychotic breakdown, and his whole life became organized around that psychotic episode, resulting in his staying in a mental hospital.

It was only during my psychoanalytic training in London that I could begin to ask the question, What was it that actually happened to my friend's brother? And could something have been done then, or before or after, to stand in the way of the psychopathology destroying his life? Of course, I will never be able to answer that question about my friend's brother, but I believe it is a question that has to be in our minds when we meet the disturbed or ill adolescent.

Following my psychoanalytic training, I began to treat adolescents as part of my psychoanalytic work, which also included treatment of adults and children. I was repeatedly faced with patients who had suddenly become ill or who were suddenly faced with a crisis: attempted suicide, anorexia, severe depression, paranoid reactions to people and things, violent attacks on others, and so on. My own disappointment grew when I realized that my adult work and my work with children somehow had not prepared me for what I was faced with in my work with the adolescent. But I felt even more alone in my work when I began to realize that so much of the literature on the adolescent and so many of the classifications of adolescent psychopathology rested wholly on the model borrowed from adult or child work. Only limited efforts were being made to understand what I believe is the specific nature of adolescent pathology. Or, perhaps, it would be more correct to say that so much of what was being described about the adolescent patient had to do with technique of work rather than with the meaning of the psychopathology and the understanding of the internal processes that brought about that pathology.

As for the development of my own thinking about adolescent pathology, the most important statements could be found in Freud's work of 1905 on the theory of sexuality and especially in his essay on transformations of puberty. Psychoanalytic theory and clinical experience have developed a good deal since that time, and perhaps much can now be added to what Freud originally said and meant, but there are certain fundamentals that are as useful today as they were when Freud first defined them.

Freud begins his essay on puberty with the following statement (a very simple statement, but the cornerstone of my work): ". . . changes set in, which are destined to give infantile sexual life its final normal shape." Later in that same essay, he talks of the process following puberty and that this process leads to what he describes as the establishment of "a final sexual organization." I want to concentrate for a moment on these changes as Freud thought about them and on the meaning that I believe Freud had in mind when he referred to a final sexual organization, because I believe that these are directly related to adult/adolescent psychopathology and they can be of much help in enabling us to define our aims of treatment. I would go so far as saying that I do not know how I could work with an adolescent without these ideas.

At puberty a process of development sets in that I believe is qualitatively different from what existed before. The presence of a physically mature sexual body forces every adolescent, whether his development is proceeding in a normal or pathological direction, to make choices that will, by the end of adolescence, result in what I believe is an irreversible sexual identity. Now, I use the word irreversible assuming that the person is not undergoing any type of therapeutic intervention. The image of the body during adolescence must alter or be altered to contain the functioning genitals both of oneself and of the opposite sex. It means in very specific terms that there is, during adolescence, an ultimate differentiation of oneself into male or female—which is not at all the same as boy or girl. And for the first time in one's life, incest is not only a fantasy but is now a possibility to which every human being must find an answer (whether it is a normal answer or a pathological one). And again, for the first time in one's life, all behavior, thought, and fantasy are now judged by our own conscience as being either a sign of normality or abnormality. For example, the boy of seven or eight may be closely tied to his mother and may unconsciously feel gratified by his passive submission to his mother. So long as he gets on well enough with friends, does well enough at school, and does not arouse the concern of his parents or teachers, then his life moves along at a more or less uninterrupted pace. But in adolescence this same person will now have to contend with his conscience, which may begin to accuse him of being homosexual or may punish him for his masturbation that may now carry with it the fantasy of submitting to a big and powerful woman. His earlier passivity has now been transformed into a sign of abnormality, and he may now begin to accuse himself and unconsciously accuse his mother for his present feelings and fantasies.

It is not at all uncommon for such adolescents to present themselves or be brought for help, but it is usually only after an acute crisis where both the adolescent and his family are surprised and bewildered by what has taken place. But what we may see in this adolescent, if he comes as a patient, is that his behavior now contains signs of what I describe as a breakdown in development. By breakdown I mean the unconscious rejection of the sexual body, the hatred of the body, and the need by the adolescent to maintain unconsciously the picture of himself as someone who is victimized, persecuted, or made helpless by forces within himself over which he has no control. By the time we see that adolescent, some compromise has already been found, and we may be confronted with a range of ways that the adolescent has found as his way of coping with the onslaught from his body and from the internal persecutors. But the point I want to make is that the breakdown in developmental process is the pathology. That is what adolescent pathology is. The various manifestations of the disorder, as we observe them in attempted suicide, anorexia, delinquency, and drug addiction, may help us trace the specific road unconsciously chosen by that adolescent both to live out the fantasy expressed in his pathology and at the same time to attack and destroy his own sexual body and the image of himself as a sexual male or sexual female.

I shall illustrate what I mean by way of talking about an adolescent who has recently begun his daily analytic treatment following a suicide attempt. This patient, whom I shall call John, is now aged sixteen. His father telephoned me soon after John had been discharged from a hospital following his effort to kill himself by drinking a bottle of paracetamol. All that John could remember was that his friends at school had begun to mock him and laugh at him. Now, whether this was a paranoid projection or not, I simply listened. I just wanted to know whether he was still in touch with what he had done. He said that as he left school he began to cry, and he then suddenly thought that there was nothing to live for. In treatment, which began only three months ago, John spent an enormous amount of time telling me stories and laughing in a loud uncontrolled way, and then suddenly he would begin to cry without knowing why. But we already have one or two possible clues into the meaning of his attempt and into the choice of wanting to murder himself with the overdose. I say murder himself because when we talk of attempted suicide we tend to forget that, in fact, it is self-murder.

Soon after treatment began, John got involved in a fight with a close friend; he said that he could have killed him. The provocation was when the friend called John a whore after John had told his friend that he had spent part of a night with a girl and that they had masturbated each other. John went completely berserk at being called a whore. He said that he could not think, and it did not matter what he did so long as he could destroy the source of that statement. A couple days after this event John came to his session with his hair changed to a different color, wearing tight jeans that showed the outline of his genitals, and telling me of his wonderful weekend, which consisted of smoking dope with a number of boys and girls. What we could establish some days later was that this wonderful weekend referred to the feeling that while smoking dope he did not know who or what he was. He had the fantasy of ripping off his penis and presenting it to his friend who had called him a whore. When John now talks of his suicide attempt, an important feature is that he feels unconsciously that he has succeeded in actually killing a part of himself and that he now carries around a dead part of himself. I do not yet know to whom the whore refers except that, in the transference, he has given me many clues to suppose that I, representing the dirty phallic mother, am the original whore and that he has to kill that whore inside himself. By so doing he will at the same time fulfill the fantasy of destroying his own male sexual body and be in the position of being able to offer his changed and, I think, now female body to his father. This feminine identification is critically important, but so is John's need to try to destroy father by continuing to get father to force John to submit to him and thereby to feel forced to attempt suicide again. And in the course of the three months a constant theme in the transference is that I should tell him that there is no hope, that I should tell him that he would be better off as a woman, that I should admire his different-colored hair. This would unconsciously be his way of telling me that he has brought the female part of himself so that I could then tell him there is no hope and he can then have a reason to kill himself. And this is, of course, a trap that one works with in the treatment of the very disturbed adolescent.

I have left out the whole question of the preparation of the treatment and what I did before I ever took John into treatment. I saw John over a number of weeks before I agreed to take him as an analytic patient. I made it clear that, with his type of disorder, I was not prepared to treat him unless he came every day. I might tell you that he is rather delighted that I have taken his pathology so seriously. In what I have said up to now I have referred to the developmental function of adolescence and to the critical contribution that this period of life makes to every individual. But by describing the period of adolescence as leading to the establishment of an irreversible sexual identity, and the pathology with which we work as being a sign of a breakdown in development, we have not yet been told anything about being able to know how to decide on the severity of the pathology that is present. Breakdown in development describes an interference in a process. This can be either a breakdown that does not at all represent damage to one's relation to the outside world, or it may be one that represents a break with reality, for example, the case of attempted suicide where there is a clear sign of the presence of severe pathology. But how do we know, and how can we apply what I have said to help us decide? Knowing about severity of pathology and being able to locate the areas of interference of development are necessary in our decision about the treatment that we choose to undertake and the aims of that treatment.

I do not rely only on the existing psychiatric categories to help me categorize what I may observe either at the time of assessment or during the course of treatment. Instead, I have in mind such things as the extent of the disruption of development, the nature of the distortion of the adolescent's relationship to himself as a sexually mature person, and the extent to which the adolescent's link with the external reality is impaired. I would define three main categories that address themselves to the various pathological processes of adolescence irrespective of the specific manifestations of the pathology: first, development that is dominated by defensive functioning; second, deadlock in development, which precipitates an acute crisis in functioning; and third, foreclosure in development where there is a premature end to the developmental process.

Defensive functioning can be divided into (1) that which allows some progress of development to take place—for example, where it appears as if there is only one specific area of the adolescent's life that is affected—

and (2) that which appears to dominate the whole of his functioning, such as his capacity to work, make new relationships, and so on.

Now, as different from defensive functioning, deadlock may be defined as the point at which the defensive process that was initially able to contain anxiety now fails to do so. There is in deadlock no possibility for development to proceed, nor is there the alternative of regressive functioning because this too is experienced as a source of anxiety. An example of deadlock in development would be attempted suicide, anorexia, obesity, the severe depressions with accompanying feelings of hopelessness, and so on. That is where the unconscious efforts to alter the image of the sexual body inevitably lead instead to greater anxiety and a greater feeling of passive submission or self-hatred.

Foreclosure means that the developmental process has ended prematurely. Foreclosure is characterized by an absence of anxiety. The main means of sexual gratification has been established without the adolescent having been able to allow for any change in earlier solutions to conflict. Here I have in mind such manifestations of pathology as the perversions, homosexual solutions, and addictions. I call them foreclosure because I would like to remind you that Freud maintained, and I think he was right, that the use of the word "perversion" should never be used before the end of adolescence. Here, I refer to those instances where the adolescent has given up doubting his answer to his developmental problem and where he feels that he does not want to give up his present answers.

There are those adolescents who present signs of perversion, homosexuality, or addiction but who at the same time experience their suffering as alien and as something linked to their sexual abnormality. This might, then, not represent foreclosure but should be considered as a deadlock in development because there is still the possibility of change in the direction of the adolescent's development and in the kind of sexual identity that is established by the end of adolescence.

The answers lie partly in the question of whether the main sexual gratifications are already lived out in his present sexual life or whether his present sexual life is primarily defensive and does not yet represent the answer that he has found to his sexual fantasies and to the kind of gratifications he seeks. For example, it may seem from my description of foreclosure that any adolescent who fits into this category should not be treated because all the signs are contrary to the possibility of success. It is often true that treatment may not get very far, and yet, I believe that it may be worth undertaking treatment even if there is the slightest possibility of change.

The example I tell you now is taken from my wife's work. An eighteen-year-old girl came to her and described her ongoing lesbian relationship. Although this had concerned the girl, whom I shall call Helen, she was primarily concerned about her isolation and her feeling that she might want to kill herself, especially if her girlfriend left her. Although my wife had made it clear that treatment would have to have the freedom to discuss anything that was relevant, for some time Helen's wish and need to continue her lesbian life was not touched at all. As far as Helen was concerned, this was not really a problem, except that she might be left. By the time Helen's girlfriend had begun a relationship with a boy and was, in fact, slowly giving up Helen, the transference had developed to the point where Helen's longing for my wife could begin to be understood and to be seen as a defensive effort by Helen to avoid the dread of wanting and being humiliated by her father. At the same time, Helen felt that life was not worth living if she was to be given up by her girlfriend. One day, on her way to her session on her bicycle, she came very close to being involved in what would have been a very serious accident. She could suddenly express her terror of her own death. This made it possible to confront Helen with the violence and the self-hatred contained in her choice of a lesbian life. Until then, there seemed little hope in the treatment—except that there were many signs during the treatment that her sexual life and the direction of her gratifications were as yet undecided. Although Helen enjoyed being held and caressed by her girlfriend, she also relied on masturbation for some gratification. The fantasy in the masturbation was not of loving or being loved by a woman but of being held and penetrated by an unknown and unrecognizable man. It was this, together with the relationship and the transference, that was the clue to the possibility that Helen's lesbian life did not yet represent a fixed and irreversible sexual organization.

I think I should add that one of the problems in assessment is that this type of contact with the unconscious usually comes in treatment and is difficult to determine during the time of assessment. Perhaps it should not be elicited early because it would be a way of destroying the adolescent's defenses. But there have been a number of instances in my own work and the experience at our adolescent center in London where such an outcome is much less likely. I refer to those adolescents who come, not because of their hatred of themselves as expressed in their sexual lives and in their object relationships, but because they unconsciously have to experience the feeling that there is no hope and that the person wanting to help is impotent. It is as if these adolescents may come to experience the unconscious pleasure from the revenge and the triumph over the person trying to help them. In such cases, it is not uncommon that their sexual lives and their gratifications have been settled well before the end of adolescence. The point I wish to emphasize here is that whether we are seeing an adolescent either for assessment or as part of treatment, it is critical not to make any decision solely on the behavior or on what it seems the adolescent wants us to believe. We must be guided instead by our own insights into the function of adolescent development and whether there is the slightest hint that the person's sexual life has not been irreversibly decided. My work with adolescents is on an individual basis, with the less seriously disturbed adolescents being treated once or twice weekly but with the more seriously disturbed adolescents, in the categories of deadlock or foreclosure, encouraged to have psychoanalytic treatment on the basis of daily attendance during the week.

At this point I want to limit my remarks to the treatment of those adolescents who have experienced a developmental breakdown. I want to concentrate on this group because work with these adolescents does not allow room for error, which means that the treatment we suggest is of great importance. Whatever treatment is suggested, it must enable the adolescent through the transference ultimately to understand why he had to have a breakdown at the time of puberty. It is only through this work that the adolescent can emotionally begin to come into touch with the meaning of the rejection of his sexuality and the attack on himself and his oedipal parent that the breakdown represents. What must also be able to be revived through the transference is the hatred of himself or herself either as a male or as a female. This kind of revival of hatred and rejection of his sexuality is what enables the process of the integration of his sexually mature body to progress again. For this to be possible, the treatment must use the experience within the transference as the primary tool for the understanding and the undoing of the psychopathology. The hatred, the blaming, the rejection of the sexual body, and the compelling need to force the analyst to take over responsibility for the adolescent's breakdown all must be experienced and lived in the transference. Unless the treatment makes this possible or, perhaps, more specifically allows for it to develop and to be understood, I do not believe that it is possible to undo the pathology and to influence the direction of the adolescent's final sexual organization. We can make all kinds of suggestions to the adolescent, but unless this is worked through in the transference it does not belong to him.

Conclusions

Although the aims of treatment that I have outlined refer to adolescents of any age, I think that it is appropriate and possible to enable a treatment process to develop with adolescents from about the age of sixteen. The younger adolescent is still too absorbed in his efforts to begin to remove himself emotionally from the oedipal parent. The time up to about the age of sixteen is characterized by the adolescent's still feeling that his body does not yet belong to him but is still the property of the oedipal parent. In such instances, individual treatment may have a difficult time and it may be better to postpone analytic treatment until the adolescent is slightly older. When I say postpone, I do not mean leaving the adolescent to himself—but not seeing him intensively. But whatever treatment is decided upon it would be wrong to compromise with the aim of the treatment—to come into touch with the breakdown and influence the direction of the adolescent's relation to himself and to the outside world as a sexual being. I am implying that to compromise with that means that you are allowing the adolescent to develop into an ill adult. Even though you may give him fancy ways of behaving, he will still be ill.

Appendix

I. THE SPECIFIC NATURE OF ADOLESCENT PSYCHOPATHOLOGY

Psychopathology in adolescence is a breakdown in the developmental functions of adolescence. Its primary interference is in the integration of the sexually mature body as part of the body image. Breakdown in development is the pathology, and it means that there must be an interference in the process of differentiation into male or female (a process that ultimately takes place during adolescence).

The breakdown that I am describing takes place at puberty. Whatever the prepubertal history of the person is, the breakdown at puberty is of a specific kind and must seriously affect the person's relation to himself as a sexual being, to objects, and to external reality in general. Such a view of pathology during adolescence does not alter with the symptomatology but seems to have relevance to the adolescent, whatever disorder he is presenting.

The period of adolescence is also a time when there is an integration of the person's past history. Breakdown will distort this integration and will, therefore, affect the person's life as an adult.

Such a view of adolescent pathology has direct bearing on our assessment and on our aims of treatment. There are specific principles of treatment that follow. These aims and principles are tied specifically to the developmental function of adolescence and to the breakdown in the person's relation to himself or herself as a sexually mature male or female.

II. HOW SUCH A MODEL OF ADOLESCENT PSYCHOPATHOLOGY APPLIES TO ASSESSMENT AND TREATMENT DURING ADOLESCENCE

A. ASSESSMENT AND DIAGNOSTIC CATEGORIES

Unsuitability of the psychiatric categories of adulthood exists. In adolescence, we are assessing something quite different, and, therefore, the categories of assessment must reflect this. There are three main categories, each referring to the extent of disruption in development, the nature of the distortion of the adolescent's relation to himself as a sexually mature person, and the extent to which the adolescent's link with external reality is impaired. These are: (1) development dominated by *defensive functioning*; (2) *deadlock* in development which precipitates an acute crisis in functioning; and (3) *foreclosure* in development, where there is a premature end to the developmental process.

Although each of these categories was elaborated in the presentation, what I mean is the following.

1. *Defensive functioning* can be divided into:

(a) that which allows some progressive development to take place—where it appears that there is only one specific area of the adolescent's life that is affected, and (*b*) that which appears to dominate the whole of the adolescent's functioning—his capacity to work, make new relationships, and so on.

2. *Deadlock* may be defined as the point at which the defensive

490

process that was initially able to contain anxiety fails to do so. There is no possibility for development to proceed, nor is there the alternative of regressive functioning because this, too, is experienced as a source of anxiety.

3. *Foreclosure* means that the developmental process has ended prematurely with the integration of a distorted body image and an inability to ward off or ignore any experiences that may create doubt in the solution found. There is an absence of anxiety. The main means of sexual gratification has been established without the person's having been able to allow for any change of earlier solutions to conflict (here I include perversions, homosexual solutions, and addictions).

B. TREATMENT

What is it that we are treating in adolescence? What should determine our choice of treatment? What do we think we can or should work toward in treatment?

1. *Aims of treatment.*—The need for the adolescent to know why he had to have a breakdown at the time of puberty. The adolescent also must come into touch with the meaning to him of the rejection of his sexuality and of the attack on himself and on the oedipal parent that this breakdown represents. The hatred of himself or herself as a male or a female must be understood, and the process of integration of his sexually mature body must be revived.

2. *Choice of treatment.*—Some doubts exist among many people about the possibility of undertaking treatment during adolescence. I consider the period of adolescence, especially the time from about sixteen to nineteen years of age, to be a most critical time for treatment to be carried out. Individual treatment is especially suitable, and other forms of treatment should be discouraged. We have to link the severity of the pathology with the intensity of the treatment. By intensity, I mean numbers of sessions each week, the place of transference and its use in the treatment, and the length of time that treatment should be continued.

3. *Some treatment principles.*—Here I refer specifically to the way in which the breakdown that took place at puberty must be a central issue of the treatment and must come into the transference for understanding and working through. Without this, it is not possible

to put the adolescent into touch with the meaning of his pathology, nor is it possible to reverse the pathological process.

It is essential to keep the treatment setting stable, predictable, changeless. This is related to the adolescent's precarious body boundaries and to his inability to allow the breakdown to develop in the transference unless there is a stability of the setting and a freedom to regress within the transference relationship.

4. *Preparation for treatment.*—Here I refer to the work of assessment, to the way in which we can use the assessment procedure to help the adolescent know what his disorder is about and what treatment is, and also how we can make use of our contact with the adolescent before treatment begins to create a framework for the treatment.

Plans, arrangements, preparation, and undertakings are of special importance; treatment may break down if such questions are not settled before the treatment begins. I refer not only to the recommendation for treatment but to discussing the adolescent's use of his available time, his school or work plans, where he will live, what happens if the adolescent needs hospital care, and the role of the parents.

28   THE RATIONALE FOR THE FAMILY
APPROACH WITH ADOLESCENTS

LUC KAUFMANN

No therapist dealing with adolescents in difficulty will dispute either the primordial role played by the family in the psychosocial development of the child or the importance of the ecosystemic context in understanding mental disturbances. However, interpretation of these relations and, in turn, conception of a clinical situation will depend on the epistemology that is taken as a frame of reference; this necessarily influences the choice and the strategy of intervention. My intention is neither to plead on behalf of family therapy or to pursue the debate among psychoanalysts and partisans of the systemic theory in terms of "verities" in a symmetric relation nor to refute the differences; rather, it is to describe a clinical situation at the level of the individual psychological process and at the systemic level involving interaction between several persons. But the question arises as to whether we can work with two epistemological frames of reference in institutions that deal with a psychiatric population from all walks of life and whose task it is to train therapists. Are these forms of approach incompatible or complementary?

The family approach may be described as a model of knowledge and treatment of mental disturbances that takes into particular account the family context. The family approach does not necessarily mean family therapy; it is more a set of therapeutic methods that include various family therapies as well as other forms of treatment—even individual psychotherapy, as I shall endeavor to demonstrate.

493

Socialization of the Child

As a living social organism, the family may be described as an open system. Its elements (parents, children) are markedly interdependent and interact among themselves and with the environment in the performance of certain functions. Its structure is never definitive but traverses a series of changes that promote the development of both the children and the parents. Like that of other living organisms, its structure is determined by the evolutive process, contrary to the situation of a traditional machine, in which the structure defines the activity (Capra 1983). The social organism known as the family has an internal flexibility and can modify certain conditions and—to a certain extent—its organization. This is possible because its elements are not too highly specialized and are able to modify their organization so as to either accomplish the same functions in a different manner or assume a new function.

The family system that develops in the course of the years is self-organizing. It has a relative degree of autonomy while yet exchanging with the environment; under certain conditions it is capable of autopoiesis. The cybernetic model of homeostasis (regulated through feedback) to which reference is frequently made within the context of family therapy is not sufficient to serve as a model of these properties. Fivaz, Fivaz, and Kaufmann (1983) propose that reference be made to a particular category of open systems, called dissipative structures, in which structure may change under the influence of external fields. I shall not present this model here, since it requires interdisciplinary competences, but I shall refer to it, and interested readers may consult the above reference for detailed descriptions and illustrations. The model permits simulation of the development in certain human systems, particularly that of a child, as an evolutive subsystem undergoing changes under the influence of the parents as the "framing" subsystem. Likewise, it allows simulation of a patient's development, as an evolutive, if blocked, system undergoing transformations during therapy (be it individual or family) under the influence of the "framing" system, that is, the therapist(s). Thus it defines therapy as a process that promotes evolution toward a greater degree of autonomy—and that is evidently limited in terms of time (Kaufmann 1983).

The model not only specifies the process of transformation (see Fivaz, Fivaz, and Kaufmann [1981, 1982, 1985] for detailed description and illustration) but also specifies the conditions that are to be fulfilled by the framing system as well as by the evolutive system to ensure a high probability of change as well as the stabilization of new structures. In this chapter I shall specify first the two fundamental conditions that the framing system (i.e., the parental or the therapeutic subsystems) must fulfill: (1) the influence of the framing system must be of a sufficient degree of constancy and greater than that of the evolutive system, and (2) the influence of the framing system must be adjusted to the developmental capacities and to the needs of the evolutive system. These two conditions define what in the psychological model is called the superior hierarchic position of the framing system. The upholding of this position by the parental system is ensured on one hand by the exercise of parental authority and on the other hand by optimal attention.

Parental authority, not to be confused with the exercise of unidirectional authority, takes effect in a system from the top downward. The attitudes and interventions of the mother and father in their parental capacity must be governed by the needs of the child as he develops, and their importance is especially crucial while the child is passing through a developmental change. The parents should pay optimal attention to (1) all communication emanating from the child, (2) how the child receives communication, and (3) the child's ability to comprehend the significance, within the context of the step in development to be taken, of "new" or "irregular" behavior. These criteria may be operationalized in such clinical terms as holding, informing, gratifying, or frustrating. The concept of the superior hierarchic position (relatively greater constancy of parental attitudes and adjustment of the measures they take) would make it possible to evaluate whether or not the parental subsystem favors the child's development (Haas, Doudin, Navarro, and Kaufmann 1985).

To fulfill these two conditions of framing, the parental system must also develop, but much more slowly. The evolutive potential of the parental system depends on, among other things, the individual experience and resources of the parents, their functioning as a couple, the type of insertion of the nuclear family into the extended family and its relations with the environment. In order to develop (at a rate different from that of the child), the parental system needs, in its turn, to be framed—and the functional family manages this need in a more autonomous manner than does the dysfunctional family. This notion of coevolution between the framing and the evolutive subsystems within the family is of considerable importance for the clinical assessment of a family being investigated or treated (Dell 1980).

During adolescence the framing conditions are more difficult to fulfill, for such various reasons as the following (see Fivaz [1984] for a detailed illustration of a functional family): (1) The family has to make major changes in its rule network in a number of domains; the parents and the adolescent must negotiate new rules that attribute control of and responsibility for certain functions to the adolescent himself (e.g., the matter of sexuality). The framing during adolescence implies a reduction in the number of direct controls, while the parents must continue caring in other forms—for example, by being present, by listening (without saying what must be done), by frustrating, and by grinning and bearing it. It is a question here of being available at the request of the adolescent and of remaining sufficiently predictable while decreasing the number of the direct measures taken. (2) The appropriate adjustment of parental attitudes and measures during adolescence becomes problematical because the parents are less well informed about their son or their daughter than they were earlier on. The world in which the child develops—this "transitional zone" he needs in order to learn through play—is now situated beyond the family frontiers (Kaufmann 1985), and the parents know it but little. (3) The parents of problem adolescents frequently missed, a generation earlier, the evolutive phase of their own adolescence and thus lack the experience, that is, the resources, for framing. They do not know how to "accompany" the adolescent. They are either unaware of the change he is undergoing or they overreact or dole out stock phrases. (4) The toleration by parents of the period of progressive separation from their adolescent children depends, far more than they realize, on their own ability to develop as individuals and as a couple.

Parental framing lasts approximately twenty years. What is it that permits functional families to retain their relative autonomy for so long a period in spite of all the influences to which they are subject? What is the structure of a human system in which processes of change alternate with periods of stabilization during which a new order is maintained for the time required—a situation termed consensual morphostasis by Wertheim (1975) and dynamic stabilization by the present model? And what has an adaptive system of this kind in common with a dysfunctional system that also continues to exist but at the cost of an interruption in its evolution (termed forced morphostasis by Wertheim and rigid stabilization by the present model)? Fivaz, Fivaz, and Kaufmann, as mentioned, propose that the stabilization of certain human systems be perceived in terms of the "resilience" property of physical systems in "phase coexistence." In these physical systems, two structures remain in equilibrium with each other in such a way that the value of a selected parameter is kept constant.

The difference between dynamic and rigid stabilization may be perceived in terms of ordered versus disordered "phase coexistence." In psychological terms, these two structures have been defined in terms of transactional modes: in dynamic stabilization agreement or conflict exists regarding the rule network, while in rigid stabilization, confusion exists regarding the rule network, a situation described in terms of paradoxical exchanges by Haley (1963) and in terms of dual-normal behavior by Fivaz, Fivaz, and Kaufmann (1981). The same model may be applied to psychotherapeutic framing as well as to parental framing.

EXAMPLE: PARENTAL FUNCTIONAL FRAMING

In order to regulate the contacts between the child and persons outside the family (= function), the latter has two different rules: R1, in which the contacts are monitored by the parents, and R2, in which the contacts are controlled by the child himself (fig. 1). Autodetermination of the family implies that its members are clearly aware of the two rules, perceive conflicts, and are capable of negotiating the allocation of the control of any given function. In the case of the dysfunctional family, its resistance with respect to external influences would be attributable to dual-norm behavior; the borderline between the two structures has become irreparable and the metarule is no longer discernible (Fivaz et al. 1983).

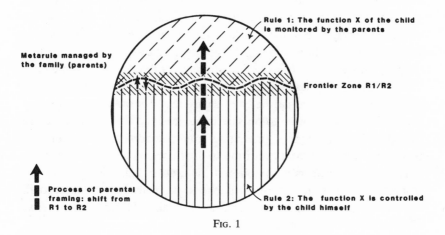

FIG. 1

497

I shall broach the subject of the dysfunctional family by focusing on symptomatic behavior—but in full awareness that the sickness and the disturbed personality are both more and other than the symptom. This approach would appear justified by the fact that it is the symptoms that bring the patients into contact with the therapists and the institutions. The family that is blocked in its development corresponds in its structure to dual-norm behavior. The symptomatic behavior of the index patient and that of other members of the family (who generally elude classical nosography) correspond to what frequently happens when two rules that are (1) of different hierarchical levels and (2) mutually exclusive (but not perceived as such by the members of the family themselves) are simultaneously enforced (Haley 1963), that is, its manifestations are unpredictable and paradoxical—and the disorder does not characterize just one member of the family but several, sometimes even the entire family. The transactions do not permit us to determine which subsystem has assumed which control function, and the various forms of behavior are no longer clearly correlated with the stages or the function given. The superior hierarchic position of the parental subsystem disappears, the framing conditions are no longer fulfilled, and the adaptive evolution of the system gives way to "pathological" evolution.

The probability of a family system's converting to the structure of dual-norm behavior is relatively greater at the time of puberty and adolescence, since the family must undertake overall change of the rules at this time. The risk of this structural accident increases when the major adjustment has not been prepared by means of progressive (and conflictual) modification of the allocation of control functions calculated to promote the child's autonomy prior to adolescence (or, more simply, when the family system has not "learned" how to change). As observation has shown, a family in which parents have overprotected the child right up to adolescence instead of framing its development sometimes corresponds to a system that "knows" but one rule—for example, "all a child's needs should be satisfied by his parents." The model indicates that such a family is sensitive to outside influences and that when these are disordered (by influences emanating from the adolescent himself, his peers, etc.), the risk of a transition to dual-norm behavior is very high. Once the transition is accomplished, dual-norm behavior reduces the system's sensitivity to external influences, particularly in relation to all information concerning the symptomatic domain. The system behaves as if it were "closed" and isolates itself, a circumstance that reduces exchanges and increases the possibility of a lasting blocking of development.

EXAMPLE OF A FAMILY SYSTEM IN DISORDERED DUAL-NORM BEHAVIOR IN RELATION TO THE SAME FUNCTION AS IN THE PRECEDING EXAMPLE

In monitoring of the child's contacts with persons outside the family, there is constant confusion between R1 (contacts that are monitored by the parents) and R2 (contacts that are controlled by the child himself). An adolescent girl, sixteen years of age, demands the right to do whatever she pleases, but her behavior (escapades, abuse of medicines, playing truant, contact with delinquents) is that of an irresponsible person and justifies the maintenance of R1. However, this rule is not applied because the parents are unable to agree on the manner of its enforcement and they appeal to the girl as arbitrator! Simultaneously, the new rule, R2, is merely invoked but not really applied either, because the adolescent fails to assume her responsibilities.

It is possible to comprehend the symptom as dual-norm behavior in different dysfunctional systems, for example, the individual, the family, or an institution. The confusion of two rules can be localized in an individual incapable of perceiving the conflict—and, as a result, unable to negotiate it. The ambiguity of certain neurotic or psychotic symptoms is well known (the instance that ought to manage the metarule but that functions only inadequately is the ego). When the disorder is within the network of family rules, not only the index patient but several other members of the family manifest dual-norm behavior.

Once the symptomatic behavior has established itself, the index patient has a well-known function in the family system—he ensures the cohesion of the system and protects it against separations that are construed as ruptures wherever the interpersonal relations are too immature to guarantee the continuity of the link (Kaufmann 1983). Thus, disturbances in an adolescent's behavior justify the family's preoccupying itself with him, and this can shelter the parents from their marital conflict. But, paradoxically, the symptom of the designated patient has another function; it announces to the world outside the family that the family is dysfunctional—it denounces it (Masson and Pancheri 1979).

499

Clinical data do not always allow us to attribute the symptom directly to this or that dysfunctional system. The symptom (phobia, obsessional ritual, ravings, escapades, delinquency, etc.) may announce an intrapsychic or family-system dysfunction. The task of the clinician is to identify the elements of the dysfunctional system by detecting the circularity in the evolution of the behavior of these elements. For various reasons it is difficult to localize this circularity: the system is an abstract construction with no body able itself to produce symptoms; the range of symptoms is limited; the circularity between the individual symptom and the family symptom is neither mandatorily nor necessarily dysfunctional (e.g., depression!); and the frontiers of a system in relation to others are not obligatorily congruent with those of the biological units (the individuals) or the social unit (the nuclear family).

It is not possible to discuss here the ways in which the clinician handles the uncertainty inherent in any hypothesis that defines and localizes a given dysfunction. I should merely like to stress that our ability to assess the correctness of a hypothesis varies but is always limited—and it is this probability that must determine our therapeutic strategy. The clinician accustomed to elaborating systemic hypotheses asks which function is controlled by what system. The probability of identifying symptomatic behavior increases when a given function is no longer controlled by the system that normally manages it but by a larger system that is, however, less well qualified for the job. The relational difficulties between an adolescent boy and girl are, for example, less well managed by the adolescent girl-boy-mother(s) system than by the girl-boy system or by the boy system all by itself; the parents' marital conflict cannot be validly administered by the mother-father-child system.

This axiom that the smallest possible system is optimal for a given function underlies all developmental framing and thus also all psychotherapeutic intervention whose aim it is to return the function in question, as far as possible and sooner or later, to the patient, be this an individual or a family. The professional or auxiliary systems (psychiatric institutions), mobilized as a result of the symptomatic behavior, tend to lose sight of this axiom and lend themselves to the extension of the dysfunctional structure to themselves. The more numerous the professionals are, the worse the coordination between them becomes and the greater the risk that the symptom will become chronic in a system that is both too big and rigidly morphostatic.

Choosing the Method of Treatment

Allow me to broach the question of the indication of the family approach by taking as my point of departure the following working hypothesis: (1) The symptomatic behavior of the designated patient is facultative in the sense that the development potential of the adolescent is more or less intact but blocked by the installation of a dysfunctional family regulation and not—or not yet or not mainly—by an intrapsychic dysfunction of antievolutive effect. (2) Restitution of the parental frame may possibly relaunch the evolutive process in the child. A temporary measure will aim at (re)mobilizing the system's resources with a view to achieving coevolution of the parental system and that of the child. The intervention in regard to the child is indirect; the therapist frames the family so that it, in turn, can frame the child.

This type of intervention has the following characteristics: (1) It is economical in the sense that, if it succeeds, it reattributes the function of socialization of the children to the smallest possible system chargeable with this function—the nuclear family. When I say economical, I am also thinking concretely of the cost in terms of money, time, and energy. (2) It allows, possibly, for exactly localizing the problem *ex juvantibus;* however, I admit that the mere disappearance of the symptom does not suffice to allow for any judgment. (3) Intervention within a family context (if it succeeds) restitutes or improves the competence and autonomy of the family, which, in turn, allows a relaunching of the development of the family system and the individuals.

EXAMPLE

A sixteen-year-old adolescent girl who played truant, indulged in escapades, and made abusive use of analgesic medicines (twenty to thirty tablets per day) for eight months was ultimately hospitalized. Even though we found that, behind her "characterial" facade, she was depressive, we sent her back and convened the family the next day, seeing them frequently in the course of seven sessions spread over three weeks. The girl tried blackmail: "If you [parents] do not let me return to England [where she had made the acquaintance of a lesbian educator], I shall continue with my escapades and go on frequenting the drug scene." We saw that the parental alliance did not function—for all manner of reasons.

During six sessions (in the course of which time the girl continued her escapades while yet attending the sessions) we attempted to get the parents to make a clear decision, in the presence of their daughter, regarding the England project. In the end, this was done. The next day the girl obtained information about the conditions governing an apprenticeship and shortly afterward commenced her training. Her symptomatic behavior, including the abuse of medicines, rapidly disappeared, not to return.

FAMILY APPROACH I: FAMILY THERAPY

This possibility, which is portrayed in figure 2, has its limitations. First, it is limited because the resources of the family are difficult to assess; generally speaking, these are underestimated, or the element of variable stress is not sufficiently taken into account. Second, it is limited by the evolutive potential of the therapeutic system—the personalities and training of the therapists; the guarantee of framing the therapeutic system by an institution; the possibility of coordinating the professionals engaged on the case; and the age, dimension, and degree of dysfunction of the preexistent "big system" formed by the patient, the family, the various institutions, and other professionals.

FAMILY APPROACH II

When the therapist reaches the conclusion that a therapeutic framing of the family (a framing that is itself aimed at making the family frame the child's development) is not feasible, the setting up of an auxiliary system

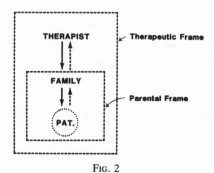

FIG. 2

to take on the family functions perhaps becomes inevitable. In order to reduce the risk of any extension of the family dysfunction to the institution, the setting up of the auxiliary system must be done in collaboration with the parents—a significant relationship must be established with them, and an exchange of information between the family, the patient, the institutions, and the therapist must be organized. The offer of real support for the parents is sometimes indicated, and it is always desirable that they be encouraged to participate in the therapeutic or educational program by entrusting certain duties to them.

FAMILY APPROACH III: INDIVIDUAL PSYCHOTHERAPY

As illustrated in figure 3 the classification of individual therapy among the family approaches is surprising only at first sight. The therapist treating an individual must inevitably touch the network of family relations—whether consciously or not. The patient is simultaneously an element of both the family system and the therapeutic system. In this version the therapist's influence on the family is indirect. The change (development) of the designated patient's relations with the therapist modifies the patient's relations with the members of his family and obliges the latter to make the changes that will enable it to leave the regime of dual-norm behavior and to take up its development afresh.

Concerning the model that is to serve as frame, the question of superior hierarchic position is crucial. The therapeutic system formed by the therapist and the individual under treatment must, in its relations with the family, be relatively more constant than that of the family; it must, in particular, not become a subsystem controlled by the family. Preference

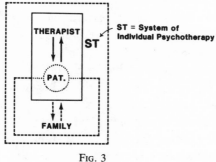

Fig. 3

503

will be given to this form of treatment when the following conditions are met: (1) The adolescent is himself motivated, demanding individual treatment sufficiently differentiated to enable him to assume the responsibility for his personal problems. (2) The members of the family (parents) are themselves also sufficiently differentiated to bear the change in the patient (the progression of his autonomy). Without wishing to make a hard and fast rule, it can be said that this differentiation is inversely proportional to the gravity of the clinical picture presented by the adolescent. (3) The therapist feels responsible for this therapeutic commitment in his relations with the other members of the family (even if he never sees them), a circumstance that implies, for example, the inclusion in the therapeutic work of the dimension of the loyalties—often formidable—of the adolescent to his parents.

According to her family, eighteen-year-old Marlyse was suffering from atypical anorexia. She was amenorrheic, had been vomiting after every meal for six months, and was losing weight. Her parents and the family general practicioner sent her to a pedopsychiatrist. The possibility of hospitalization was envisaged but refused by the patient and her family, and the pedopsychiatrist advised the girl's mother to come directly to us.

Marlyse was the youngest of the four children of a businessman who successfully runs a small enterprise. He is also a municipal councillor, a calm, circumspect man, an authority not to be questioned. The girl's mother, a teacher's daughter, has been busy and in a constant hurry from morning till night for the last twenty-five years and has acquired an enormous reputation as a worthy woman. The two eldest children, a son at the university and a daughter at teachers' college, now live at home only part of the time; the third child, who has a trade, and the youngest, the index patient, live with their parents. No one in the family has ever done anything remotely wrong; everything is ordered, balanced, and apparently thoroughly solid.

The first discussion between the family and the two therapists showed that the family was going through a crisis sufficiently serious to force it to take steps. The atmosphere was tense. The youngsters, if somewhat awed, were nevertheless accessible, and they talked—with the exception of Marlyse, who was dressed all in black, thin, almost "extinguished," pitiful—and all-powerful. Her mother, gentle and sad, kept her eyes on the floor. The father, ambivalent and very much put out, was visibly isolated. With the help of the siblings, the family and the therapists, in their first session, broached what, according to several members of the family, was the heart of the problem—the father-Marlyse conflict. It should be pointed out here that they were discussing this for the first time. The previous year Marlyse had had a friendship (platonic?) with a boy, and the relationship had not won her father's approval. She had been sent to Germany "to learn the language," where, in fact, she had been thoroughly exploited as an au pair in a family. She had been largely left alone with a baby while her young mistress, expecting a second child, went out with the master of the house. Marlyse was miserable and spoke of her difficulties when she returned home at Christmas. But her father insisted that she return to the German family and complete her commitment. She became even more miserable, was pursued by nightmarish ideas, began worrying about her mother, lost her appetite, and started vomiting. The moment she returned to her own family in April (to begin an apprenticeship), the vomiting became worse.

The hypothesis formulated by the therapists after two sessions took into consideration the individual psychological problems of the parents, the marital problem, and the family system, including the extended families of the father and mother. We were very much interested by the intensity of the link between Marlyse and her father. But taking the framing model as our point of departure, we asked ourselves the following question: What family constellation and what type of family transactions prevent the Marlyse-father relationship from developing spontaneously? And we found that there was difficulty (1) for all the children —and not only for Marlyse—in leaving their parents to themselves in the "parentification"; (2) in the loyalty, both invisible and misunderstood, of Marlyse to her mother; and (3) in the laws ruling the interactions, as imposed by the narcissistic and vulnerable father. (The law of the father is that one does not comment on relationships, that it is futile to express emotions, and that one must not attach too much importance to futile matters such as these.) We were, moreover, aware of the fact that, the more the children and their mother entered into the therapeutic alliance, the more the father bridled in protest and was maneuvered to the edge of the "action." As the work focused on the relationships advanced and we tried to trace back to the extended family, it seemed as if the father would sabotage the therapy—Marlyse simultaneously defended his authority and vomited more than ever.

505

We then dramatized the situation somewhat. Saying that we needed accurate information and stressing their competence, we asked the parents to decide between them what Marlyse should eat and to bring to each session a precise daily report on the frequency of her vomiting, including the state of the lavatories. (The parents were able to inform themselves about Marlyse's vomiting by observing the state of toilets—which her mother then cleaned.) We chose this directive measure to bring the parents closer together, to revalorize the father, and to decrease Marlyse's power. It should be noted that we imposed one rule (that what Marlyse ate be controlled by her parents) to ensure that the difference between this and the more appropriate rule (that Marlyse herself controlled what she ate) be marked. The result was that the lavatories remained clean, the vomiting diminished both in frequency and in quantity, and Marlyse began to gain weight.

The work continued. The father (perhaps identifying himself with the aggressor) anticipated our projects. Before we got around to suggesting it, he invited Marlyse to dine with him alone at a restaurant. She was delighted. And he invented a kind of "behavioral therapy": for every day that there is no vomiting he buys his daughter a rose at the flower shop. Marlyse succeeded in keeping these roses alive for several weeks. At the same time she changed—she dressed differently, and she was becoming more beautiful, more vivacious. The siblings' organization started changing, for we noted that there was the risk that the brother and the two sisters would tend to redelegate the function of "parentification" to Marlyse—that is, the probability that she would be the one to stay at home with them was put into words. This and the children's suggestion that we meet for a session without the parents prompted us to organize a sesson with the children alone, followed by a session in which the parents and the children watched an audiovisual recording of this session. This procedure brought the conflict between the father and the therapists, together with the marital conflict, into the open, thus enabling us to. demonstrate the fundamental problem—namely, the nonadjustment of the parents' attitudes and measures toward their more or less grown-up children. A key change will, of course, be suppression of the rule of indirect communication between the children and their father. So far, paternal communication had always passed via the mother, a circumstance that kept the father isolated and increased the mother's power. In a final phase, which has not yet been completed, the family broached the problem of separation. Once again we were beaten to the post. Marlyse arrived at the tenth session with two poems, one of them a very subtle acknowledgment of both the roses and her father's love; the other, describing the painful therapeutic sessions, was a lyrical aimed at the departure of the children. The reports show that Marlyse now vomits only on Sundays, which she spends at home. She can explain that she does not know, on Sundays, whether she may pursue her own interests or whether she should consider mummy and daddy. Prior to the session, Marlyse had addressed her father directly, asking his permission to go and live in an apartment with a girlfriend. And her father, a sensitive man, correctly evaluating the situation, gave his consent. The family therapy entered its final phase; the control of the symptom by report was entrusted to Marlyse herself as of the time that she left home to go and live with her friend. The vomiting ceased, and the menstrual cycle rees-tablished itself. The family, in agreement with the therapists, deemed itself capable of taking charge of its own problems and left quite happily, after having received careful instructions as to how to reestablish contact with us if the request of one of its members ever made this necessary.

Conclusions

These brief reflections on the choice of therapeutic method are rather too theoretical, while at the same time leaving the reader inadequately informed in regard to the "specific" indications of family therapy. Catamnestic research in this domain is rare; its methodology is a riddle; and results are significant only in a local context. Inclusion of the existing family relations in the therapeutic considerations in respect of an adoles-cent presenting clinical problems appears to me to be always indicated. However, if the choice of the form of approach depended only on the patient, his family, and other systems involved, treatment "made to measure" could be applied. But the therapeutic context, personality, and training necessarily also condition this choice. Even if one has an identity as a psychotherapist, one cannot work miracles. Hence there is the need to postulate polyvalent institutions with several options at their disposal that, like any other evolutive system, coordinate the work of subspe-cialists.

REFERENCES

Capra, F. 1983. *Wendezeit*. Bern: Scherz.

Dell, P. 1980. Researching the family theories of schizophrenia: an exercise in epistemological confusion. *Family Protocols* 19:321–335.

Doudin, P.-A.; Haas, C.; Navarro, C.; and Kaufmann, L. 1985. La communication dans des familles "fonctionnelles" et "dysfonction-nelles" avec enfants adolescents. III. La mise en relation des communications verbales et non-verbales. *Archives suisses de neurologie, neurochirurgie et de psychiatrie* 136:69–80.

Fivaz, E. 1984. Approche systémique de l'adolescence. *Archives suisses de neurologie, neurochirurgie et de psychiatrie* 134:229–239.

Fivaz, E.; Fivaz, R.; and Kaufmann, L. 1979. Therapy of psychotic transaction families: an evolutionary paradigm. In C. Müller, ed. *Psychotherapy of Schizophrenia*. Amsterdam: Excerpta Medica.

Fivaz, E.; Fivaz, R.; and Kaufmann, L. 1981. Dysfunctional transactions and therapeutic functions: an evolutive model. *Journal of Marital and Family Therapy* 7:309–320.

Fivaz, E.; Fivaz, R.; and Kaufmann, L. 1982. Encadrement du développement, le point de vue systémique: fonctions pédagogique, parentale et thérapeutique. *Thérapies familiales et pratiques de réseaux, Bruxelles* 4:63–74.

Fivaz, E.; Fivaz, R.; and Kaufmann, L. 1983. Agreement, conflict, symptom: an evolutionary paradigm. In J. Duss von Werdt and R.-M. Welter-Enderlin, eds. *Zusammenhänge III*. Zürich: Institut für Ehe und Familie.

Haas, C.; Doudin, P.-A.; Navarro, E.; and Kaufmann, L. 1985. La communication dans des familles "fonctionnelles" et "dysfonction-nelles" avec enfants adolescents. II. Communications non-verbales. *Archives suisses de neurologie, neurochirurgie et de psychiatrie* 136:55–67.

Haley, J. 1963. Strategies of psychotherapy. In *Voices*. New York: Grune & Stratton.

Kaufmann, L. 1983. L'autorité du psychothérapeute dans la perspective de la théorie systémique. *Archives suisses de neurologie, neurochirurgie et de psychiatrie* 133:119–129.

Kaufmann, L. 1985. Les communications agressives comme frein au processus évolutif de la famille. *Series paedopsychiatrie* 6:39–49.

Masson, O., and Pancheri, E. 1979. Thérapie de famille, son choix dans le traitement des adolescents. *Acta paedopsychiatrie* 44:149–161.

Wertheim, E. S. 1975. The science and typology of family systems. II. Further theoretical and practical considerations. *Family Protocols* 14:285–309.

29 THE DEVELOPMENT OF PERSONAL INDIVIDUALITY: LIMITED TREATMENT GOALS IN A PSYCHOANALYTIC HOSPITAL

BRIAN J. MUIR

> Surely some revelation is at hand;
> Surely the second coming is at hand.
> [W. B. Yeats, "The Second Coming"]

The admission of an adolescent to a mental illness hospital is a painful and catastrophic experience for the patient and his family. It is an experience charged with despair, hope, rage, fear, and guilt, and all concerned must struggle with these feelings over long periods of discouragement and occasional optimism. It follows, then, that if the hospital experience is to be a constructive and fruitful one, these powerful emotions must be carefully attended to, contained, held, and detoxified so that internal dynamic changes and maturation can take place.

In this chapter I want to describe the social system and inpatient community at The Cassel Hospital as a setting within which an intensive residential treatment program for adolescents ranging from fifteen to twenty years of age takes place. These adolescents are ill enough to need to be in hospital and are all diagnostically within the borderline and sometimes the psychotic category. The hospital cannot contain and does not admit primarily addicted, delinquent, or brain-damaged young people. The Cassel has been firmly committed to applying psychoanalytic principles to our inpatient treatment program for young adults, adoles-

cents, and families for nearly forty years, and its psychoanalytic affiliations go back even further.

Although during recent years there has been some very important
literature published in America on the psychoanalytic hospital, with
detailed descriptions of its social network (Fromm-Reichman 1947;
Kernberg 1976; Novotny 1973), and although Main in Britain (Main
1946, 1974, personal communication) has also singularly contributed, the
earliest writing on the subject was by Simmel (1929), who published his
work on the psychoanalysis of inpatients in his Tegel Klinik in Berlin.
Many of his early and penetrating insights into the special problems
posed by the psychoanalytic therapy of narcissistic, impulse-ridden inpatients are still applicable today, despite the fact that his particular experiment seems to have encountered many difficulties. We have had to await
the psychoanalytic studies of hospital society such as have emerged from
the Menninger Clinic, Chestnut Lodge, and The Cassel Hospital to be
able to create and maintain a social milieu as a context in which psychoanalytic therapy can take place.

Usually, in applying psychoanalytic principles to hospital treatment,
the milieu has been regarded by most authors as an adjunct to support the
psychotherapy (Adler 1973, 1977). Although I believe this to be true of
the more integrated patient, I think that in the hospital treatment of
borderline adolescents—particularly in its earlier stages when there is
greater need for containment of regressive behavioral disturbances and
for limit setting—the true situation is the other way around, that is, the
psychotherapy is an adjunct to the milieu, interpreting and giving meaning to the patient's experience in the society of the hospital community. It
is, I believe, a fundamental mistake to underestimate the importance of
either modality.

It is within the context of this developmental background of the inpatient setting that the intensive treatment of borderline and some psychotic adolescent patients proceeds. The particular psychoanalytic
theoretical orientation of the hospital is that of the British object relations school of Klein, Winnicott, Balint, and Bion.

The Setting

The total patient community comprises twenty-four young adults (the
majority experiencing difficulties characterizing late-adolescent develop-

ments and individuation as well as diagnostically borderline and narcissistic personalities), twenty-four family members (mothers, fathers, and young children), and eight to ten adolescents. The family members and adolescents constitute one unit or "firm," whereas the young adults constitute two units of twelve. Each unit is headed by a consultant psychoanalyst and a nursing officer, with an administrative officer as adviser and backup. These professional staff have no personal caseload. The length of stay for adolescents ranges from eighteen months to two years.

The whole hospital is run along therapeutic community lines, with clear role definition, lines of responsibility, and social structure. The culture is permissive and enquiring but with high expectations of social participation, self-responsibility, and cooperative endeavor by way of work groups, daily unit meetings, and community meetings that are built around significant areas of communal life, for example, reception of new patients, rooming, cooking, cleaning, and limit setting.

These particular conditions have direct and detailed consequences in everyday management and administration in supporting the treatment program. Administrative staff are thus in some measure clinically involved, working immediately alongside patients, backing up a setup that can allow for the possibility of error or failure and hence of learning from experience. Thus, although the social structure of the community is clear, it is permissive enough to provide a degree of ambiguity that necessitates thoughtful participation by the patients.

In this setting the adolescents are offered three-times-a-week psychoanalytic psychotherapy, which aims to focus on the here-and-now experience of the adolescent's life in the hospital, with all its multiple transferences. Psychotropic medication is used only occasionally, in circumstances of overwhelming anxiety, manic overactivity, or severely disturbed behavior, when the human holding capacities of the community and nursing staff become overtaxed. The reason for administering medication is always openly and actively discussed by staff and patients.

The adolescent unit is separate from the rest of the hospital only in terms of staff organization, there being no geographical or physical separation. Nor is there any physical containment, that is, there are no closed wards or locked doors. These features are at variance with the tendency over the last twenty years or so to hospitalize adolescents in "pure culture," isolating them from older patients and children and usually employing closed units. Indeed, Masterson (1972) and Rinsley

(1967a, 1967b) specifically state that such conditions are mandatory for a satisfactory treatment engagement and to protect hospitalized adolescents from the disturbing or corrupting influences of older patients. Although our patients are selected on the basis of considerations of suitability for the setting and some capacity for positive motivation and self-appraisal—and hence are perhaps a somewhat less disturbed group than the patients Masterson and Rinsley described—it has nevertheless been our experience that certain positive advantages accrue from a mixed culture and an open institution. Our adolescents often derive much support from older patients, particularly from those who are parents, and make insightful use of understanding adult difficulties. Similarly, experience with younger children in the hospital can be conducive to the adolescent patient getting into better contact with his own infantile aspects. Problems do arise, of course, but usually they are of a kind that enhances therapeutic possibilities.

A feature of the psychopathology of virtually all our adolescent patients is a problem in the relationship to one or both parents, and this can, of course, take many forms. But since the theoretical basis for the psychotherapy that is provided stresses the patient's difficulties as being bound up with the real parents and their internalized representations—reenacted in transferences within the hospital setting—and since it is well known that adolescents are capable of massive denial when separated from an area of conflict, it has been a deliberate policy that adolescents go home for the weekend, and only when it is adjudged clinically appropriate are they allowed to spend the weekend in hospital.

Work with Parents

A singularly important and essential part of the initial therapeutic contract established with the adolescent and his parents before admission is an agreement with the parents that they will attend weekly meetings with the adolescent-unit social worker to explore the dynamics of the marriage and of their relationships with the adolescent patient. The parents must also undertake to attend regularly a weekly evening parents' and adolescents' group convened by the social worker and nursing staff. This arrangement helps to ensure that parents retain parental responsibility and that communication between home and hospital is maintained. The dynamics of the group are difficult and very complex, and the staff involved require considerable toughness and sophistication to manage the multiple manifestations of guilt, rage, blame, and scapegoating, in which primitive splitting and projective processes are rife. This group is not a psychotherapy group as such but focuses on the task of staff and parents in sharing the difficulties they experience in common regarding the care and management of the adolescent patients. Discussion is often charged with high anxiety but centers around such ordinary issues as schoolwork, pocket money, weekend plans, acting-out behavior, and so on. Frequently, however, management of impulsive behavior is further helped by one or more conjoint family meetings with the nurse, therapist, and social worker, and such meetings are usually indicated when the working alliance with either the adolescent or the parents is fragile (Shapiro, Shapiro, Zinner, and Berkowitz 1977).

It is now well known that in all cases of hospitalized borderline and borderline-psychotic adolescents the adolescent disturbance is also a symptom of pathology of moderate or severe degree in the family, with one or both parents frequently, but not always, manifesting borderline features of personality disturbance themselves. The adolescent patient is frequently unconsciously perceived by one or both parents as representing a disowned and feared aspect of themselves. Such mechanisms have been well described by many authors, but Zinner and Shapiro (1972) specifically give a very clear and useful account. Thus, any major change in the adolescent may, if the family is not prepared, impose new and perhaps intolerable strains. We have not infrequently noted that the mother becomes depressed and occasionally suicidal in response to clinical improvement in her child—or even earlier, as a result of the separation incurred by admission of the adolescent to hospital.

With the adolescent spending weekends at home, the family can better adapt to progressive change in the adolescent with treatment, thereby avoiding the situation in which hospitalization helps to render the problem virtually inaccessible to therapy and likely to reappear after discharge. Masterson (1972) and Rinsley (1965, 1967b, 1971) both assert that severe curtailment of contact between the adolescent inpatient and the parents is mandatory, especially during the earlier phase of treatment, in order to minimize the toxic effect of family pathology and to facilitate engagement with the treatment program and the emergence of the "abandonment depression" underlying the behavioral disturbance and acting out. It has been our experience, however, that careful work from the beginning with parents about weekends and about their feelings and fears regarding the hospitalization helps much to ameliorate guilt and hostility and minimizes the problem of loyalty conflicts. The expectation that the family have a responsibility for the adolescent at weekends, if this arrangement is clinically possible, carries with it the need for the setting described (the parents' and adolescents' group), in which parents have opportunities for adequate contact with the hospital, for talking about their anxieties, and for reality testing to set against their often paranoid distortion about the hospital and the staff. The group enhances under-standing of what the hospital is trying to do. In this way parents can be helped to evolve a cooperative working relationship with the hospital that will enable them to satisfy their wish to show the hospital—and, more important, their child—that they are willing to make some effort to facilitate the treatment.

The Psychopathology of the Borderline Adolescent

The literature on the subject of the psychopathology of the borderline personality is now very large, and I do not intend here to attempt more than a brief recapitulation. More attention has been paid to the specific syndrome as such by American authors such as Kernberg, Masterson, Rinsley, and Adler, to name but a few, while British authors have approached the problem from the point of view of encountering and analyzing these primitive mental mechanisms in most if not all patients who present to us for "mending," to use Winnicott's (1960, 1972) term. The writings of Klein, Bion, Fairbairn, and Winnicott have of course been major early contributions, but many of the more recent works have further developed the field. In particular, Rosenfeld (1978) has stressed the potential usefulness of allowing the development of a transference psychosis in the analyses of these patients and paying particular attention to the part played by the primitive, sadistic superego and the presence of confusional states.

Most of these authors agree that an inborn constitutional propensity for excessive primitive aggression is a feature of borderline patients, but there now is a clear consensus also that the borderline has suffered severe traumatization in early infancy in the form of subjection to extremes of hunger, frustration, and abandonment. The mothers of these patients are intolerant of spontaneous gestures or self-assertive moves toward inde-pendence in their infants and respond by emotional withholding or withdrawal. They reward, however, any signs of clinging dependency, compliance, or renunciation of autonomy. They blow "hot and cold," experience of which Winnicott (1951, 1952) described as being "perhaps the worst thing that can happen to a human infant." This mode of relating by mother to baby essentially implies an impaired capacity in the mother to recognize her baby as a separate human person and is well described by Mahler as a distortion of the separation/individuation phase of infant psychological development.

The normal developmental pathways that the adolescent has to negotiate under the impact of a rising tide of sexual feelings involve some considerable measure of regression to infantile modes of mental functioning—primitive splitting of self and objects into good and bad, idealization and devaluation, denial omnipotence, and primitive projective identification.

When either conditions of excessive primitive constitutional aggression or excessive frustration and trauma exist during infancy, the adolescent's capacity to differentiate between his self and object images—and to integrate them in appropriate ways—is severely impaired. Whole object relationships have virtually no existence, and the depressive position (Klein) or capacity for concern (Winnicott) cannot be sustained or even reached. The patient is entangled in the primitive world of the paranoid-schizoid position—a world of primitive good and bad, fusion and confusion, intense loneliness and abandonment—and is full of hate, rage, and despair about himself and his objects and, accordingly, feels remorselessly attacked by a primitive, sadistic superego. Escape from this torment is only by way of fusion and compliance—thus negating identity—or by means of omnipotence and manic denial. These patients are often chronically confused as to whether they are good or bad, big or little, male or female, inside or outside. Although often apparently in touch with reality, they achieve this either by gross manipulation of their environment and other people or by scotomatizing whole areas of reality perception. Their sense of personal identity is fragile and precarious and shifts wildly and continually, the varying states of mind having little or no contact with one another. The world of objects is experienced as being highly dangerous and is constantly scanned for signs of rejection, intrusion, or hostility (Carter and Rinsley 1977). The libidinal dependent or needy self becomes highly aggressive and feels attacked as it is blamed for the states of helpless rage and envy that the dependency creates. This is the beginning of a primitive narcissistic organization in the ego that is antilife as its attacks on the confused, loving, and destructive self cause feelings of emptiness, ego weakness, lack of desire to do anything, and, consequently, apathy and despair (Rosenfeld 1978).

516

There is a constant vacillation between fusion and a sense of isolation akin to feeling "lost in space," a state of mind one of our patients described as "being in a black hole." This limbo or "neither here nor there" state of mind has been described by Rey (1977) as a "claustrophobic agoraphobic dilemma."

The borderline adolescent has grossly impaired peer-group relations, usually experiencing himself as a social outcast as his hesitant attempts to become part of a group are confounded by his propensity to attract the projections of the psychotic parts of all the other group members. His frustration tolerance is minimal, and he is therefore vulnerable to intense, explosive actions and behavior or, alternatively, to despair, apathy, and negating compliance. The group affiliations he does manage tend to be those with a perverse, addictive, or delinquent orientation.

The Treatment Process

Masterson (1972) and Rinsley (1965, 1967b, 1971) both describe three stages of the treatment process with hospitalized adolescents. Masterson's stages of "testing," "working through," and "separation" very much coincide with Rinsley's stages of "resistance" (to treatment), the "definitive" or "introjective phase," and "resolution." By including the notion of "limited" treatment goals in the title of this chapter, I am intending to convey my agreement with these authors that much work ideally remains to be done in outpatient psychotherapy after these goals—or so it is to be hoped—have been achieved. The aim of the hospital treatment is to free the adolescent from the pathological vortex of his family group and all the projections, confused ego boundaries, and primitive affects that abide there. It is to help him separate from it with some basic sense of autonomy and personal identity and self-esteem that is at least sufficient to allow him to function at an adequate enough level at college, university, or work, that will allow him to live away from home and with some degree of confidence that the school failure, suicidal depression, or severe phobic and paranoid states that brought him into hospital will not return. Much ground might yet remain to be covered after discharge, however, to consolidate the gains and to guide him through the pains of later genital-oedipal conflicts toward a reasonably well-functioning heterosexual adulthood.

Masterson's and Rinsley's formulations of three stages of treatment are confirmed by our own observations of adolescent inpatients at The Cassel Hospital. The act of admitting an adolescent to the hospital provokes the

517

escalation of a multitude of primitive and often overwhelming fantasies, affects, and anxieties, in the parents as well as in the adolescent. The separation arouses a sense of imbalance in the dynamic status quo of the family as a group and of the individuals within it. It confirms the adolescent's worst fears that he is bad, evil, and unlovable and fit only to be "put away" and abandoned. It causes grief and pain, guilt and rage, and inevitably a regression to more primitive modes of functioning. Amid this welter of anxiety and painful affect, hope is also present, but it is usually idealistically and unrealistically colored, with subsequent disillusionment and disappointment inevitable. In addition, for the adolescent, the provision of board and lodging, nursing care, and a psychotherapist to talk to imply a permission to abdicate any personal responsibility and an entitlement to be totally cared for and looked after. This regression often results in the patient appearing to become much more ill, with further loss of whatever little capacity there is for verbal and symbolic communication and a resort to create behavioral modes of expression that can become extremely bizarre and intolerably demanding. It is clear that the hospital, by providing the setting that it does, to some extent invites or elicits this state of affairs, and, although individual adolescents' pathologies and depressive manifestations may differ widely (from clinging, shadowing, or pestering to disturbing intrusiveness, self-mutilation, suicidal attempts, violence and window-breaking, drug taking, or running away), the primary task and function of the staff is to ensure as much as they can—and, if possible, without recourse to psychotropic drugs—that these behaviors are contained in human modalities and understood in ways that can gradually and nonpunitively be fed back to the patient.

Now, of course the social setting of the hospital cannot cope with these manifestations beyond certain limits and the containing structure needs, in human interpersonal terms, the support of firm and good authority that is capable of appropriate confrontation and limit setting. The capacity for containment, which depends on personal flexibility and tolerance combined with firmness is a matter of individual staff (and often patient) attributes, but it can be maintained in "good enough" repair, utilizing both preservation and conservation, by daily staff meetings chaired jointly by a nursing officer and consultant psychoanalyst. Detailed feedback and reporting of the minutiae as well as the larger aspects of the adolescent's life over the previous twenty-four hours help to minimize the exploitation by the adolescent of latent staff splits (as classically described by Main 1957) and to facilitate a shared understanding of the patient. We regard it as mandatory that these meetings be attended by *all* staff concerned with the patient, that is, nurse, therapist, social worker, teacher; and the ability of the staff group to function in a thoughtful cooperative way is an accurate analogy of Bion's (1970) concept of "container" and "contained." Gold (1983) applied these concepts to the wider problem of the therapeutic community, stressing the difficulties involved in the depersonalizing effects of the larger group, with all the enhanced tendencies such a group provides for more primitive projective processes to operate (Main 1974).

Technical Modifications Required for Inpatient Psychoanalytic Therapy

It should be clear that the two notions of transference to the institution as a whole (i.e., to the building as well as to various human beings living and working within it) and of the patient's free associations—consisting of more than his utterances and behavior in the consulting room—are singularly important. Thus, the key feature distinguishing individual psychotherapy with inpatients is that the reality of the objects of multiple split transferences occurring outside the consulting room are known directly to the therapist. In outpatient work, the therapist does not usually have firsthand knowledge of the significant events, people, and material reality in the patient's life. He only knows what the patient tells him, drawing it into the transference and interpreting it as such. In inpatient work he either knows or can find out about the realities and can check the patient's perceptions against his own and other staff members' accounts. The therapist can choose either to ignore these "extraneous" sources of materials or to utilize them to advantage in furthering the treatment.

For example, a nurse may report an adolescent's inability or refusal to engage in assigned household tasks, such as keeping one's bedroom clean, taking part in the general care of the servery or other work groups, or avoiding community meetings. The therapist, having at the time of admission established that part of his contract with the patient will be that he has full and regular communication with the nurse, will indicate in a nonaccusatory but enquiring way that he is in receipt of this information. He may decide to interpret or not, but if he does, relevant interpretations may have to do with the exploitation of a providing maternal figure; manifestations of a dirty, neglected, or unwanted part of the self in relation to a maternal figure; or paranoid anxieties involving projected jealousy and envy leading to self-impoverishment and consequent work difficulties. In this way, the various problems of adulteration of the traditional therapist/patient dyad by the intrusion of other persons and extraneous factors tend to fade away and become useful enrichments of the therapeutic process.

The question of privacy and confidentiality, which is so important in psychotherapy, does, however, pose some immediate problems in the inpatient setting, despite the fact that there is an explicit contract on the part of all staff members to preserve confidentiality. Clearly, behavior is not a problem, because it becomes public property in the community very quickly, but certain verbal communications may require more sensitive handling. For example, an adolescent girl, previously having revealed it to no one else in her life, told her therapist that her father had some years earlier attempted to engage in incest with her. At the time of this revelation she was doing fairly well in treatment and her parents had a constructive relationship with the hospital. The patient's confidence was kept between her therapist and herself and the psychoanalyst supervisor, an act of judgment that proved correct, since she did well after discharge.

What, then, is likely to happen if the therapist attempts to do orthodox psychotherapy keeping interpretation of the transference solely to himself? In my experience, the majority of inpatients under these conditions will form a false or compliant engagement with the therapist—viewing the therapeutic process as an absorbing and gratifying exercise in self-study—but will be devoid of any real intent to change through genuine understanding. They will undertake to enter this kind of compliant and insincere relationship as payment of a kind, which they feel qualifies them to remain in the hospital, in which they have usually carved out a very firm niche that enables them to perpetuate their illness.

There are some dangers involved in interpreting the transference hospitalwide, and the unintentional fostering of aggressive acting out is one of these. The danger is minimized by careful joint nurse-therapist supervision, but it may be brought about by the patient feeling rejected by the therapist if the latter does not acknowledge and interpret negative and positive feelings toward himself as well as to the institution, the building, and others in it. It is particularly important that strong feelings that are clearly experienced primarily toward the therapist not be deflected from the person of the therapist to others in the hospital. This is especially tempting to younger and less experienced therapists working with adolescents whose affect is primitive and intensely uncomfortable.

Because of the limited nature of the treatment goals in terms of facilitating the separation of the adolescent from his family and his individuation, the therapist must be wary of the danger of omnipotent and unrealistic expectations in himself, in nursing staff, and in the patient and his family. He and the nurse should be asking themselves and the adolescent at intervals, Why is this adolescent still in hospital? In other words, it is important that the focal nature of the treatment goals, formulated in terms of the patient's individual and family psychopathology, should not be lost sight of. A corollary of this stance is that often some painful truths will have to be confronted and accepted. These are truths about permanent damage that cannot be undone, but that, if faced with courage, may make possible a more creative adaptation to real life and more realistic expectations of oneself in that life.

Conclusions

I have described an inpatient social system as a context for intensive milieu and psychotherapeutic treatment of borderline adolescents. I have indicated the usefulness of a mixed social setting, as opposed to the more traditional adolescent unit, and have drawn particular attention to three areas of work: these are intensive work with parents, intensive scrutiny and supervision of the nurse-therapist relationship, and, last, certain technical modifications that I believe to be essential for the practice of inpatient psychotherapy.

REFERENCES

Adler, G. 1973. Hospital treatment of borderline patients. *American Journal of Psychiatry* 130:–32–36.

Adler, G. 1977. Hospital management of borderline patients and its relation to psychotherapy. In G. Hartocollis, ed. *Borderline Personality Disorders: The Concepts, the Syndrome, the Patient*. New York: International Universities Press.

Bion, W. 1970. *Attention and Interpretation*. London: Tavistock.

Carter, L., and Rinsley, D. B. 1977. Vicissitudes of "empathy" in a borderline adolescent. *International Review of Psychoanalysis* 4(3): 317–326.

Fromm-Reichman, F. 1947. Problems of psychotherapeutic management in a psychoanalytic hospital. *Psychoanalytic Quarterly* 16:325–356.

Gold, S. 1983. Projective identification: the conformer and reverse as concepts in applied psychoanalysis. *British Journal of Medical Psychology* 56:279–287.

Kernberg, O. 1976. Towards an integrative theory of hospital treatment. In *Object Relations Theory and Clinical Psychoanalysis*. New York: Aronson.

Main, T. F. 1946. The hospital as a therapeutic institution. *Bulletin of the Menninger Clinic* 10:66–70.

Main, T. F. 1957. The ailment. *British Journal of Medical Psychology* 30:129–145.

Main, T. F. 1974. Some psychodynamics of large groups. In L. Kreeger, ed. *The Large Group*. London: Constable.

Masterson, J. F. 1972. *Treatment of the Borderline Adolescent: A Developmental Approach*. New York: Wiley.

Novotny, P. C. 1973. The pseudo psychoanalytic hospital. *Bulletin of the Menninger Clinic* 37:193–199.

Rey, H. 1977. The schizoid dilemma and the space-tune continuum. *Bulletin of the British Psychoanalytic Society* 1:12–43.

Rinsley, D. B. 1965. Intensive psychiatric hospital treatment of adolescents. *Psychiatric Quarterly* 39:405–429.

Rinsley, D. B. 1967a. The adolescent in residential treatment: some critical reflections. *Adolescence* 2:83–95.

Rinsley, D. B. 1967b. Intensive residential treatment of the adolescent. *Psychiatric Quarterly* 41:134–143.

Rinsley, D. B. 1971. Theory and practice of intensive residential treatment of adolescents. *Adolescent Psychiatry* 1:479–509.

Rosenfeld, H. 1978. Notes on the psychopathology and psychoanalytic treatment of some borderline patients. *International Journal of Psycho-Analysis* 59:215–223.

Shapiro, E. R.; Shapiro, R. L.; Zinner, J.; and Berkowitz, D. A. 1977. The borderline ego and the working alliance: indications from family and individual treatment in adolescence. *International Journal of Psycho-Analysis* 58:77–89.

Simmel, E. 1929. Psychoanalytic treatment in a sanitarium. *International Journal of Psycho-Analysis* 10:70–89.

Winnicott, D. W. 1951. Transitional objects and transitional phenomena. In *Collected Papers: Through Paediatrics to Psycho-Analysis*. London: Tavistock, 1958.

Winnicott, D. W. 1952. Psychosis and child care. In *Collected Papers: Through Paediatrics to Psycho-Analysis*. London: Tavistock, 1958.

Winnicott, D. W. 1960. The theory of the parent-infant relationship. *International Journal of Psycho-Analysis* 41:585–595.

Winnicott, D. W. 1972. The use of an object and relating through identifications. *International Journal of Psycho-Analysis* 50:711–716.

Zinner, J., and Shapiro, E. R. 1972. Splitting in families of borderline adolescents. In J. Mack, ed. *Borderline States in Psychiatry*. New York: Grune & Stratton.

PHILIPPE JEAMMET

Adolescent psychiatry today—which adolescents ought to be treated and how? At the close of this meeting, can we believe that such an ambitious question has been answered? I suppose not, if what was expected was a systematic evaluation of the treatments to be prescribed and an inventory of methods.

As a matter of fact did we only focus on psychiatry? Was this meeting not devoted primarily to psychopathology? Several interventions from the floor appeared to support this view, emphasizing the gap between those treatment procedures mentioned by the speakers, which might seem to be ideal but unrealistic, and the actual possibilities of most services and staffs, with their budgetary restrictions in the majority of countries. Consider a psychiatric unit faced with the task of dealing annually with the problems of hundreds if not thousands of adolescents. What can Laufer's model of a consultation center with its four or five weekly psychoanalytic sessions mean to them? I am all the more sensitive to such issues, since, in the adolescent and young-adult psychiatry unit to which I belong, we treat each year some 400–500 patients who are either fully hospitalized or in daytime treatment centers and conduct 8,000–10,000 consultations.

Nonetheless, in my view, this meeting has contributed to the demands of these adolescents, demands so varied in their expression yet so fundamentally similar. If no answer has been provided (since no exhaustive and unequivocal conclusion could be expected), at least some elements of primary importance as to the direction our responses might take were discussed.

This conference has abundantly illustrated what is at stake in the psychic processes at play during adolescence and their fundamental importance in the organization of the personality. As Kestemberg has said, "If childhood is when the pieces are set up, the game is played during adolescence." More than is the case for any other stage of life, the way we look at the adolescent is not without its consequences. It contributes toward the organization of his or her self-image and personal identity. Hence our view of the mental functioning of adolescents—and of the psychic processes at play during that period—cannot help but influence our attitudes toward them and affect their future. In psychiatry perhaps even more than in other fields, no view of the other is neutral, and the view taken of adolescence is less neutral than that taken toward any other age. This view is formed by the knowledge we have and therefore by our basic psychopathological model. Psychiatry cannot avoid considerations of psychopathology. I shall not reopen the issues raised by those classifications, such as DSM-III, that claim to be neutral, objective, and to have no concern for etiology or even for psychopathology. I do not deny the utility of DSM-III in specific instances, in an epidemiological study, or in an assessment of a therapeutic method. However, it becomes a dangerous utopia when it pretends to offer an objective panorama of pathology. To pay exclusive attention to behavior and symptoms is necessarily to be party to their defense functions and to fail to understand what they are intended to mask—all the more so at adolescence, a period when personality is in process of organization and the adolescent is in quest of both personal identity and of a self-image in whose organization these symptoms play a part.

To consider the adolescent exclusively from a psychiatric point of view is deliberately to ignore the problems underlying the organization of personality, problems that these disorders reveal. Indeed, all the speakers have warned us against the danger of that kind of attitude. In this regard, I essentially accept the importance of what Laufer calls the "breakdown" of development and accept even more fully what he characterizes as being the "foreclosure" of this development, which results in a scar that may prove to be permanent, cutting the adolescent from a part of himself and his vital forces. This results in rejection of a particular part of his body, essentially its sexual dimension, closing him off to particular types of emotions and ways of relating to others. In other words, it is during adolescence that denials and splits that cut off the adolescent from a significant part of his potentialities may take root in the form of character traits and a stable organization of the ego.

The content thus denied will no longer be available to the adolescent. Rather, it will be the object of countercathexes, projective expulsion, and/or active ignorance in the event that such content appears in another member of the family. Emotionally deprived mothers will permit their babies to cry, unconcerned by the baby's distress and apparently not hearing them. Only after adequate psychotherapy will they be able to identify their own emotional needs and underlying depression. It is because they become aware of their own depression that they are able to experience empathy for their child, to perceive its suffering, and to hear its sobs, as has been described by Fraiberg.

Such potential consequences, however, are not likely to be analyzed and taken into account unless a theory enables one to understand their importance and significance. Supposing that such a theory were formulated, would we thereupon be in a position to apply appropriate therapy? Could we succeed in getting the adolescent to undertake the desirable measures to avoid such risks? Of course not. Nevertheless, however unsatisfactory the proposed therapeutic procedures, it seems to me that, given the potential risks, it is quite a different thing to be party (possibly unwittingly) to this closure and denial mechanism than it is to know how to find and develop in the adolescent whatever may minimize the closure process and keep alive and accessible to the therapist the potentialities for opening and change. However, this knowledge is not possible unless we can base our work on a model of both what is involved and what is most important at adolescence.

Purely psychiatric, symptomatic, and behavioral observations are scarcely enough to clarify matters for us. To illustrate this, I shall briefly report the case of a woman, well established professionally, married, with two children, who, at the end of her adolescence, was diagnosed as going through a psychotic breakdown and was treated with electric shock. She recovered from her breakdown, which did not recur, and subsequently was socially and professionally successful. The reason that I mention this woman is that I met her as the mother of two daughters who at adolescence were themselves diagnosed as, in one case, undergoing a psychotic development verging toward schizophrenia and, in the other, having a severe behavior disorder of a hypomanic psychopathic type with largely psychotic functioning. Furthermore, this mother is noteworthy for her paradoxical attitude toward her children. She insists on the fact of their illness while at the same time totally denying the worth of their treatment, which she does not trust, disparages constantly, and interrupts repeatedly. Her jealousy of the care from which her children benefit has been more and more overtly expressed, thus far culminating in her crying out one day, "When *I* fell ill, no one ever took the trouble to talk to me or asked me what was wrong. A few electric shocks and that was that." At the same time she seeks contact with the staff and has them understand that she desires assistance, which she simultaneously quite effectively sabotages.

Looked at purely in terms of the symptoms and from the mother's perspective, the results of her own therapy were excellent and there is every reason to be pleased with the treatment given her when she was adolescent. However, looked at from the side of the children and in terms of the mother's success in her personal life and with regard to emotional life and the ability to interact, our evaluation is necessarily quite different. One wonders what might have been the development had the mother benefited from another kind of listening at adolescence. What if someone had helped her not to disavow either the envious and hateful traits of her personality or her emotional needs? History cannot be rewritten, but one cannot help but think that subsequent developments might have been different. However this may be, this example shows to what degree the evaluation of the needs of the adolescent as well as of the results to be expected will vary depending on the model that, at least implicitly, guides our assessment.

The arguments put forth by the various speakers in the course of this colloquium concern more than individual or family modes of treatment for adolescent disorders. In addition to their therapeutic value, these procedures may be considered as models likely to guide our attitudes toward these patients and to play a part in the organization of the ongoing life of our institutions, as illustrated by the work done at Cassel Hospital and by the chapter by Muir.

These chapters make clear the degree to which adolescence represents what Blos calls this "second individuation process" that either (1) returns to the vulnerability and conflicts of childhood and the oedipal period and attempts to work them out within the dynamics of adolescence or (2) on the contrary, uses them to petrify a developmental process cut off at that point. All the authors, but especially Laufer and Kestemberg, show how symptoms and behaviors at that age act as powerful personality organizers. From very divergent perspectives, psychoanalytical and system theory join in emphasizing the importance of the phenomena of opening up: opening up the family system, negotiating a new family space, questioning of preexisting hierarchical relationships; displacement of cathexes; appearance of a divergence between prior ideals and the actualization of current drives; and divergence between the new sexual body and the psyche and between this body and the pregenital body.

These changes constitute an element of fragility. The awareness of these divergences and of the specific risks that they involve for the adolescent is what accounts for the careful attention given by caregivers to the maintenance, at any cost, of cathexes with the adolescent that are active but tolerable, maintained at a distance, and respectful of his ideals and his conservation of a positive self-image. Kestemberg has drawn our attention to the danger of abetting the adolescent in his defensive attempts at decathexis and withdrawal from interpersonal relations. The symptoms are the building blocks of this kind of defense, becoming substitutes for object relations and thereby masking and ossifying the conflicts.

It seems to me to be possible to draw some lessons from the models of psychopathological understanding of the adolescent that have been put forth in these chapters.

1. Whatever our place in the adolescent aid network, our role cannot be limited to responding to symptomatic emergencies. The encounter with the adolescent is always a rare opportunity that must be used to render him or her secure as far as possible, arouse the desire to be concerned with what is going on within, and not serve to reinforce denial.

2. At a time when economic difficulties push state authorities to minimize therapy-oriented interventions and to be satisfied with immediate symptomatic improvements, the problem of professional training is important. The briefer the intervention, the more sophisticated the training of the staff should be. Such training involves a thorough knowledge of the dynamics of the individual and family behavior. Without underestimating the interest—and, quite often, the inevitability—of brief interventions, the comments we have heard clearly establish that therapeutic avarice is inappropriate in the case of adolescents. Therapeutic responses will strongly influence the future of the adolescent. Long and intensive treatment often appears to be the one alternative likely to modify the course of development and to safeguard the future of the patient. Long-term

treatment is all the more valuable in that the personality is still malleable and attitudes have not yet become fixed. In some instances, such treatment may require a long-term stay in an institutional setting. Muir showed the beneficial character of such therapy, and we have had the same experience with it. Making do with some adaptive patchwork is all the more regrettable since appropriate treatment often enables the adolescent to make full use of all his potentialities, something that is no longer possible when, for example, a chronically psychotic mode of functioning has become established.

3. The pathology of adolescence tends to evolve toward an increase in the number of behavioral disorders. Addictive pathologies (e.g., drug addiction and alcoholism) affect family relationships and result in role confusion, an effacement of intergenerational barriers, a decrease in parental authority, and conflict avoidance. This in turn may induce role confusion in therapists insofar as they are led to become substitutes for the parents and to play a role in which educational and therapeutic attitudes are not always kept clearly distinct. Only a deepening of our understanding of psychopathology will allow us to escape the dilemma and adopt an unambiguous attitude.

4. Emphasis has been placed, particularly by Kaufmann, on the adolescent's right to suffer. In my view this is of central importance, because such an acknowledgment constitutes the first step toward understanding the crisis that the adolescent is experiencing and the conflicts that he faces—and hence is a first step toward contributing to help him work them out rather than deny them by encapsulating them in symptoms or in behavioral disorders. Now, this right to suffer, which implies neither indifference nor a waiting, purely passive attitude, runs counter to the right to health proclaimed by society. Dangerous shifts in meaning may occur that lead to the view that the right to health calls for the immediate elimination of any suffering, whether it takes the form of either behavioral or physiological disorders (such that one episode of insomnia, for example, calls for the immediate administration of sleeping pills). We are familiar with the social pressure in this direction, that is, the search for a quasi-mechanical response and the prescription of drugs for all difficulties and suffering. Thus, it is perhaps not surprising that drug addiction more and more represents a mode of response that society makes available to adolescents. The medical world itself does not always escape the risk of assuming that the priority is to eliminate suffering rather than to consider what this difficulty has to offer as a way of identifying the patient's

conflicts, a response that can thereby favor the development of the denials mentioned previously.

If we now turn to a more detailed consideration of these chapters, we find discussions in them of five relatively different types of functioning that, over and above the common features that I have stressed, point to a number of differences and discrepancies among them, which may seem somewhat puzzling. However, I think that these differences, which are explicated in an excellent fashion, represent rather well my own ambivalence about the treatment of adolescents. Without trying to achieve a synthesis that would, I fear, considerably dampen the originality of each position and mask the fundamental theoretical differences between some of these views, I must note that I feel that the very discrepancy in their presentations helped me to become conscious of the kind of problem that I am currently faced with in my practice with adolescents. For example, I believe that in having shown the important role played by the therapist as a protective shield, Masterson has noted that our priority should be to deal with the pregenital archaic elements that allow the subject to avoid the excitation of the oedipal confrontation.

During the discussion, Masterson made it quite clear that the adolescents he had in treatment were of course confronted with oedipal conflicts, but I think it is not a distortion of his view to say that he believes that the oedipal conflict no longer acts as the organizer but rather as a stimulant of the psyche and personality in such cases. Any confrontation with gender differentiation is a source of excitation that disorganizes the adolescent. Given this, one has to deal with the adolescent at another level, at a more repressive, less stimulating, more bearable level, one that in a second phase may enable us to tackle the oedipal element. Thus, I think that Masterson has given appropriate emphasis to something that we feel frequently about this kind of patient, that is, the significance of the part played by caregivers and institutions as protective shields when such are needed.

This being said, I personally would not agree that one keeps the various levels as distinct as he suggests. Dealing with a human being, and above all with an adolescent, one may not work the way archaeologists do, saying "Let us deal first with one level, and once it has been thoroughly investigated, we will deal with the one beneath." What I in fact experience in my practice is that we have to maintain the uncomfortable position of dealing with both levels simultaneously, passing from one to the other continuously. Some adolescents will protect themselves from oedipal confrontation by means of preoedipal regressive elements and vice versa; others will preserve actively cathected object relations in a narcissistic form or, conversely, mask essentially narcissistic positions under apparent objectification. Silence about one of the levels is never neutral but is to be understood as a condemnation of that level, whose conflictual character is thereby reinforced.

Laufer emphasized the quite crucial question of the part played by the sexual body, the body undergoing changes at adolescence, and pointed to the significance of the repetition of prior conflicts in the here and now of adolescence. It is often difficult to know how to treat the role played by the body. I have the impression that Laufer has succeeded in being at ease in discussing sexuality with adolescents without seeming to be seductive and apparently without risking a reinforcement of the excitation just mentioned. Perhaps, as Ladame suggested, it is because of his own style. Laufer also laid great emphasis on the work of the conscious and on the work of representation. I have had the feeling that for Laufer it is very important that the adolescent relive strong emotions in the transference, but he accompanies the adolescent by verbalizing at length what is going on and also by allowing the adolescent to verbalize what is happening to him.

Some of Laufer's comments suggest a pedagogical and normative attitude in the therapist. The importance that he accords to the work of the conscious differs somewhat from what tends to be the case in France and possibly from Kestemberg's view as well. Kestemberg has emphasized instead the importance of economic factors during adolescence as well as the usefulness of providing the adolescent with a substitute object that can become an object he may utilize and manipulate. As I understood her, Kestemberg often considers it more important to let the adolescent use her—to behave in such a way that the adolescent may use her—than to interpret what is going on. The need to induce a relationship that is both active and tolerant is given priority, given the risk that the adolescent may experience deobjectification and encapsulation in mechanical symptoms. She thus is led to talk of the relationship rather than of the framework. A relationship that permits cathectic displacement and, therefore, an opening to differences that little by little become tolerable, that is, cathectic displacements that do not necessarily involve their reproduction—I think that is what she showed in the report on her adolescent patient.

One gets the impression that, through repetition and little by little, in the framework of the transference differentiated cathexes come into being and are perceived differentially rather than massively and globally, as was the case in the first phase of therapeutic work. Kestemberg's main objective is to enable the adolescent to reexperience the pleasure of functioning at intellectual and interrelational levels, including object relations, and to ensure that this is no longer a defensive pleasure in relation to some unbearable relationship but rather a pleasure that involves implicitly the presence of an object that has now become tolerable. She thus is led to stress the importance of everything that relates to the person's narcissism and totality. Unlike Laufer, she appears to me largely to resort to elements that are implicit. Her perception of the kind of changes that have taken place is grounded in structural changes, as revealed by the type of object relations, by the ability to fantasize, and through dreams. These changes need not always be verbalized. Compared to that of Laufer, her practice includes fewer systematic attempts to furnish a clarification of what is going on, possibly owing to her concern to spare the adolescent an overly stressful confrontation with the identification process and his dependency. Here we find, at the economic level at any rate, the protective-shield effect that Masterson attempts to induce using different procedures. Excessive concern with having the adolescent understand what is happening may give him the feeling that we are influencing him and that he must either submit to us or rebel against us and refuse to accept the interpretation. If we deliberately choose to leave the adolescent in the dark regarding a significant part of what is experienced, the unspoken may be followed by elucidation, in deferred action at a later stage. By that time, the adolescent is assumed to have gained a sound personal, narcissistic foundation via his work, his emotional cathexes outside analysis, and his professional cathexes.

As Kaufmann has shown, adolescence is a period when the family is strongly involved, and that may often entail work with the family, which raises the question of how to articulate the individual and the family approach.

Muir has shown, and I entirely agree with him, the importance of the repetition of what occurs in institutional treatments. Even if we do not function the way Muir does, possibly owing to a lack of appropriate means and training, we can see from the example that he has reported that such repetition is important and probably inevitable. I think that we would be greatly mistaken to consider that such repetition does not occur during brief hospitalization (in the use of purely chemotherapeutic treatment, for example). Indeed something is actually repeated then too, but it may be something masochistic that serves to confirm to the adolescent his shortcomings and damaged personality.

All of this underlines the importance for the adolescent of the encounter on the one hand and of personal variables—and perhaps the charisma of the therapist (mentioned by Ladame), as well as perhaps the gender of the therapist—on the other hand. It has often struck me that in the examples Laufer cited he talked of a boy as being his patient and of a girl as being his wife's patient. Maybe we should not neglect the possibility that this involves some elements of primary homosexuality, in Kestemberg's sense of the term, which, even if implicit, is nonetheless very important.

How shall we pose the problem of evaluation? We are all faced with the frequent need to evaluate, to make diagnoses, if only to have available comparative ideas as to the development of the patient. We are often confronted with an inescapable contradiction, of which we must become conscious if we are not to behave too mechanically and thereby produce too serious consequences. We need criteria, but these very criteria may hinder our comprehension. In this regard, I am struck by the excessive extension of the concept of borderline. Organizations with conflicts essentially at the neurotic level are labeled as being borderline. For example, if hysteria in the form depicted in the beginning of the century is now rare, it nonetheless still exists. But it takes pseudopsychotic forms too readily labeled borderline, with ensuing therapeutic and countertransferential consequences. Given the well-known mimetic ability of the hysterical patient, there is the risk that a number of such patients will thereby become psychotic. On this matter, I would like to ask Masterson a question. It seems to me that a certain borderline triad is found in all adolescents. Is there any adolescent who is not faced with a separation anxiety? On what grounds are we then to establish a diagnosis? When we look into this in more detail, we see that borderlines are spoken of in a way that no longer specifies them with regard to the adolescent. It is termed a problem of borderline, and whether the patient is an adult or an adolescent makes no difference. The adolescent loses his specificity, just as is the case when, confronted with an authentic psychosis, the therapist considers that he or she is dealing primarily with a psychotic and not so much with an adolescent. However, before deciding that we are confronted with a borderline or an authentic psychosis, we should think twice, because this may affect both our attitudes and the identification models proposed to the adolescent.

Finally, I would like to discuss the relative importance each participant assigns to identifications. It seems to me that this issue was not discussed and remained at an implicit level. If I understand Masterson, he maintains that one cannot speak in terms of identification as long as it is still the object of too great an excitation and that one must also first resolve the problem of separation in a way that may seem somewhat categorical, but that I think is nonetheless important and useful. As for Laufer and Kestemberg, I wonder if there are not some elements that are shared by the theories of the central masturbation fantasy and the sexual body. Laufer speaks in terms of the body and of the masturbation fantasy, but does this not inevitably refer back to the underlying parental identifications? How does he articulate the two? Does he think it would be useful at some point to interpret the integration of the body with its physical experience as being part of the process of identification? On this subject I think that Kestemberg and Laufer also say similar things in seemingly different ways, notably concerning the risk of seeing the adolescent encapsulate himself in reified autoerotic behavior that progressively loosens the traces of the initial relationship with living objects.

I would like to end on a point raised by Ladame that we have failed to mention—the importance of bifocal therapy, which we often use precisely to resolve some of the contradictions alluded to previously. Bifocal therapy consists of one therapist's following the adolescent with the appropriate frequency while another therapist has the hierarchical responsibility (to use Kaufmann's terms) to establish the link with the family, the external world, and the institution.

THE AUTHORS

BARTON J. BLINDER is Associate Clinical Professor of Psychiatry and Director, Eating Disorder Programs and Research Studies, University of California, Irvine.

DAVID DEAN BROCKMAN is Clinical Associate Professor of Psychiatry, University of Illinois College of Medicine; and Training and Supervising Analyst, Faculty and Council, Institute for Psychoanalysis, Chicago.

KRISTIN CADENHEAD is a medical student and psychiatric research assistant at the University of Texas Medical Branch, Galveston.

KATHARINE N. DIXON is Assistant Professor in Psychiatry and Director, Eating Disorders Program, Ohio State University, Columbus.

AARON H. ESMAN is Professor of Clinical Psychiatry, Cornell University Medical College; Faculty Member, New York Psychoanalytic Institute, New York; and a Senior Editor of this volume.

SHERMAN C. FEINSTEIN is Clinical Professor of Psychiatry, Pritzker School of Medicine, University of Chicago; Director, Child Psychiatry Research, Michael Reese Hospital and Medical Center; and Coordinating Editor of this volume.

ENRIQUE J. FRIEDMAN is Assistant Clinical Professor, Department of Psychiatry and Human Behavior, University of California at Irvine School of Medicine.

DAVID M. GARNER is Associate Professor in Psychiatry, University of Toronto; and Director, Research Division, Department of Psychiatry, Toronto General Hospital, Ontario, Canada.

DAVID B. HERZOG is Assistant Professor of Psychiatry, Harvard Medical School; and Chief, Child Psychiatry Consultation Service, Massachusetts General Hospital, Boston.

KENNETH I. HOWARD is Professor of Psychology, Northwestern University; and Senior Research Consultant, Department of Psychiatry, Michael Reese Hospital and Medical Center, Chicago.

LAURA LYNN HUMPHREY is Assistant Professor, Northwestern University Medical School, Chicago.

PHILIPPE JEAMMET is Professor of Adolescent Psychiatry, University of Paris; and a Special Editor of this volume.

CRAIG JOHNSON is Associate Professor of Psychiatry and Co-Director, Eating Disorders Program, Northwestern University Institute of Psychiatry, Chicago.

LUC KAUFMANN is Associate Professor, University of Lausanne; and Director, Centre d'Etude de la Famille, Lausanne, Switzerland.

EVELYNE KESTEMBERG is Director, Center for Psychoanalysis and Psychotherapy, Mental Health Association, Paris.

FRANÇOIS LADAME is Director, Unité de Psychiatrie de l'Adolescence, University of Geneva; and a Special Editor of this volume.

MOSES LAUFER is Director of the Centre for Research into Adolescent Breakdown and the Brent Consultation Center, London.

HAROLD LEITENBERG is Professor, Department of Psychology, and Clinical Professor of Psychiatry, University of Vermont, Burlington.

JERRY M. LEWIS is Clinical Professor of Psychiatry, Family Practice and Community Medicine, Southwestern Medical School of the University of

Texas at Dallas; and Psychiatrist-in-Chief and Director of Research and Training, Timberlawn Psychiatric Hospital.

LORETTA R. LOEB is Assistant Clinical Professor of Psychiatry, Oregon Health Sciences University, Portland; and Faculty, Psychoanalytic Association of Seattle.

JOHN G. LOONEY is Staff Child Psychiatrist, Timberlawn Psychiatric Center; Research Psychiatrist, Timberlawn Psychiatric Research Foundation, Dallas; and a Senior Editor of this volume.

KAREN L. MADDI is Research Associate, Eating Disorders Program, Northwestern University Institute of Psychiatry, Chicago.

JAMES MASTERSON is Adjunct Clinical Professor of Psychiatry, Cornell University Medical College, New York.

JAMES E. MITCHELL is Associate Professor of Psychiatry, University of Minnesota Medical School, Minneapolis.

BRIAN MUIR is Director of Psychotherapy, Melbourne Clinic, Richmond 3121, Victoria, Australia.

RICHARD L. MUNICH is Associate Professor of Clinical Psychiatry, Cornell University Medical College; and Director, Extended Treatment Services Division, The New York Hospital–Cornell Medical Center, Westchester Division, White Plains, New York.

DANIEL OFFER is Chairman, Department of Psychiatry, Michael Reese Hospital and Medical Center; and Professor of Psychiatry, Pritzker School of Medicine, University of Chicago.

ERIC OSTROV is Director of Forensic Psychology, Department of Psychiatry, Michael Reese Hospital and Medical Center, Chicago.

RICHARD L. PYLE is Assistant Professor of Psychiatry, University of Minnesota Medical School, Minneapolis.

DONALD B. RINSLEY is Clinical Professor of Psychiatry, University of

Kansas School of Medicine; and Associate Chief for Education, Col-
mery-O'Neil Veterans Administration Medical Center, Topeka, Kansas.

JAMES C. ROSEN is Associate Professor, Department of Psychology; and
Clinical Professor of Psychiatry, University of Vermont, Burlington.

ELISA G. SANCHEZ is Resident in Psychiatry at The University of Texas
Health Science Center in San Antonio.

JOHN L. SCHIMEL is Clinical Professor of Psychiatry, New York University–Bellevue Medical Center; and Associate Director and Training and
Supervisory Psychoanalyst, William Alanson White Institute of Psychiatry, Psychoanalysis and Psychology, New York.

KENNETH M. SCHWARTZ is Consultant Psychiatrist, Whitby Psychiatric
Hospital, Whitby, Ontario; and in private practice, Toronto, Canada.

ALLAN Z. SCHWARTZBERG is Associate Clinical Professor of Psychiatry,
Georgetown University School of Medicine, Washington, D.C.; and a
Senior Editor of this volume.

JAMES C. SHEININ is Clinical Associate Professor of Medicine, Pritzker
School of Medicine, University of Chicago; and Attending Physician,
Division of Endocrinology and Metabolism, Michael Reese Hospital and
Medical Center.

HERMAN SINAIKO is Associate Professor of Humanities and Dean of Students, University of Chicago.

ARTHUR D. SOROSKY is Associate Clinical Professor of Psychiatry, University of California at Los Angeles; and is a Senior Editor as well as a
Special Editor of this volume.

MAX SUGAR is Clinical Professor of Psychiatry, Louisiana State University;
Director, Children's Unit, Coliseum Medical Center, New Orleans; and
a Senior Editor of this volume.

B. TIMOTHY WALSH is Assistant Professor of Clinical Psychiatry, College of

Physicians and Surgeons, Columbia University; and Research Psychiatrist, New York State Psychiatric Institute, New York.

FRANK S. WILLIAMS is Director, Family and Child Psychiatry, Cedars-Sinai Medical Center, Los Angeles; and a faculty member, Southern California Psychoanalytic Institute.

C. PHILIP WILSON is Assistant Clinical Professor of Psychiatry, Columbia College of Physicians and Surgeons; and Senior Attending Psychiatrist and Lecturer, St. Luke's–Roosevelt Hospital Center, New York.

CONTENTS OF VOLUMES 1–12

541

BARAN, A., *see* SOROSKY, BARAN, AND PANNOR (1977)

BARGLOW, P., *see* WEISSMAN AND BARGLOW (1980)

BARGLOW, P.; ISTIPHAN, I.; BEDGER, J. E.; AND WELBOURNE, C.

Response of Unmarried Adolescent Mothers to Infant or Fetal Death (1973)   2:285–300

BARISH, J. I., *see* KREMER, PORTER, GIOVACCHINI, LOEB, SUGAR, AND SCHON-FELD (1971)

BARISH, J. I., AND SCHONFELD, W. A.

Comprehensive Residential Treatment of Adolescents (1973) 2:340–350

BARNHART, F. D., *see* LOGAN, BARNHART, AND GOSSETT (1982)

BEDGER, J. E., *see* BARGLOW, ISTIPHAN, BEDGER, AND WELBOURNE (1973)

BENEDEK, E.

Female Delinquency: Fantasies, Facts, and Future (1979)   7:524–539

See also LOONEY, ELLIS, BENEDEK, AND SCHOWALTER (1985)

BENSON, R. M.

Narcissistic Guardians: Developmental Aspects of Transitional Objects, Imaginary Companions, and Career Fantasies (1980) 8:253–264

BERGER, A. S., AND SIMON, W.

Sexual Behavior in Adolescent Males (1976)   4:199–210

BERKOVITZ, I. H.

Feelings of Powerlessness and the Role of Violent Actions in Adolescents (1981)   9:477–492

The Adolescent, Schools, and Schooling (1985)   12:162–176

BERLIN, I. N.

Opportunities in Adolescence to Rectify Developmental Failures (1980)   8:231–243

Prevention of Adolescent Suicide among Some Native American Tribes (1985)   12:77–93

BERMAN, S.

The Response of Parents to Adolescent Depression (1980)   8:367–378

BERNS, R. S., *see* KREMER, WILLIAMS, OFFER, BERNS, MASTERSON, LIEF, AND FEINSTEIN (1973)

BERNSTEIN, N. R.

Psychotherapy of the Retarded Adolescent (1985)   12:406–413

BERTALANFFY, L., VON

548

NAME INDEX

Kaplan, A. H., 109, 113
Kaplan, A. S., 231, 238, 439, 444
Kaplan, B. H., 123, 137
Kaplan, N. M., 413, 419
Karol, C., 307, 310
Kaslow, F. W., 196, 197, 200
Kassirer, J. P., 413, 418
Katz, J. L., 256, 271, 335, 357, 406, 407,
    409, 410, 417, 420, 421
Katzman, M. A., 235, 238, 242, 243, 244,
    245, 247, 252, 403
Kaufman, M. D., 281, 310
Kaufman, M. R., 232, 240, 313
Kaufman, L., 449, 452, 453, 494, 495, 496,
    497, 499, 508, 529, 532
Kay, J., 412, 419
Kaye, W. H., 236, 238, 411, 418, 425, 427
Keesey, R. E., 263, 271, 367, 386
Kellam, S. G., 124, 136
Kelly, J., 392, 403
Kelly, M. L., 342, 355, 369, 386
Kenfrick, J., 231, 238
Kennedy, H., 157, 162
Kennedy, K., 99
Kernberg, O. F., 94, 96–97, 99, 100, 103,
    107, 113, 285, 286, 307, 310, 511, 515, 522
Kestemberg, E., 449, 452, 525, 527, 528,
    531, 532, 533, 534
Keys, A., 263, 271
Kiecolt-Glaser, J., 394–95, 396, 397, 398,
    399, 401, 402
Kipnis, D. M., 407, 417
Kirkley, B. G., 342, 355
Kirschenbaum, D. S., 257, 270, 272, 315,
    317, 320, 325, 331
Kirshbaum, W. R., 232, 233, 238, 256
Kirsner, D., 159, 162
Klein, M., 24, 25, 27, 291, 310, 93, 511, 515,
    516
Klerman, G. L., 443, 444
Klinefelter, H., 411, 419
Klose, G., 411, 419
Koenig, L., 135, 316
Kohut, H., 31, 42, 94, 96, 97, 99, 159, 261,
    271
Koslow, S. H., 410, 418–19
Kramer, M., 422, 427
Kramer, S., 293, 310
Krasner, J., 392, 403
Kream, J., 409, 410, 420

Kris, E., 64, 65, 83
Krupinski, J., 122, 136
Kumahara, Y., 406, 419
Kuperberg, A., 256, 271
Kupfer, D. J., 410, 418–19, 443–44
Kurash, C., 328, 332

Lacan, J., 86–87, 93, 99
Lacey, J. H., 358, 360, 364, 371, 372, 382,
    386–87, 394–95, 397, 398, 400, 401, 403,
    414, 419
Ladame, F., 531, 533, 534
Laffer, P. S., 255, 270, 334–35, 355, 410,
    419, 424, 427, 435
Laing, R. D., 18, 27
Lake, M. D., 431, 435–36
Lamberg, B. A., 426
Lang, P. J., 355
Langner, T. S., 22, 27, 28, 122–23, 139
Lantz, S., 431, 436
Larkin, J. E., 259, 271
Larson, R., 121, 136, 234, 235, 238, 255,
    267, 271, 338, 341, 355, 372, 376, 386,
    428–29, 435
Lasch, C., 10, 19, 27
Laufer, M., 101, 112, 217, 449, 450, 451,
    452, 524, 525, 527, 531, 532, 534
Lawson, J. S., 352, 356
Lazovik, A. D., 355
Leary, T., 16
Lee, H. B., 78, 83
Lee-Brenner, K., 396, 403
Leehey, K., 409, 421
Leighton, A. H., 22, 27
Leighton, D. C., 22, 27
Leitenberg, H., 226, 267, 272, 333, 338,
    351, 356, 357, 361, 383, 388
Lentz, R., 372, 387
Leon, G. R., 316, 319, 330
Leslie, S. A., 124, 137
Levin, J., 409, 410, 420, 421
Levin, P. A., 414, 419
Levin, T. M., 190, 197, 199
Levine, S. V., 189–90, 198, 199
Levinson, D. J., 189, 199
Levy, P. L., 407, 417
Lewis, J. M., 3–4, 29, 33, 35, 42, 43
Lewis, L., 234, 238, 242, 252, 258, 260, 261,
    271, 334, 355, 391, 403

SUBJECT INDEX

Abandonment depression, in borderline patient, 471

Action vs. behavior, 59

Addictive personality, and bulimia, 284

Adolescence
uniqueness of, 455–56, 481–82, 525
views of, and treatment, 480–81, 488

Adolescent experience, nature of, for child, 30

Affective disorder. *See* Depression

Affect regulation, and bulimia, 264–65

Age, and medical effects of eating disorders, 406

Aggression, excessive primitive, 515, 516

Amenorrhea
and anorexia, 407, 409
and bulimia, 423–24

Anal phase, 201
danger situations in, 203
and obsessive-compulsive neurosis, 204, 213

Analyst, as parent and teacher, 120, 167–70, 176–77. *See also* Therapist

Anorexia, 222, 226, 232
and bulimia, 369, 391
cognitive and behavioral therapy with, 360
described, 406
distinguished from bulimia, 333–34
group therapy for, 392, 393
medical problems with, 405–14
mortality rate from, 223, 224
psychodynamics of, 280–82
research on, 222–23
see also Eating disorders

Anorexics, families of, 321–27

Anticonvulsants, in treating bulimia, 437–39

Antidepressants, in treating bulimia, 288–90, 410, 432–33, 439–43. *See also* Medication

Anxiety, and vomiting in bulimia nervosa, 338–41

Anxiety neurosis, in case example of brief therapy with college student, 152

Autonomy, development of, and family structure, 36–37, 41

Beck Depression Inventory, 352

Behavioral disorders, 529

Behavioral exercises, with bulimics, 377

Behavioral therapy, with bulimics, 341–54

Behavior vs. action, 59

Bifocal therapy, 534

Binge eating, as bulimic behavior, 243–44. *See also* Bulimia

Binge-purge cycle, 317

Biological factors, and bulimia, 253–56. *See also* Genetics

Body image
and bulimia, 261, 284–85, 359
in parents of eating disorder patients, 299

Body weight
and amenorrhea, 409, 423
and anorexia, 407, 408
and bulimia, 423–24
and bulimia nervosa, 366–70

Borderline disorders, 23–24, 450
extension of concept of, 533–34
and hospitalization, 511
and narcissistic personality, 98
and object representations, 89
and parents, 514
psychopathology of, 515–17
treatment of, 517–19

Borderline triad, 467–79
clinical picture of, 477–78
origin of, 477
psychodynamics of, 470–71
therapeutic management of, 478–79

Boundaries, problems with, in bulimic families, 323, 326

Diagnosis, problems in, 4–5, 100–111
  of bulimia, 242–46
  and characteristics of adolescence, 101–4
  and developmental breakdown, 490–91
  and familial factors, 109–10
  and sociocultural factors, 108–9
  and therapist's conceptual framework, 104–6
  and therapist's personality, 107–8
Dialogues, 44–60
Diary keeping, in treatment of bulimia, 397
Dichotomous reasoning, in bulimia nervosa, 373
Diets, pattern of, in bulimic families, 318–19
Directed associations, 185
Discipline, need for, 9
Dissipative structures, 494
"Divergent" thinking, 63, 64, 65
Divorce rate, and sociocultural changes, 20
Dominant-submissive parental relationship, 34
  and stress, 35, 39–40
Dreams, sand symbolism in, of anorexics, 292
Drug use, 16–17
  and self-image and delinquency, 128–29
DSM, utility of, 525
Dual-norm behavior, of dysfunctional family, 498–99
Dysfunctional families, 34–35, 498–500

Eating Attitudes Test, 352
Eating disorders, and cultural context, 221, 224, 233, 234. *See also* Anorexia nervosa; Bulimia; Bulimia nervosa
Eating disorders, medical aspects of, 405–16
  blood problems, 412
  endocrine problems, 409
  electrocardiographic changes, 413–14
  fluid status, 411–12
  general problems, 406–8
  hypothalmic problems, 408–9
  metabolic abnormalities, 409–10
  potassium levels, 412–13
  renal function, 413
Ego factors, in bulimic child, 283, 284, 285
Endocrine abnormalities, and anorexia, 409
Environmentalism, 14–15

Ethnoreligious groups, 8–9
"Euthyroid sick syndrome," 409
Excessive primitive aggression, in borderline patients, 515, 516
Exhibitionistic behavior, in families of bulimics, 279
Extrafamilial relationships, 9–10
E.T., 88–89

False-self borderline disorder, 469
Familial factors, and diagnosis, 109–10
Families
  of bulimics, 431
  of gifted and creative children, 64
  structure of, 494
  variables in, and impact of adolescence, 31
Family Adaptability and Cohesion Evaluation Scale, 317, 321
Family approach, 532–33
Family Assessment Measure, 319
Family competence, 33–34
Family dynamics, in bulimia, 315–30
  diets in, 318
  food or nurturance, 317–18
  hostility in, 319–20
  loss of control, 319
  and normal families, 321–27
Family Environment Scale, 317, 321
Family history, and bulimia, 431
Family involvement, and treating bulimia, 393
Family profiles
  of anorexic patients, 276
  of bulimic patients, 276–80
Family relationships, and self-image, 128, 130, 135
Family structure, 32–42
  and adolescent development, 36–37, 41
  and the adolescent, 3–4, 29–42
  and bulimia, 256–58
  and competence rating, 33–34
  competent but pained, 34, 38–39
  dysfunctional, 34–35, 39–40
  healthy, 33–34, 37–38
  importance of traditional, 8–9
  and sociocultural climate, 19–20
  and stress, 35–36, 37–38, 38–40
Family system, and development of bulimia, 226